The Edge

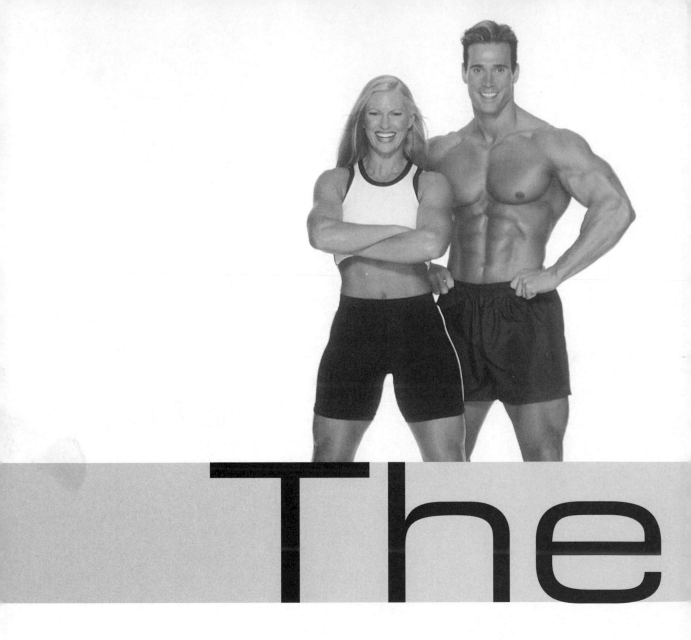

The

Ben Weider and Joe Weider
with Daniel Gastelu

Edge

Avery
a member of
Penguin Putnam Inc.
New York

This book is not intended for use as a substitute for consultation with a qualified medical practitioner, health practitioner, or fitness professional. Before beginning any diet and exercise program, you should consult a physician. All matters regarding your health require medical supervision. If you have symptoms of any illness, or if exercise-induced injury occurs, it is essential that you see your doctor without delay. You are unique, and your diagnosis and treatment must be individualized for you by your own doctor. This book provides information about exercise, nutrition, and dietary supplements and the ingredients they contain. But no book can replace the personalized care that you may need. You are encouraged to work closely with your doctor and other health-care professionals to achieve optimum health. The publisher, authors, and authors' agents shall not be liable or responsible for injury, loss, or damage occasioned to any person acting or refraining to act as a result of any information or suggestion in this book, whether or not such injury, loss, or damage is due in any way to any negligent act or omission, breach of duty, or default on the part of the publisher, authors, or authors' agents. The brand names included in this book are not intended to be product endorsements. A product's inclusion in this book does not imply that it is any better than products not included in this book. The opinions expressed in this book represent the personal views of the authors and not of the publisher.

Most Avery books are available at special quantity discounts for bulk purchase for sales promotions, premiums, fund-raising, and educational needs. Special books or book excerpts also can be created to fit specific needs. For details, write Putnam Special Markets, 375 Hudson Street, New York, NY 10014.

AVERY
a member of
Penguin Putnam Inc.
375 Hudson Street
New York, NY 10014
www.penguinputnam.com

Copyright © 2002 by Ben Weider and Dan Gastelu

Library of Congress Cataloging-in-Publication Data

Weider, Ben.
    The edge : The Weider guide to ultimate strength, speed, and stamina / by Ben Weider
and Joe Weider, with Daniel Gastelu.
      p.   cm.
    Includes bibliographical references and index.
    ISBN 1-58333-126-3
    1. Physical fitness.   2. Exercise.   3. Nutrition.   4. Physical education and training.
    I. Weider, Joe.   II. Gastelu, Daniel.   III. Title.
    RA781 .W377   2002   2001045998
    613.7—dc21

Printed in the United States of America
10 9 8 7 6 5 4 3 2 1

This book is printed on acid-free paper. ∞

Book design by Lee Fukui

Acknowledgments

The authors wish to thank the following people for their participation in the preparation of this book: Per Bernal, Mike O'Hearn, Gea Johnson, David Marsh, Vince Scalisi, Lisa Clark, John Duff, Laura Shepherd, and Christopher Mariadason.

Contents

Preface

Congratulations on your purchase of a book that has obviously been written with great care and attention to the needs of athletes and fitness enthusiasts everywhere.

I respect Ben and Joe Weider enormously and consider them to be the founders of strength conditioning and sports nutrition for modern athletes. They are largely responsible for the boom in fitness worldwide, and their International Federation of Bodybuilders now has 172 countries as members.

The Edge will show anyone interested in sports and fitness how to use the best training methods to build muscle, strength, endurance, and speed, and the way to use sports nutrition products to supply the energy required to become a champion.

As president of the International Sports Medicine Association, I am readily in contact with numerous training organizations and athletes throughout the world. Using sports supplements is permissible and helpful to athletes in all sports. However, they should be used with caution to ensure they do not contain banned substances or elements that may convert to a drug in the body. Your purchase of this book shows that you wish to compete on an even playing ground, as a natural athlete.

Good luck as you begin your fitness program or, if you are at the competitive level, as you strive to improve your performance. The Weider method of training is highly efficient and should help you achieve your goals.

Dr. Eduardo Henrique De Rose
President, International Sports Medicine Association

Foreword

At Weider Health & Fitness, we are always on the leading edge of breakthrough weight-training and nutrition concepts. Our understanding of exercise physiology and nutrition is continually evolving. You probably already know that weight training is beneficial, but you question whether or not the same programs apply to everybody. We answer those questions when we discuss the Variable Weight Training approach. Variable Weight Training acknowledges that, based on different sports performance goals and personal fitness objectives, the types of exercises, the weight used, the number of reps, and the number of sets need to vary for optimum results. In Variable Weight Training, the key word is *variable*—one size does not fit all. Taking this approach puts you in control and allows you to settle into a weight-training program that best suits your personal needs.

When it comes to nutrition, the same rules apply. While everyone should follow the principles of healthy eating, each person has specific nutritional requirements that are unique to their body type, lifestyle, and gender, as well as the types of sport and physical activity they perform. The Dynatrition approach solves this problem for you. With Dynatrition, you will start to experience the results you want while eating many of the foods you love. These new scientific discoveries reveal the

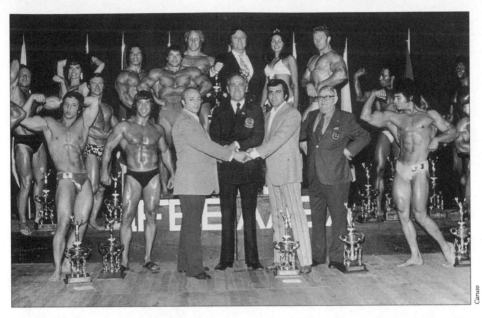

By the 1970s the Weider Triangle Method was being used by professional bodybuilders to build strong, lean, and massive physiques. As bodybuilding became more popular, other athletes and fitness enthusiasts began to turn to the bodybuilding masters, Ben and Joe Weider, for guidance on building champion physiques using muscle-building weight-training and nutrition techniques. Ben Weider is pictured center, bottom row, and Joe Weider is pictured center, top row.

proper proportion of protein, carbohydrates, and fats your diet should include, while taking into account which foods are best for bodybuilding, energy, weight loss, health, and longevity. We also take the guesswork out of which supplements to purchase by showing what works best for different purposes—from building muscle to losing unwanted body fat. And if you are interested in sports nutrition, we have included our updated "Commandments of Sports Nutrition" to ensure your athletic success. Following the Weider Triangle Method of Peak Athletic Performance and Fitness will bring you to new levels of fitness success.

Ben Weider & Joe Weider

The Edge

Introduction

GET THE WEIDER PERFORMANCE-FITNESS EDGE

You have in your hands a powerful tool that guarantees success. *The Edge* contains proven exercise and nutrition methods that help you achieve peak fitness and perform better as an everyday athlete. The Weider program makes you healthier, extends your life, and guarantees a more attractive body. Ben Weider and Joe Weider are your personal coaches to fitness excellence throughout *The Edge*. Joe Weider is known as the father of the modern fitness movement, which he started in 1940. Ben Weider joined him in business in 1945, and together they created the Weider Health & Fitness empire, which includes Weider Publications, Weider Nutrition International, and the International Federation of Bodybuilders. Their credentials say volumes about what they can teach you. Ben and Joe have worked with some of the most famous sports figures and bodybuilders in the business. The secrets of their success have been tested in the laboratory by scientists and proven in the field by champion athletes.

Now they show you how to turn your body into the performance machine you want, using training and nutrition methods perfected over the past six decades and proven to work by millions of professionals and fitness enthusiasts in more than 170 countries. *The Edge* delivers the new Weider performance-fitness plan, which

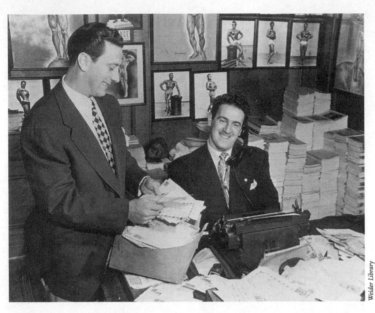

Weider Library

Fitness and bodybuilding legends Joe Weider (left) and Ben Weider (right) are pictured here during the 1950s in the early days of publishing magazines and books about muscle building. From this humble beginning, they built an international fitness empire and remain a major driving force behind the health and fitness movement.

includes their variable technique training, and vital-life nutrition, to give you a competitive edge in sport and in other areas of your life. These training concepts detail advancements that you won't find in other books about fitness and nutrition. They allow you to achieve your goals quickly and effectively but in a way that is sustainable.

If you are an athlete and your goal is to build a better body to be superior at your sport, this book includes the best exercise and nutrition plans for you to do so. If you are simply interested in transforming your body to look and feel your best, you too will find just the right plans. And if you want to lose weight, you'll learn how to do that as well, while improving your body, energy levels, and health at the same time.

What motivated the Weiders to write this book now is that despite the availability of information on exercise and nutrition, they still see many people falling victim to fads. In fact, it was no surprise when a recent review by the U.S. Department of Agriculture determined that most of the popular diet books being sold on the market are unhealthy and could actually cause more harm than good. It was also no surprise to read that the diet the experts found worked best had the same characteristics as the Weider nutrition plans they have followed their entire lives.

The same is true for the exercise gimmick quagmire. They see people of all fitness abilities getting caught up in training routines that are ineffective and potentially harmful. This situation is especially tragic because many people have a strong desire to make changes and commit to a program, but they are led down the wrong path by quick-fix promises. Fitness is not a trend like fashion, it's a science.

As you flip through these pages, you will discover that this book offers the best of both worlds: quick training and nutrition tips backed by expansive reference chapters to improve your understanding of health and athletic performance. The Weiders will cover their

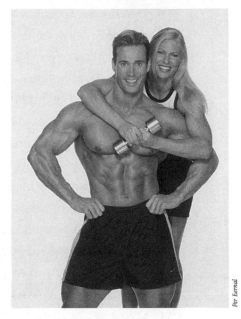

Michael O'Hearn and Gea Johnson.

proven, cutting-edge training and nutrition programs; if you start using them today, you'll notice results tomorrow. The foundation of the program is the revolutionary Weider Triangle Method of Peak Athletic Performance and Fitness. *The Edge* takes you through the easy-to-follow steps of this famous method, which has been expanded here to include advanced training and nutrition programs for anyone interested in a performance-based fitness regimen, from competitive athletes to weekend fitness enthusiasts, to the coaches and health professionals who support them. Special Weider performance tips provide vital insights to becoming your personal best.

The step-by-step training and nutrition plans are easy to follow because they are loaded with detailed photographs and illustrations to make your fitness quest that much easier. The models for the exercise section are natural world-class bodybuilders Michael O'Hearn and Gea Johnson. Mike has won several bodybuilding and powerlifting titles including Mr. Universe, Mr. International, and NPC Super Heavyweight, and he is the three-time California Powerlifing Champion. Gea Johnson, known as the World's Greatest Female Athlete and America's First Miss Fitness, is a world-class heptathlete and a nationally ranked Olympic lifter. More information about Mike and Gea can be found at the end of this book.

The Edge details an expanded model of the legendary Weider Triangle Method that includes a new concept of fitness we call "performance fitness." Performance fitness allows everyone, no matter what your goals, to achieve your personal best. It shows you how to develop personalized programs to enhance your body, fitness level, and overall health.

The goal of *The Edge* is to enhance your fitness knowledge and understanding of more complex exercise and nutrition issues, so the book is packed with information about body form and function, muscle types, sports and fitness supplements, performance nutrition, and natural alternatives to drugs sometimes used in sports. There are powerful alternatives to anabolic steroids and diet drugs, and we show you how to take advantage of these safely and effectively. The Weiders show you how to select the best supplements by knowing which ingredients work best for your fitness or sports performance goals. How you train influences your body composition, which in turn determines how you should eat. It's not enough to just eat a balanced diet. Making a few adjustments to the foods you eat can mean the difference between winning or losing, or getting that hard lean body you are training to develop.

It's hard to believe that exercise and health experts once shunned the idea that weight training and proper nutrition could have beneficial effects on physical performance and longevity. In fact, it was only within the past decade that the medical community recognized that resistance training and supplementation with calcium and vitamin D is the most effective way for men and women to build stronger bones and reduce their chances of developing osteoporosis and bone fractures later in life. Science continues to confirm what the Weiders knew sixty years ago. But you don't have to wait for the rest of the world to catch up, because the most current research for you to benefit from is right here.

The list below includes just some of the key benefits that the Weider Fitness Revolution will deliver:

- Increased muscle mass and strength.

- A youthful metabolism.

- A lean, well-proportioned body.

- Increased aerobic capacity.

- Fast reflexes and increased speed.

- High antioxidant blood levels.

- Increased hemoglobin level and red-blood-cell count.

- Ideal insulin function and maintenance of blood sugar levels.

- Healthy cholesterol levels.

- Normal blood pressure.

- Flexibility.

- Strong bones.

- Lowered risk of developing many diseases.

- Reduction of depression and anxiety.

- Sharper mental focus.

- Happier outlook on life.

- Best sports supplement ingredients.

So let's get started. The Weider Edge for peak performance is your ticket to fitness success.

—Daniel Gastelu

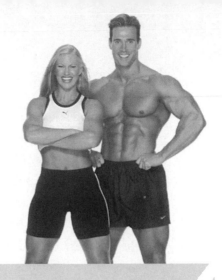

The Weider Triangle Method
of Peak Performance

erhaps your best efforts seem to be failing and you have begun to question the feasibility of your goals and even your ability to attain them. It's only natural.

The good news is that in our experience, *you're* not the problem. The problem is with the methods and products you have been using. Gimmicks don't work, but you can succeed and you will succeed, using the Weider Triangle Method. This method utilizes training and nutrition programs that are proven to work. It gives

you the tools you need to fine-tune and customize your performance-fitness program to attain the results you want and get that competitive edge.

Since its development, the model has evolved to a new point, and we updated it to include the most discoveries about health, exercise, bodybuilding, fitness, nutrition, and sports performance. Today, more people are engaged in fitness activities for the sake of health, and looking and feeling better, than

So you want to build a strong, youthful, attractive body?

Are you ready to commit and work hard, but you're not sure what to do, or whether what you are already doing is working?

After looking through this book, and looking at the Weider Champion Hall of Fame photos on page 22, you know it is possible to get what you want. If they did it, so can you. Right?

they are for athletic competition. We've taken this shift into consideration as we fine tune the Triangle.

Unfortunately, we still see people making plenty of mistakes as they try to get fit, and competitive athletes make some of the very same mistakes. From yo-yo dieting, to cutting out entire groups of healthy foods, to exercising too much too quickly, to taking dangerous diet pills—we've seen it all. People are confused! They succumb to bad advice, loads of it. They hear tips in the gym or they discover theories in quick-fix books. Some of these authors will have you believe they've made a major discovery, only to hook you into following their unbalanced approaches.

Fortunately, in response to this sad state of fitness affairs, we are here to provide the fitness-minded public a solution in the form of the new Weider Triangle Method. We are here to help lead you to fitness success.

WHAT IS FITNESS?

Before getting into the particulars of the Weider Triangle Method, it seems appropriate to review exactly what we mean by fitness. Fitness means different things to different people. It's a matter of degree, extent, and magnitude. What works for one person in terms of results and enjoyment does not necessarily work for another. Just as a marathon runner and a power lifter will have different views of what fitness is, so do people training to attain their ideal weight and shape. Laborers need a different level of fitness than do office workers. To some, fitness might mean a slim build. They look and feel good and can run to catch a train without becoming winded. To others, it might mean they are able to lift heavy weights. To you, it may mean being able to swim for an hour.

Generally, to be fit means more than simply being able to perform your daily activities with ease. Real fitness implies something more, and it is usually associated with above-average strength and stamina. This is what *The Edge* is all about—it's about attaining real health. The health component of fitness is always important to keep in mind, because in our experience we see people who exercise following unbalanced training and nutrition programs that are actually causing long-term harm. This is especially true for people who are exercising to lose weight. It is just as easy to lose weight sensibly by adopting an exercise regimen, and you will be better off in the long run. Just because someone looks thin does not mean that they are healthy or in peak athletic condition. This brings us to the introduction of a new concept in fitness science, the concept of "performance fitness."

WHAT IS PERFORMANCE FITNESS?

While developing fitness is great, developing fitness with more specific performance goals in mind is even better. Performance fitness is a concept built into the WTM. Performance fitness is a new way of looking at fitness. It's a way that makes you aware that there are many facets of fitness, and that in order to achieve performance fitness you need to consider these physical, mental, and biochemical factors. Just as astronauts have to run through their systems checklist before taking off into outer space, you need to perform your own systems check on a regular basis to keep your personal fitness goals on track. It is about developing your fitness for performance needs. It's about setting goals, and following a program of training and nutrition to reach them. But it's also about setting a cross-section of goals to attain well-rounded results.

The checklist that follows at the end of this chapter will get you thinking about the different components of performance fitness. If you're going to stick to a program and get results, it's crucial that you consider all these elements, such as physical, mental, and biochemical factors (such as your cholesterol level). We encounter many people who spend all week long weight training every day and eating a very healthy diet, only to pig out on the weekends, stuffing themselves full of junk. Then there are people whose fitness salvation is running, and run they do, every day. But their diets are garbage. Exercise alone isn't enough, because performance fitness always starts with good nutrition.

If you do not clearly identify your fitness goals, how can you make any progress? For example, if you don't realistically have time to train, then should you really try to do a race? If your goal is to build strength to be a great tennis player, your program is obviously going to be much more intensive than someone who wants to be a little faster on the court during the weekly recreational basketball game, or someone who just wants to look better in the mirror. Training should not run you down; it should enhance your performance. So knowing your performance-fitness goals and how to best achieve them is vital to the Weider performance-fitness philosophy.

Once your goals are established and you have a plan in place, another consideration for achieving peak performance is to include everything in your life that will help you reach your goals, and exclude everything that will detract from them. It sounds simple enough, but in spite of this obvious correlation, even the best athletes can score low when it comes to proper strength training and sports nutrition programs. Attaining peak performance means developing the "right" new habits; constantly learning about new discoveries; mastering the art of setting clear and realistic goals; effectively planning to achieve your goals; employing intelligent nutrition and training methods; having perseverance to develop athletic and fitness excellence; and finally the reward—becoming a champion.

THE PURSUIT OF PERSONAL EXCELLENCE

The Weider Triangle Method allows you to be your personal best and achieve your goals. This success model applies to attaining athletic performance and personal fitness goals, and it can be applied to other areas of your life.

First, by following the Triangle approach, you will quickly develop a healthy and functional body. You will also see improvements in your mental fitness, and you will develop good habits, which include planning and scheduling to integrate your fitness goals into your life. In time you will begin to realize that being positive and believing in yourself will help you stick to your plan and accomplish your goals.

Second, you must then start to identify bad habits, the ones that detract from attaining your goals. This could include bad eating habits, poor time management, substance abuse, or lack of motivation.

Third, work on your skill and technique. Become a master of them. Strive for perfection.

Fourth, always think positive thoughts. Focus on your daily and long-term goals every day. Create daily mantras to repeat every morning and in the evening, to keep your mind focused on what matters most to you and free from extraneous thoughts.

THE WEIDER TRIANGLE METHOD OF PEAK ATHLETIC PERFORMANCE

THE TRIANGLE

The Weider Triangle Method combines three crucial components: strength from weight training and bodybuilding; energy from sports nutrition; and technique

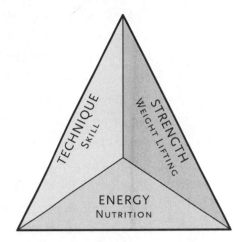

The Weider Triangle Method of Peak Athletic Performance and Fitness, developed by Ben and Joe Weider, underscores the importance of weight lifting for strength, nutrition for energy, and technique training for building skills. Only when all three legs of the triangle are followed in a balanced program can peak athletic performance and ultimate fitness be achieved.

from skill training and practice. These components are integrated to produce reliable improvements in athletic performance and personal fitness. No one component can work without the other two. Without technique, there is no skillful movement. Without strength, there is no effective body movement. And without sports nutrition there is no growth, energy, or recovery. By integrating the three components of the Weider Triangle Method, we have a system that is proven to succeed.

The Triangle is unique in tailoring weight training and nutrition needs to your chosen sport. Specificity is important. For example, we know from viewing sophisticated video and computer skill analysis techniques developed over the past twenty years that even one finger out of place can impede performance. This knowledge is important for your goals, too. The Triangle shows that precision leads to optimum fitness.

1. STRENGTH

In sports, strength makes a critical difference between two athletes of equal skill. Once trainers concentrated on the specific muscles used in a given sport, but now we know that it is the strength of the whole body that counts. Functional power comes only from a complete program of weight training and physical conditioning. During the past several decades, more and more people have turned to bodybuilding and weight training to improve their body build and strength. We have continued to review the latest advances in this form of training for your utilization and to benefit your athletic and personal fitness objectives. This includes the newly developed Variable Weight-Training approach, which breaks the barrier of the antiquated one-size-fits-all weightlifting approaches you may have already tried, with limited success.

In recent decades, there have been significant advances in exercise science, especially in the area of using weight training to improve athletic performance and personal fitness. Not long ago coaches and trainers thought weight training for the whole body produced "muscle-bound" athletes with big, slow muscles. But correct muscle building techniques do just the opposite, and instead will result in building faster, more flexible athletes. Muscle building not only improves athletic performance, but also extends an athlete's career and contributes to general health and longevity. These athletic muscle-building techniques have been modified to also meet the needs of fitness enthusiasts—people looking to reshape their bodies for personal fitness and improved appearance.

By using the Variable Weight-Training approach you can target the exercise frequency, intensity, and duration to best meet your specific goals. For years, we have researched the science of weight training—which exercises, frequency, sets, and reps work best to build the massive physiques of bodybuilders, powerlifters, and other strength athletes? These variables can be manipulated to create a continuum of muscle and strength development results. For example, it is well established that lifting heavy weights for a low number of repetitions stimulates muscle growth and strength. But now we know that exercising with lighter weights for higher repetitions also stimulates muscle growth and strength, particularly muscle strength-stamina—strength that can be sustained for long periods of time rather than quick bursts only. This new approach increases the benefits that weight training has to offer, and allows you to fine-tune your training that much more. The science behind this phenomenon is described in chapter 3. The Variable Weight-Training approach is the new frontier of muscle development, strength, and bodybuilding.

2. ENERGY (SPORTS NUTRITION)—THE DYNATRITION APPROACH

When we first developed the triangle we used the term "energy" as the base, because energy is the result that most people want. Good energy production drives the body, but it comes from good nutrition. Sound sports nutrition, based on your biochemical individuality, is a key component of the Triangle, as it feeds your body what it needs to build energy. You need top-notch nutrition to fuel your exercising muscles, and also to rebuild and maintain them. Your body needs both the raw materials of energy and all of the energy-producing cofactors to work correctly. So in our model, energy is a result of good sports nutrition, intertwined with the other two factors of the triangle.

It is crucial for you to understand the physiological dynamics of nutrition for peak performance to gain the best possible competitive advantage in sport, as well as the body build you want for the rest of your life. Great advances have been made in nutrition designed for the athlete and applied to a particular sport. Unfortunately, separating the truth from the fiction can be a full-time job. Be wary of advice that comes from profit-driven organizations and businesses that do not explain the research behind their ideas. Even government nutrition standards, like the Recommended Dietary Allowances, are limited in application and often misleading and inappropriately applied to people who exercise frequently. In fact, the committee that determines the RDAs states that these recommendations do not apply to individuals with special nutrition needs, and certainly not to athletes. The most cunning advertising methods are used to sell junk food under the guise of optimum nutrition, especially by attaching them to a paid athlete's endorsement. We help you overcome the effects of these subjective advertisements and learn that most of the promises that seem too good to be true probably are, and may not need to be part of your performance nutrition program.

We educate you on the proper use of supplements in chapter 11, the Nutritional Supplement Review (page xx), and explain how to avoid arbitrary use of vitamin and mineral supplements as practiced by many athletes today. Many new supplements, along with natural alternatives to common drugs used in sports, can be used for improving training, strength, endurance, and athletic performance when you know the right ones and the optimum combinations. Sports supplements can also contribute to longevity, weight loss (see page 247), and more.

To encompass all of these nutrition elements, we introduce a new term to describe this concept of sports- and performance-fitness nutrition: Dynatrition. Dynatrition is a new aspect of the Triangle. We cover this thoroughly beginning on

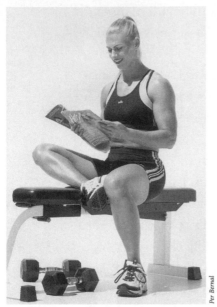

Per Bernal

page 157, but it's so easy to follow that you can begin using it with your very next meal. In order for you to master nutrition for sports, we include the new Commandments of Sports Nutrition (see chapter 6). These Commandments will help keep you on your performance-based eating program. The Commandments of Sports Nutrition were introduced many years ago and were way ahead of their time. You will see that they are time-tested and contain advanced nutritional wisdom that independent medical research studies continue to support.

3. TECHNIQUE

When it comes to attaining peak athletic fitness for performance, even the top athletes with the best team of experts working with them do not always reach their full potential, because they lack certain performance-enhancing skills. Technique applies to everything you do, including your strength-building and nutrition programs. Mastering skills sometimes takes time. So mastering good technique is about mastering winning skills. Chapter 10 provides guidelines and insights on how to master your skills. It also presents one of the most advanced sports training methods ever developed, called periodization. The information in this chapter will help keep your efforts focused on results-building activities.

GOAL SETTING—GETTING THE RESULTS YOU WANT

Begin with the end in mind—your goal. Make it a mantra that guides your daily decisions about eating and recreation. If you do not clearly list your goals, establish strategies to attain them, and establish a system to review your progress, then how can you succeed? Yet in our experience, poor planning is the most common failure of all. Use the performance-fitness planning table below to establish your particular goals, then chart a course to achieve them. Set realistic goals. Write them down. Review them weekly, add new ones, and make adjustments to them as required.

PERFORMANCE-FITNESS GOAL PLANNING SUMMARY TABLE

Body Composition Fitness. Keep track of this on a weekly (for athletes) or monthly (for fitness exercisers) basis. Your percentages of body fat and lean body mass can be determined by trainers or at home with skinfold calipers. Body composition is related to health and longevity. Knowing your percentages of body fat and lean body mass will allow you to keep better track of changes in your muscle mass and fat loss.

	WEEK 1	WEEK 2	WEEK 3	WEEK 4	WEEK 5
Body Weight					
% Body Fat					
% Lean Body Mass					
Measurements:					
Neck					
Forearms					
Upper arm					
Chest					
Waist					
Hip					
Thigh					
Calf					

PERFORMANCE-FITNESS GOAL PLANNING SUMMARY TABLE

Psychological Fitness. Your mind controls your body. Always think positive. Adopt can-do thinking. The way you feel can also be an indication of poor nutrition, over-training, or too much stress in your life. Keep track of your mental energy levels, physical energy levels, mood, concentration, and sleep patterns. If you have a lot of negative thoughts, ask yourself why and try to take actions to correct this trend. Evaluate whether you are experiencing the following attributes and actions with "yes" or "no."

	Week 1	Week 2	Week 3	Week 4	Week 5
Positive mental outlook, "can-do attitude"?					
Good mental energy and alertness?					
Good physical energy?					
Mood positive?					
Mood depressed (doldrums)?					
Concentration good?					
Good night's sleep (seven to nine hours)?					
Nervous or edgy?					
Anger outbursts?					
Good winning physical-fitness habits?					
Good eating habits?					
Taking your supplements every day?					
Time for daily rest and relaxation?					
Time for vacations and weekly day off?					

PERFORMANCE-FITNESS GOAL PLANNING SUMMARY TABLE

Medical Fitness. Getting regular medical exams is vital for monitoring your health. Get a physical at least once a year and always before beginning a new exercise program. Take nutritional and prescribed medical actions to correct medical problems. In addition to maintaining good health for peak physical performance and health, monitoring these parameters will also help prevent common degenerative disease conditions, such as diabetes, cardiovascular problems, arthritis, osteoporosis, dementia, and more.

	MEDICAL EXAM 1	MEDICAL EXAM 2	MEDICAL EXAM 3	MEDICAL EXAM 4	MEDICAL EXAM 5
Pass routine medical exam?					
Good blood pressure?					
Good cholesterol levels?					
Good blood-sugar levels?					
Good reflexes?					
Good vision?					
Good hearing?					
Good resting heart rate?					
Good exercising heart rate?					
Good lung capacity?					
Good posture?					
Well nourished?					
Good bone health?					

PERFORMANCE-FITNESS GOAL PLANNING SUMMARY TABLE

Physical Fitness. Maintaining physical fitness is vital to health and will obviously improve athletic performance. Below are some key parameters to keep track of. Consult your doctor, coach, or trainer on periodically conducting physical fitness tests to verify that you are in good working order.

	TEST 1	TEST 2	TEST 3	TEST 4	TEST 5
Good flexibility?					
Good agility (ability to move body around with speed and accuracy)?					
Good balance (ability to maintain equilibrium while stationary or moving)?					
Good coordination (ability to use senses, together with body parts, in performing body movements accurately)?					
Good reaction time (response time between stimulus and reaction to it)?					
Good sports performance motor skills (sport-specific movements and performance)?					
Good aerobic fitness as related to aerobic and oxidative conditioning (ability of circulatory system and respiratory system to supply oxygen to muscles during prolonged physical activity)? *Note: sports and fitness goals specific.*					
Good anaerobic fitness condition?					
Good muscle strength?					
Good muscle power?					
Good muscle speed-strength?					
Good stamina-strength?					
Good endurance-strength?					

PERFORMANCE-FITNESS GOAL PLANNING SUMMARY TABLE

Daily Schedule. Do you have the time each day you need to be healthy, improve physical conditioning, and enjoy life? Prioritize, and make the time to do what you need to do each day. If you are short on time, figure out how to maximize the time you spend on household tasks by sharing responsibilities with your spouse/family/roommates. Advance planning of shopping trips and meal preparation can help save hours per week.

	Week 1	Week 2	Week 3	Week 4	Week 5
Sleep					
Personal hygiene					
Meals					
Shopping					
Exercise					
Career					
Rest and relaxation					
Social					
Family					
Self-improvement					

Once you get started, refer to these goals often, as often as it takes to keep you headed in the direction you desire. Men should aim for a body fat range between 8 and 14 percent, and women should aim for a body fat range between 11 and 19 percent. Of course, all body composition analysis methods have a margin of error as high as plus or minus 5 percent, so don't take them too seriously. What you see in the mirror is usually the best indicator of your body composition status.

LET US LEAVE YOU WITH THIS MOTIVATING THOUGHT.

We are the biggest advocates and followers of the Weider Triangle Method. It has given us many rewards, more then we ever dreamed of. Besides the obvious health payoff, being super-fit enabled us to take on a world of opportunities and achieve many successes in our personal lives and careers. Building the most successful fitness company in the world took plenty of planning and persistence, trial and error. We share this only because we want you to know our "secrets" so you too can achieve your fitness goals. And if you believe strongly in yourself and in your dreams, you can surely achieve them. It worked for us, and it worked for millions of champions all over the world.

But whatever your goals are, we want you to be healthy and happy along the way to achieving them and becoming a champion in your own right. Believe in yourself and persistence will win the day.

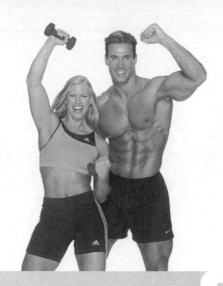

Strength and Muscle Building

2

Take a close look at the photos of men and women in this book, and you'll see that the human body has the ability to take on a wide variety of muscular-development and physical-performance potential. When training for a particular sport or personal fitness goal, the type of training you do is of paramount importance. It is not enough to just build muscle unless you address specific objectives and link weight training to your specific goals.

Peak physical condition means different things to different people. For athletes, it means being best at their sport. They have to develop a body that is specific to that sport. For personal fitness, it means looking good, feeling good, and being healthy. It means training away the flab until you have an attractive, shapely body. Whatever your personal bodybuilding goal is, physical conditioning starts by understanding how different resistance training methods affect your body's form and function.

It is easy to see the differences in body type between a marathon runner and a sprinter. While they are both runners, each has trained with very specific goals in mind, and their bodies develop accordingly. The sprinter is conditioned for quick, powerful bursts of energy and therefore he has thicker, larger muscles. The marathon runner needs to sustain his energy for long distances and so his muscles

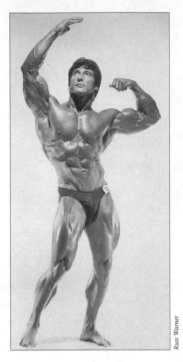

Russ Warner

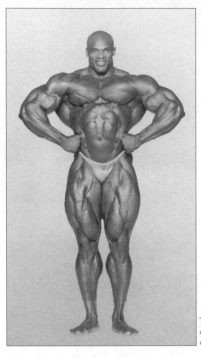

Per Bernal

Top left: Frank Zane, Mr. Olympia, 1977–1979.

Top right: Ronnie Coleman, Mr. Olympia, 1998–2000.

Bottom left: Rachel McLish, Ms. Olympia, 1980, 1982.

Bottom right: Cory Everson, Ms. Olympia, 1984–1989.

Meet some of the men and women who have won a place in the Weider Hall of Fame. They include Mr. Olympia winners Frank Zane and Ronnie Coleman, and Ms. Olympia champions Rachel McLish and Cory Everson. All used Weider weight-training and nutrition techniques to build their Olympia physiques. You can use the same techniques to build your muscles and reduce body fat to suit your particular needs with the Variable Weight-Training Approach and Dynatrition.

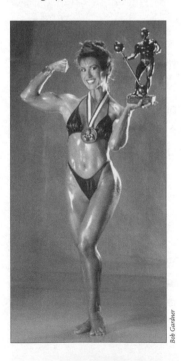

Bob Gardner

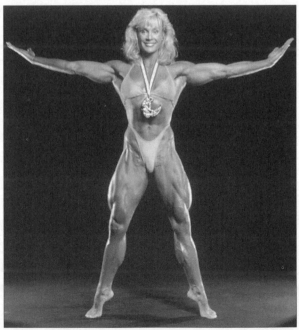

Bob Gardner

are smaller and leaner. Tailoring your training to these different sports performance goals is very important. This is one reason for development of the Variable Weight-Training approach. If you are involved in a sport, you need to follow a strength and bodybuilding program specific to your sport and body type.

If your goal is building a better body for personal fitness, your weight-training program will be less demanding than that of a competitive athlete, but it still needs to be exacting. The point is that the right weight-training program can help you look good, feel good, and have a healthy body, without weight training the way you would need to for maximum athletic performance. You need to make sure that your weight-training program yields your desired results. This is important to keep in mind. Very often we see people training for personal fitness by following programs designed for competitive athletes or competitive bodybuilders. These people usually spend too much time weight training and end up overdoing it to the point of diminishing returns. On the other hand, we often encounter competitive athletes who are following weight-training programs not suited for their particular sports. Let's see what the different training methods can accomplish and which one is right for you.

MUSCLE BUILDING, STRENGTH TRAINING, AEROBICS, AND MORE

What's the terminology all about? Fitness experts use a variety of related terms to describe the process of building up the body. Our favorite term is bodybuilding, because it encompasses the broader notion of training to build up your body. When you hear the term "bodybuilding" you might envision men and women who have achieved a body build of gigantic proportions. In this sense, "bodybuilding" refers to the sport and its related competitions. Bodies like these don't come easily. It takes many years of daily weight training to achieve massive muscles, not to mention the right genes.

But bodybuilding also refers to a type of training that gives people well-proportioned, lean bodies. These people train with weights, eat right, and live a healthy lifestyle. A common denominator to all bodybuilding is weight training (weight lifting, resistance training, or the like). Now, if you are an athlete reading this book, you hunger for strength. You know that being stronger can improve your athletic performance. But if you are reading this book to achieve personal fitness goals and improve your body build, you still may not be sure about how strength training will benefit you. You may still be thinking that you will develop massive muscles like the competitive bodybuilders. Trust us—this won't happen unless you really want it to, and even then, it takes nearly a full-time commitment. When your body is untrained, it is not very good at using the food you eat for energy and muscle building. The untrained body is good at being lazy and building fat. But as you start to exercise and build more muscle, your body responds at the cellular level to build up substances needed to use body fat stores and ingested foods for energy more effectively. Your muscles develop, your circulatory system improves and actually grows larger, and many other changes start to occur so your body is better suited to handle the new stimulus in your life: exercise. You actually transform your body from a soft, untrained fat-building machine into a strong, firm, and shapely fat-burning machine: a better body that will perform best for you now and later on in life.

Think about how important strength is in your daily life. During the day, you need strength to lift things, to do chores around the house, and maybe even to perform well on your job. Every time your muscles contract and relax to move your body around, strength is exhibited. Another remarkable benefit of bodybuilding is that it keeps your body looking young. Just take a look at some of the photos in this book and in magazines you read, and compare the bodies of both young and old champions. If you look at their bodies from the neck down, you will be amazed to discover that the body of a 60-year-old is as youthful-looking as that of a 20-year-old. Weight training actually has a youth-promoting effect on the outside *and* inside of your body. From a function standpoint, your nervous system, circulatory system, joints, muscles, endocrine system, and digestive system all benefit when you weight train to build a stronger body, but the added muscle also does wonders for your skin and metabolism.

Our method of strength training is rooted in bodybuilding, and it will turn your body into a functional body that will not only suit your specific needs, but also look attractive and balanced. While it is true that in most sports certain muscles are used more than others, it is also true that building up both your primary and secondary muscles will result in better performance. Total bodybuilding will also prevent imbalances in muscle groups. Muscle imbalances often lead to a reduction of flexibility, with one group of muscles overpowering the other, which can lead to injury. Bodybuilding prevents and corrects these problems.

Now, when you think "bodybuilding" you should also think weight training, which is the method of choice for building larger and stronger muscles. Exercising with weights is also called resistance training. Resistance training takes on many forms, such as calisthenics, participation in a sport, manual labor, and weight training. Even movement performed in aerobic exercise classes is a form of resistance training. But as it turns out, building strength and muscles is best accomplished by exercising with barbells, dumbbells, and weight-lifting machines and devices.

STRENGTH: THE CRITICAL DIFFERENCE

In the 1940s, when we first popularized bodybuilding and weight training in our magazine *Your Physique,* we could not get scientists to write articles for us, as they did not believe back then that weight training would enhance performance. Over the years all that has changed, and our health and fitness magazines are filled with articles written by world-renowned health, fitness, and sports scientists—hundreds of them. The names on our advisory board read like a who's who of the most prestigious universities.

In the midst of all this science there is still some confusion, however, regarding weight training. Old myths do a disservice to athletes and fitness enthusiasts. In order to help set the record straight, here is a review of four of the most commonly encountered myths and misconceptions about weight training.

Myth #1
"Weight training makes you muscle-bound and restricts your range of movement, making you unable to use your muscles like a normal person."

Actually, weight training helps you maintain flexibility as you age. Weight training develops and liberates muscle.

There is no doubt that unbalanced weight training may lead to a tightening or shortening of muscles. That is why it is crucial to follow a balanced weight-training program, designed for your specific goals.

Myth #2

"Weight training causes people to grow big muscles that slow them down."

The opposite is true. Weight lifting will actually develop your muscles to contract faster, which will be enable you to move faster. For example, after following weight-lifting programs, football players of today are far more muscular than teams of 20 years ago, and they are also faster in the 40-yard dash. The classic weight-lifting athletes, Olympic weight lifters, tend to be the fastest of all athletes over short distances (20 to 30 yards), even faster than sprinters, because they have a greater amount of fast-twitch muscle fiber, which is conditioned to generate explosive muscle contractions. (See chapter 3 for details on muscle fibers.)

We have found that the basic physics principle of *power = strength × speed* holds true for the human body as well as objects in motion. If you move a weight at a faster speed, then power is increased. The more raw strength you have in a muscle, even if that strength was built using slow movements, the faster you can move a given weight. When you train so as to move weights at high speed, you also tend to increase the size of your muscles, thereby further enhancing your capacity to exhibit speed of movement. You also stimulate new neuromuscular links, so that muscle fibers previously unused are brought into the normal range of function. Weight training, especially at high speed, leads to faster, not slower, muscles, and faster athletes all around.

Myth #3

"Weight training only builds muscle tissue."

Weight training not only builds muscles, it also builds connective tissues, bones, the nervous system, and the cardiovascular system. For example, a shot putter's putting arm and a javelin thrower's throwing arm have much stronger bones than in their nonthrowing arms. It is not because that was their stronger arm to begin with. If they stop the sport or change to another event involving both sides of the body evenly, the bone strength eventually becomes equal on both sides.

More evidence comes from Dr. Jon Block at the University of California in San Francisco. He measured bone density in men under 40 years of age. He showed that men who did weight training had greater bone density than those who did aerobics, and both groups had greater bone density than a group who did not exercise.

Other recent studies confirm that weight-bearing exercise increases bone strength even in older people and prevents loss of calcium from bone.

The message is clear. Weight training strengthens bones in men and women. This benefit is very important in our society, where osteoporosis has become epidemic in older people. Think how much suffering could be prevented if more people started regular weight training. Stronger bones will also help prevent sports injuries and enable the athlete to reach peak performance fitness.

Myth #4
"Weight training does not produce cardiovascular health."

Wrong. While aerobic exercises, such as long-distance running or biking and aerobic training classes, are good for developing a healthy heart and circulatory system, so is weight training. While it is true that aerobic exercise will provide additional benefits, weight training definitely contributes benefits of its own to promoting cardiovascular health. Weight training also builds strong bones and connective tissues better than aerobic exercises.

Scientific studies have demonstrated that weight training will improve cardiovascular fitness in addition to increasing muscle size and strength. In their evaluation of athletes who use Olympic-style weight training, M. H. Stone and coworkers reported that weight training can produce significant and positive changes in some cardiovascular parameters. These included better oxygen-carrying ability, lower resting heart rate, and reduced systolic blood pressure. Additionally, lean body weight increased significantly and body-fat percentage decreased significantly. Stone also reported other benefits of weight training based on observations of bodybuilders, including positive changes in serum lipids, improved glucose tolerance and insulin sensitivity, and improved short-term high-intensity endurance. A recent study by W. J. Kraemer and coworkers examined the benefits of weight training combined with bench-step aerobics on women's health. These researchers observed the effects of adding a multiple-set upper and lower body weight-lifting exercise program to 25 minutes of bench-step aerobics, compared to the effects of exercising only with bench-step aerobics. Kraemer found that adding weight training improved peak cardiovascular fitness, increased upper and lower body power, lowered resting heart rate, and improved body composition changes, when compared to exercising with bench-step aerobics alone.

Medical researchers even report about how weight training is effective in promoting cardiac rehabilitation. D. E. Verril and P. M. Ribisl observed that cardiac event patients following weight-training programs experienced improvements in muscular strength, cardiovascular endurance, body composition, bone density and mineral content, and self-confidence. As a result of weight training, these patients were able to return to their daily activities sooner. In another study, Y. Beniamini and coworkers reported similar improvements that weight training produced as part of an outpatient cardiac rehabilitation program. They discovered that when weight training was added to a standard cardiac rehabilitation aerobic exercise program, the weight-training patients lost more body fat, gained more lean tissue, and had greater improvements in treadmill exercise time. They concluded that weight training also reduces cardiac risk factors from these added results.

The scientific evidence for the health benefits of exercise is impressive. The Center for Disease Control and the Surgeon General report that regular physical activity—which, keep in mind, includes both aerobic exercise and weight training—improves health in the following ways:

- Reduces the risk of dying prematurely.

- Reduces the risk of dying from heart disease.

- Reduces the risk of developing diabetes.

- Reduces the risk of developing high blood pressure.

- Helps reduce blood pressure in people who already have high blood pressure.

- Reduces the risk of developing colon cancer.

- Reduces feelings of depression and anxiety.

- Helps control body weight.

- Helps build and maintain healthy bones, muscles, and joints.

- Helps older adults become stronger and better able to move about without falling.

- Promotes psychological well-being.

Furthermore, the American College of Sports Medicine recommends a combination of aerobic and resistance training and flexibility exercises for developing and maintaining cardio-respiratory and muscular fitness and flexibility in healthy adults.

WEIGHT TRAINING AND PERFORMANCE FITNESS

Almost all elite athletes today use some type of weight training to enhance their power and athletic performance. Over the last twenty years, research has produced precise programs applying weight training to particular sports. In fact this research has been so successful that it has now become a branch of the sports science in its own right.

While weight training will improve athletic performance in many ways, here is an example that applies to numerous sports: the vertical jump. How high an athlete can jump straight up is obviously important in basketball, volleyball, and high jumping. It is equally important, however, in football, tennis, martial arts, long jumping, triple jump, javelin, and other sports. And many people don't realize its importance in shot putting, discus, and even Olympic weight lifting, where the high pull in the snatch depends on the athlete's power to jump up from a crouched position against the resistance of the weight.

It used to be believed that jump height only depended on technique and leg speed, and that running was the best way to get the leg speed. We know now that running, especially over long distances, actually reduces the vertical jump. We also know that the vertical jump depends on technique plus the power of muscle contractions and the recruitment of large numbers of muscle fibers in the shortest period of time. The power and recruitment of muscles are rapidly increased from weight-training exercises. In fact, we now know that the primary requirement for the vertical jump, even before technique is taught, is muscle strength gained by weight training.

As we have stressed before, this strength has to be gained throughout the body, not just in the legs. You have to strengthen the whole of what is called the "jumping chain" of muscles that includes the legs, midsection, chest, back, shoulders, arms, and neck. Only an overall weight-training program will do it. Examples of weight-training programs are presented in the following chapters. The next chapter, however, presents important scientific insights about the form and function of your muscles, and how different exercise frequency, intensity, and duration affects the development of strength and muscle size.

EXERCISE AND ARTHRITIS

As more people are living longer, degenerative diseases are increasing rapidly. About 40 million Americans suffer from arthritis. Research in nutrition and exercise demonstrates that for many this condition is preventable by living a performance-fitness lifestyle, and it is even curable using dietary and exercise techniques. Evidence that exercise can provide benefits for people with arthritis is so compelling that the United States government health authorities have published information for patients and doctors to encourage them to work together to use exercise as an effective treatment for arthritis, along with nutrition and drug therapies.

Proper exercises performed on a regular basis are an important part of arthritis treatment. Years ago doctors advised no exercise, fearing that activity would cause more damage and inflammation. However, modern research has found that not exercising causes weak muscles, stiffer joints, reduced mobility, and lost vitality. Regular exercise and moderate physical activity are beneficial in decreasing fatigue, strengthening muscles and bones, increasing flexibility and stamina, improving cardiovascular health, and promoting a general sense of well-being. The amount and form of exercise should depend on which joints are involved, the amount of inflammation, how stable the joints are, and whether a joint replacement procedure has been done. A proper program will usually require working with a physical therapist under the close supervision of a doctor.

Three main types of exercise for people with arthritis include:

- Range-of-motion exercises, which involve moving a joint as far as it will comfortably go and then stretching it a little further to increase and maintain joint mobility, decrease pain, and improve joint function. Range-of-motion exercises can usually be performed every other day.
- Strengthening exercises involve resistance exercises to build up muscle tissues and stabilize weak joints. Strength exercises are usually performed a few times per week or more depending on your condition.
- Endurance or aerobic exercises include walking, swimming, and bicycling for 20 minutes or more at a time. Aerobic exercises tone up the body and, in particular, strengthen the circulatory system, heart, and lungs. This type of exercise should be done for 20 or more minutes a day, three or more times a week, as your condition permits.

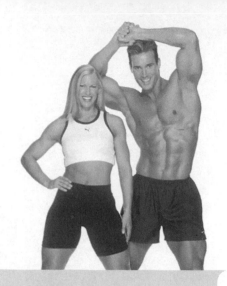

Weider Variable Weight-Training Approach for Muscle Building, Athletic Performance, and Fat Loss

n this chapter and the next one, we'll take you through a short course in the science of weight training. Familiarize yourself with some of these terms and concepts and you'll not only understand the Variable Weight-Training approach better, but you'll also be more comfortable in the gym. We want you to know some basic muscle physiology and biomechanics, and the underlying reasons how and why certain types of exercise condition your body in different ways. Don't be intimidated by the scientific terminology. It's not that complex and you should be able to identify the major muscle groups, so you can have an intelligent conversation with a trainer in a gym. This will further guarantee your success.

Then in chapter 4 we'll present Variable Weight-Training programs that you can begin using immediately, followed by a demonstration of core weight-training exercises.

MAJOR MUSCLE GROUPS

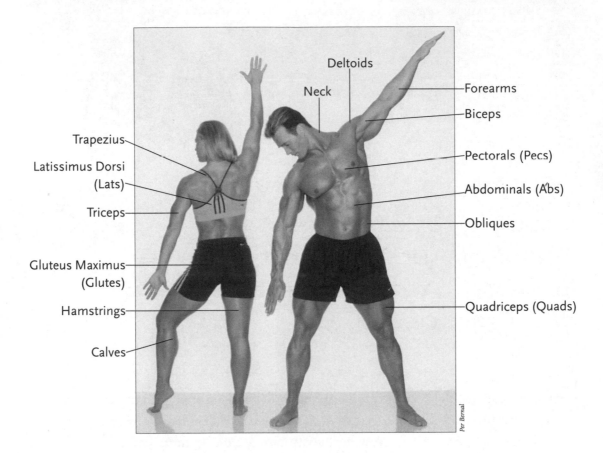

Deltoids

Neck

Forearms

Biceps

Trapezius

Latissimus Dorsi
(Lats)

Pectorals (Pecs)

Triceps

Abdominals (Abs)

Obliques

Gluteus Maximus
(Glutes)

Hamstrings

Quadriceps (Quads)

Calves

Per Bernal

PUTTING AN END TO WEIGHT-TRAINING CONFUSION

Confusion about weight training still abounds. We've visited thousands of gyms in some two hundred countries and we always find dedicated individuals who train ineffectively with weight-lifting equipment. There are a few reasons for this. First, it's human nature to want to do it yourself. So, armed with a little bit of knowledge, people try to copy the experts and make up their own weight-training programs. In most cases these programs are not based on science or proven principles. We're not saying that you should not or could not customize your own weight-training routine. By all means, do so when you're ready, but first make sure that you are following a program that is both safe and effective to get the best results for your exercise effort.

Another common mistake is that people try all sorts of crazy exercise variations, which in most cases put them at risk and lead to injury. They put themselves in extreme positions, attempting to shock or "isolate" the muscles in contorted ways. Don't do this. In the end, a contorted weight-training program is counterproductive; it will lead to injury and yield inefficient results. Stick to the key weight-training exercises we show you in the following chapters. These are the weight-training exercises that are proven to work; use them.

You may have asked yourself, Why are there so many different weight-training programs published in books and magazines? Perhaps it is because there are so many different types of machine and free-weight exercises, not to mention the different muscles we have learned to isolate. Some programs are better than others. The good ones are based on solid exercise science. They offer variety for the reader to help them achieve their personal goals. As you get more advanced in your training, you will be ready to add some new exercises so reading how others have achieved their performance-fitness goals may help you to stay on target, or enable you to discover something new to try. But when you take a close look at the exercises, repetitions, and sets, there is an underlying similarity among effective weight-training methods.

The key to effective weight training is to follow the best routines that will help you achieve your specific goals, within the least amount of time. You do not have to spend years experimenting. Chapter 4 has weight-training exercises and programs that get results, without wasting time. And you may be surprised to know that for personal fitness you only need a total of a few hours a week for developing and maintaining improved strength and body build.

Keep in mind that professional strength athletes use the same weight-training equipment as everyone else. Everybody follows the same principles of exercising different muscle groups using repetitions and sets. Different body parts may be trained the same days or on different days. Weight-training sessions are followed by periods of rest for those muscles exercised, which is needed to give the muscles you exercised time to recover and grow.

PROGRESSIVE OVERLOAD

When weight training at any intensity and duration, the key is to work each set of repetitions to failure or near failure. This in turn stimulates your muscles to grow and develop to accommodate the workload. So if you are training with 300 pounds in the bench press for six repetitions, or 150 pounds for 32 repetitions, work the muscles to failure to apply the adaptive stress they need to develop size and strength. As your muscles develop in response to various workloads, you need to periodically increase the amount of weight you are training with if you want more gains in muscle strength and size. Guidelines for this are provided in chapter 4.

If weight training is so standardized, then why do different people get such varying results? When you compare the bodybuilders of past and present, or any group of strength athletes, it is interesting to note that these champions followed scientific weight-lifting programs "of the day" to build their massive physiques. Then why are there such differences in the size of their physiques? Some of the gains you see in today's strength athletes stem from a new understanding of muscle anatomy and physiology and better nutrition science. We've made huge advancements in sports supplements, and we have refined the strength and body-building diet, which consists of high carbohydrates, moderate protein, and low fat.

What you may find surprising is that there have been only a few advancements in the weight-training equipment used by professional strength athletes. Free weights are still the instrument of choice for most of their exercises. They offer the best stimulus for muscle growth, provide a full range of motion, and usually recruit other muscles in the body for stability. However, research also indicates that combining free-weight exercises with exercises performed on machines is also beneficial. Machines offer convenience, especially when selecting a workload to exercise with. Ultimately, the weight-training exercises you use will reflect a balance of what best suits your goals and what is available to you.

SPECIFIC TRAINING YIELDS SPECIFIC RESULTS: KEEP YOUR GOALS IN MIND

Today championship bodybuilders can develop massive muscles using a more diversified scientific weight-training program—one that's not necessarily longer or harder, but smarter. This is due in part to a new understanding of anatomy and physiology and how growth occurs at the microscopic and biochemical level.

With this new knowledge, weight-training programs for other athletes can be aimed at stimulating the different types of muscle cells, called muscle fibers, that make up your muscles. If you want a strong, lean, slim, muscular body, or a massive, lean, muscular body, the secret is in your muscle fibers.

MUSCLE FIBERS

Your muscle is composed of two types of muscle fibers: slow-twitch and fast-twitch. Fast-twitch fibers are selectively recruited when heavy workloads are demanded of the muscles, and strength and power is needed. They are recruited for high-intensity, short-duration work. They contract quickly, yielding short bursts of energy, and are recruited in high amounts during brief, intense exercises such as sprinting, weight lifting, shot putting, or even swinging a golf club. But these fast-twitch muscle fibers exhaust quickly. Pain and cramps settle in rapidly as they become vulnerable to lactic acid build-up, a by-product of their own metabolism.

Slow-twitch muscle fibers produce a steadier, low-intensity, repetitive contraction, characteristic of endurance activities. They are capable of sustaining workloads of low intensity and long duration, such as long distance running, swimming, and cycling. Athletes of high-intensity sports such as weight lifting, wrestling, and sprinting tend to have a greater percentage of fast-twitch muscle fibers. Athletes of low-intensity sports, such as long-distance running, tend to have a higher percentage of slow-twitch muscle fibers.

There are several points of interest to the athlete. The first is that when you train, the intensity and duration will influence the physiology of muscle tissue and development of muscle fibers. The long-distance runner tends to develop slow-twitch muscle fibers, while the power lifter develops fast-twitch muscle fibers. One reason the fast-twitch muscle fibers increase in size is to increase the capacity to store more adenosine triphosphate and creatine phosphate (ATP and CP). ATP is the body's primary energy molecule and CP is a compound that replenishes ATP. ATP and CP are needed for explosive energy that lasts only a few seconds. The second reason is that the physiological conditioning of muscle tissue determines which fuel source is used. Power athletes need more muscle glycogen to fuel their muscles, while endurance athletes need both muscle glycogen and fatty acids. One reason power-lifting athletes tend to carry excess fat is because their diets tend to be high in fats, and their mode of training does not burn much fat. The excess fat develops into large fat stores.

From a strength and bodybuilding development standpoint, low-intensity, long-duration exercise provides certain fitness benefits but does not build up much muscle mass or strength. In fact, it can have the opposite effect. To illustrate this, think of how a marathon runner is built, compared to a sprinter. They both run fast, but the marathon runner is conditioned to run as fast as possible for a long period of time—usually about a maximum of 12.5 miles per hour. The marathon runner has well-developed slow-twitch muscle fibers but underdeveloped fast-twitch muscle fibers. Some long-distance runners actually develop bodies that make them look undernourished.

Sprinters, on the other hand, have trained their bodies to move as fast as possible over a very short distance—100 meters under ten seconds, for a maximum speed of about 22.5 miles per hour. This takes explosive muscle power and a higher output of energy per second. To develop the capacity to do this, the sprinter needs to build up fast-twitch muscle fibers, which have the capacity to get really big, and generate explosive muscle contractions for a short period of time before fatigue sets in. Visually sprinters are more muscular and shapely than long-distance athletes. And while athletes with highly developed fast-twitch muscle fibers mostly draw upon carbohydrates for energy, they are still able to maintain a low percentage of body fat because these larger muscles need more total calories per day for energy. Sprinters and other strength athletes have the timeless classic body of champions depicted in early Greek and Roman art—the body type that comes from weight lifting.

The point of this excursion into anatomy and physiology is to show you that your body has the ability to respond and develop differently depending on the type, frequency, intensity, and duration of exercise. For the sake of this book, heavy-intensity weight training means using heavy workloads (weights) and expending a lot of energy in a short period of time. When you exercise at heavy intensity, your duration will be limited because muscle fatigue occurs quickly from this type of physical exertion. Light-intensity weight training means using light workloads that allow you to perform more repetitions for longer periods of time. Medium-intensity weight training means using weights somewhere between heavy and light, with the number of repetitions per set also in the middle range. When following a weight-training program using a variety of heavy-intensity, medium-intensity, and light-intensity workloads, you will actually be stimulating increases in strength and muscle growth in all of your muscle fiber types.

A CLOSER LOOK AT FAST-TWITCH MUSCLE FIBERS: DYNAMIC MUSCLE-BUILDING POSSIBILITIES

Because your muscles are composed of both fast-twitch and slow-twitch muscle fibers, there are some dynamic muscle-building possibilities. But the story gets even more interesting because there are actually two primary types of fast-twitch fibers in your muscles. One type, called type IIb (or fast-twitch glycolytic), can be trained to grow to massive proportions and has the ability to store a great deal of immediate energy in its cellular liquid that can then be used to fuel extremely powerful muscle contractions. This immediate energy is used up quickly under extremely heavy workloads, and fatigue sets in within a few seconds when exerting maximum effort. The other type of fast-twitch muscle fiber is called type IIa (or fast-twitch oxidative glycolytic), and it is conditioned from weight training with middle-intensity workloads, for a wide range of reps.

Development of type IIb muscle fibers is important to people who are involved in sports that require extreme bursts of muscle contractions, such as competitive weight lifting, powerlifting, sprinting, football, baseball, shot put, goal keepers, and the like. Your fast-twitch muscle fibers can be developed to perform over a range of heavy- to middle- to light-intensity workloads. The extent to which you need to develop the type IIb muscle-fiber energy systems depends on your performance goals and what energy systems are needed to be best at your activities.

When type IIb muscle fibers are exercised correctly they get quite large and store a high resting level of ATP and CP; as ATP gets depleted, the CP is used to quickly make more. This is one reason why loading up with creatine supplements results in increased strength and longer workouts. At just about the same time, glucose molecules in the muscle fibers are quickly split in half, which produces more ATP—this allows for the burst of strength you can generate during the first few seconds of resistance training with weights. When weight training with a lighter workload, for more repetitions, this is an important means of generating energy for muscle contractions. But lactic acid builds up quickly, faster than it can be cleared away, and muscle fatigue occurs. Lighter workloads with higher reps develop type IIb and type IIa muscle fibers. But type IIa muscle fibers have the capacity to develop and perform over a range of intensities and duration. As the workloads are reduced, a weight-training set can last more than a minute. This is important to realize, because it is your underlying energy system that you are actually training to build up the capacity of your muscles to develop and to store more energy, to accommodate different types of workloads.

Slow-twitch muscle fibers burn glucose more slowly and completely than fast-twitch muscle fibers, and also use more fatty acids for energy. This means activating the slow-twitch muscle fibers will burn fat more readily. As described above, high-intensity exercise uses primarily glucose from muscle tissue and glucose circulating in the bloodstream as supplied from the liver. Therefore, this type of exercise is not very effective in burning body fat. Studies show that by varying the amounts of anaerobic and aerobic exercise, you can achieve a diversity of body composition and performance results.

Aerobic and anaerobic metabolism are occurring all of the time, but different workouts will employ one type of metabolism more than the other. How your body uses the different energy systems is what makes the difference. Let's look at an example. If you were to lift a one-pound weight for several minutes, the slow-twitch muscle fibers in your arm muscle would be supplying most of the energy to do this type of low-intensity, long-duration work. But if you chose a 30-pound dumbbell and began to do reps, within a few seconds your type IIb fast-twitch muscle fibers and anaerobic energy systems are doing the primary work. At this level of all-out effort, however, all of your muscle fibers are working to some extent.

THE INTENSITY-DURATION MUSCLE-FIBER CONNECTION

So, what does all this talk about fast-twitch and slow-twitch muscle fibers have to do with you? It opens up new possibilities to how you can use weight training to develop your body best for your sport or personal fitness goals. Let's face it, it's hard pumping heavy loads of iron. But probably you don't need to. Very few athletes need to lift very heavy weights for a few repetitions like powerlifters and Olympic weight lifters do. When you think about using weight training to improve

MUSCLE FIBER TYPES SUMMARY

Type I (also called Slow-Twitch, Slow Oxidative [SO])

Type I muscle fibers have a high oxidative metabolism capacity. They are highly fatigue-resistant, with less capacity for exercise-induced muscle growth, and highly resistant to exercise-induced structural damage. They will increase in size with weight training, but not as much as fast-twitch muscle fibers. They are best conditioned using high-repetition training with lighter weights and slow continuous tension movements. With progressive long-duration training, slow-twitch muscle fibers develop higher density of mitochondria, which increases their ability to produce energy from fatty acids. They are small in diameter, with high capillary density and low glycogen content, compared to fast-twitch muscle fibers.

Type IIa (also called Fast-Twitch Oxidative-Glycolytic, Fast Oxidative Glycolytic [FOG])

Type IIa muscle fibers have oxidative-glycolytic metabolism capacity. They are moderately fatigue-resistant, have a high capacity for exercise-induced hypertrophy, and have moderate resistance to exercise-induced structural damage. Important for sustained stamina-strength. They respond best to medium-repetition training using moderate weight and fast concentric movements, but slower eccentric movements. They are medium in diameter, with intermediate capillary density and intermediate glycogen content.

Type IIb (also called Fast-Twitch Glycolytic, Fast Glycolytic [FG])

Type IIb muscle fibers have a high capacity for glycolytic metabolism, low oxidative capacity, and are highly susceptible to fatigue. They can be trained to store a ready-to-use supply of immediate energy in the form of ATP and CP. They have a great capacity for exercise-induced muscle growth and susceptibility to exercise-induced damage. Well-developed type IIb muscle fibers have the capacity to generate explosive strength and power. They respond best to high-intensity, explosive concentric movements using heavier weights, and a slow eccentric movement. When fully developed they have the largest diameter, high glycogen content, and low capillary density.

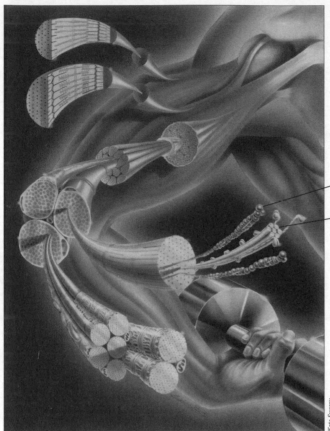

Muscle Fiber Details. Muscles are composed of fibers that are bundled together. These bundles are then grouped together to make up a particular muscle. Notice that the muscle fibers contain the thin myofibrils, the thick myosin filaments, and thinner actin filaments, which cause muscles to contract and relax.

Thin Filament

Thick Filament

Kate Sweeny

your sports performance, will being able to squat 1,000 pounds once help you much? Even in power sports like football, there is a need to develop muscle that not only produces powerful muscle contractions, but can also produce these contractions over and over again.

For fitness exercisers who want to increase muscle size and strength for health and physique reasons, lifting heavy weights for a few repetitions is not needed. Most weight-lifting exercisers will do much better using a diversity of medium- to light-intensity workloads for a wide range of repetitions. This will develop larger muscles that have strength-stamina.

When you take a look at a professional competitive bodybuilder, you see several types of athletes in one. Most bodybuilders have developed all of their muscle fibers, in particular both types of fast-twitch muscle fibers. As they get stronger,

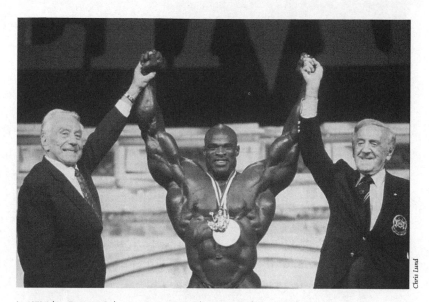

Chris Lund

Joe Weider, Ronnie Coleman (2000 Mr. Olympia), and Ben Weider.

they get bigger. Even their warm-up sets contribute to building strength and muscle, in particular type IIa and type I muscle fibers. To illustrate the magnitude of type IIb and type IIa muscle-fiber development, let us take a look at some impressive statistics from bodybuilding legend Arnold Schwarzenegger. In a recent article in *Muscle & Fitness* magazine, Arnold was reported to be able to lift the following weights and repetitions in the bench press: 500 pounds for one rep, 405 pounds for eight reps, 315 pounds for 25 reps, and 225 pounds for 60 reps. From a muscle-fiber development standpoint, Arnold's ability to lift such an impressive amount of weight for a variety of repetitions is a direct reflection of his diversified muscle-fiber development. We think most people would be satisfied with being able to bench-press 225 pounds for one repetition. But being able to bench-press 225 pounds for 60 repetitions demonstrates the strength-stamina potential that well-developed fast-twitch muscle fibers have to offer, especially type IIa muscle fibers. Ronnie Coleman, the 2000 Mr. Olympia champion, is reported to display similar diversified muscle-fiber development and wide-ranging weight-lifting abilities. In fact, in one of his favorite exercises, the dumbbell lateral raise giant set, he is reported to lift (without stopping) 30-pound dumbbells for 25 reps, then 40 pounds for 15 reps, then 50 pounds for 10 reps, and then 60 pounds for 8 reps. He performed two of these giant sets about twice a month and produced drastic gains in shoulder-muscle development. This again demonstrates how Variable Weight Training can be used to stimulate total muscle-fiber development.

MUSCLE-FIBER RECOVERY

There is another side to the muscle-fiber story: time for recovery. When you are training with heavy workloads for a few repetitions to develop type IIb muscle fibers, these muscle fibers break down and need a few to several days to fully recover. When weight training with medium workloads targeted at developing type IIa muscle fibers, you are using muscle fibers that are more resistant to exercise-induced damage, but they still need a few days to recover. When using light workloads for higher repetitions, less muscle damage occurs and less rest is needed.

In practice, this means that it is best to alternate the intensity of your weight-training sessions from workout to workout. After a heavy-intensity weight-training day, you need to wait several days for your type IIb muscle fibers to fully recover. But in the meantime, your muscles can endure medium- and light-intensity weight-lifting sessions. There are some individual dynamics concerning recovery from weight-training sessions to consider also. Some people may recover more quickly than others. In general, young people recover more quickly than older people, and men recover more quickly than women. So while we can provide you with weight-training programs to follow, as you become more advanced, you will need to fine-tune your weight training to best suit your individuality.

STRENGTH-TO-BODY-WEIGHT RATIO

Most people don't need to overdevelop their type IIb muscle fibers for a few reasons. First, it takes a tremendous amount of high-intensity training (lifting extremely heavy weights for only a few to several repetitions at a time) to develop them. Second, most people don't need to exert this huge amount of force in their daily life or recreational activity. And finally, there comes a point where an increase in maximum strength will result in an increase of body weight that is not practical. This is where the concept of strength to body weight is important. Massive type IIb muscle fibers are generally too big and fatigue too quickly, making them impractical for competing in many sports and performing daily chores. Most people want more strength and to improve their body build, but they don't need to build the massive physique of a powerlifter, bodybuilder, or football lineman.

Even sports that require massive strength and power don't really require you to develop your body to a point of maximum power. For example, football linemen need strong, massive bodies to generate explosive muscle contractions and overpower their opponents. But if a lineman were to spend the time in the gym lifting just like a powerlifter and were able to generate enough force to squat 1,000 pounds for one repetition, he would do extremely well only for the first few plays. A lineman needs to maintain that level of explosive strength off the line, however, over perhaps more than 60 plays during a game. After that first few plays he would fatigue because he did not spend time developing the other fast-twitch muscle fibers, type IIa, which give us the ability to produce powerful muscle contractions over and over again.

Even in a strength sport like boxing, where explosive power for the knock-out punch is key, muscle stamina and endurance is also important. Boxers are in the ring slugging it out for three minutes at a time, contracting their muscles over and over again as if they were performing a combination weight-lifting giant set and short run around the track. Then they only get a minute of rest, and have to perform again for three minutes of all-out, sustained effort. While powerlifters and bodybuilders are extremely strong athletes, I think you will agree that unless they knocked a well-trained boxer out early in the first round, their ability to generate explosive muscle contractions in the second round would greatly be reduced, and continue to be reduced each round thereafter.

In fact, true "cross training" is employing different types of exercise or sport activities to train your different energy systems and muscle fibers. Under these terms, the triathlon is not really cross-training, because all of the sport activities are aerobic, long distance. None of them require maximum development of the fast-twitch muscle fibers or anaerobic energy systems. A good example of a cross-trained athlete is a decathlete. In the decathlon all of the energy systems need to be developed to excel at the different events. For example, the shot put requires very short-lived, extremely explosive strength. Other anaerobic strength events in the decathlon include the 100-meter sprint, long jump, high jump, 110-meter hurdles, discus, pole vault, and javelin, which need well-developed fast-twitch muscle fibers, both types. The 400-meter run tests the athlete's type IIa muscle fiber development. This event then ends with a grueling 1,500-meter aerobic run, which also relies on the anaerobic energy systems early in the race and at the end-of-the-race sprint to the finish line, but also requires a well-developed level of high-intensity aerobic performance-fitness.

FOOD AS FUEL

Your nutrition will also have an important impact on the optimal development of the different muscle fibers and energy systems. As fast-twitch muscles fibers are larger and break down more easily, when you develop more of them you need to eat more protein to maintain and rebuild them. Also, because fast-twitch muscle fibers use mostly carbohydrates for energy during exercise, and less fat, strength and bodybuilding diets need to be lower in fat. The supplements a strength athlete takes will have some similarities to those taken by other types of athletes, but there will be important differences. When you start thinking at the cellular and biochemical level, it is easy to understand how the dynamics of your body are shaped by different types of exercise and nutrition programs. We'll discuss food and supplement needs for different athletes more in chapters 7 and 11.

MAINTENANCE—USE IT OR LOSE IT

It is a well-known medical fact that disuse of your body will lead to premature aging and premature death. Weight training your entire body on a regular basis will keep your muscles in good working order. It will stimulate growth and development and keep you looking younger longer.

Another important point to remember in the "use it or lose it" principle is that this is a lifelong commitment. There are no quick fixes to weight loss or three-month miracle exercise programs. Once you achieve your strength and bodybuilding goals, this does not mean you stop weight training. You need to stick with it to experience lifelong benefits. So, when you reach your particular goals, continue weight training for maintenance. This may mean cutting back on the days and sets of weight-training exercises you perform. But try to exercise each muscle group at least once or twice a week for maintenance of strength, muscle size, and the other health benefits of weight training.

SYMMETRY

Remember to work your entire body, all muscle groups. People sometimes favor arms over legs, or shoulders over abs, but disuse of just one muscle group can have potentially crippling effects, or severely limit your range of motion and physical performance potential. For example, if certain muscles in your lower back are not exercised and stretched on a regular basis, they can become shortened over time and can squeeze the discs that cushion your vertebrae. Muscles may spasm and, eventually, a herniated or ruptured disc could occur, causing severe back pain and life-long back problems that can require surgery.

Even well-trained athletes need to make sure they don't ignore certain muscles. This is especially true among athletes who engage in sports that are asymmetrical, like baseball or tennis. Even during the season, when your weight training has to be focused on just a few primary weight-training exercises as directed by your coach and trainer, it is wise to perform the basic total-body weight-training exercises for your other muscles. Use a middle- to light-intensity workload for a few sets to keep them in good condition.

Chapter 4 includes the weight-training routines to get you on your way to improving strength and bodybuilding. It also reviews some important related terminology and concepts related to weight lifting, like reps, sets, rest, and recovery. You will also discover one of the most important muscle groups to keep in shape are often underdeveloped.

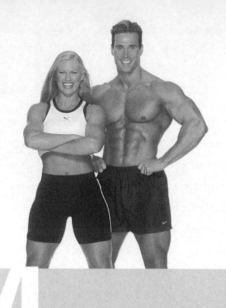

4

The Strength and Bodybuilding Makeover: Exercise Programs

In the pages that follow we present examples of a variety of weight-training programs for you to follow, depending on your current level of physical conditioning and performance-fitness goals. These programs are primarily designed for adults who want to improve their strength, muscle mass, and body build, including both competitive athletes and fitness enthusiasts. Use them with your sport-specific weight-training programs in the off-season and developmental season to help round out your muscular development and stimulate growth all of your muscles—not just the ones you may be using for your sport. (See chapter 10 for some guidelines on year-round athletic training and weight lifting.) Competitive strength athletes will find the weight-training programs useful in off-season training, but they are not intended for competitive powerlifters, Olympic lifters, or bodybuilders. You'll need to follow specialized, advanced programs under the supervision of a specialist.

SOME PERFORMANCE-FITNESS CONCEPTS TO KEEP IN MIND

• Your weight-training routine should be appropriately tailored to match your performance-fitness goals.

• Build your program gradually, especially if you are a beginner. Advance carefully from beginner to intermediate to intermediate/advanced levels as your fitness and strength improve.

• One size does not fit all. As you advance, fine-tune the programs to suit your needs.

• Once you achieve your desired strength and muscle-building goals, adjust your routine to maintain your gains.

Regardless of whether you are a competitive athlete, beginner, or well-trained fitness exerciser, if weight training is new to you, we recommend that you start by following the beginner's weight-lifting programs described below. You may be able to advance to the intermediate programs quickly, depending on your level of fitness. If you are experienced in weight training, then use this period as a new beginning to identify your strong areas of muscular development and areas of underdeveloped muscles. Also, this is a good time to work on improving your all-around flexibility and building up strength in the often-neglected midsection of your body (abdominal, obliques, and lower back). You can also work on achieving proper weight-lifting technique, including working the muscles through their full range of motion, and proper deep-breathing technique.

Below are some terms and concepts you should review to get the best results from your weight-training program.

BREATHING

While breathing is an automatic function, most people we encounter do not breathe correctly. Try to notice if your breathing is shallow and in the chest, instead of deep and in the abdomen. When you breathe, your diaphragm expands downward into the abdominal region. In order to make room for the expanding diaphragm, you need to expand your abdomen, allowing maximum expansion and inhalation of the lungs. This in turn maximizes oxygen intake and carbon dioxide elimination. Good deep breathing is crucial if you want to make any improvement.

The best way to see if you are breathing correctly is to lie down on the floor on your back, and place a book over your navel. Now breathe normally. If you are breathing correctly, your abdomen should be expanding like a bellows, moving the book up and down. If your breathing is shallow, and up in the chest, then the book will not move up or down that much, if at all. If this is the case, then you need to do some breathing exercises.

If you failed the book test, then each day, lie on the floor and practice breathing deeply, and pushing the book up and down with your lower abdomen. During the day, while in the car, or at home, try singing along with your favorite music. When you sing, you naturally breathe deeply from your lower abdomen. In fact, this is one of the reasons why people feel better after they sing along with a song. The deep breathing has relaxing effects. Deep breathing is clinically proven to reduce stress and destructive hormones, such as cortisol, a hormone associated with stress. In fact, when you exercise, you are forced to breathe deeply. This is one of the reasons why exercise is de-stressing. As you practice your deep-breathing exercises, you will become more aware of how daily stress tightens your chest and makes your breathing shallow. When this occurs, try some deep breathing.

During your weight-lifting exercise sessions, keep these basic rules of breathing in mind.

- Breathe out during the muscle contraction phase of the repetition, and breathe in during the phase of the repetition where your muscles are elongating.

- Never hold your breath during the repetition.

- Keep your mouth open to equalize pressure in your chest, and exhale and inhale completely during each repetition. This will also keep your body well oxygenated, and enable to you to perform more work during your exercise sessions.

You may encounter some advanced breathing techniques used by strength athletes, such as temporarily holding your breath. Unless you are a competitive athlete trained in these special breathing techniques, do not use them. Follow the general rules of breathing discussed above.

FLEXIBILITY AND STRETCHING

Flexibility is an often-neglected but very important component of peak athletic performance and fitness. If the muscles become tight and inflexible, then blood flow is impaired, which in turn impairs muscle contraction and function. Also, as muscle tension builds up over the years, it causes problems in your spine and joints. So, improving and maintaining good muscle and joint flexibility is essential.

We recommend that you get in the habit of stretching once or twice a day, before and after your weights session and on non-weight-training days. Take a look at the basic stretching routine illustrated by our model, Gea Johnson (pp. 50–55). When you stretch, do so slowly, and hold the stretch for a few seconds while maintaining good breathing. Do not force yourself into these positions. It may take you time to develop this level of flexibility, so be patient. Also, everybody has a different range of flexibility, so not everyone will be as flexible as Gea.

In addition to these examples, you may want to join a yoga class to learn some new stretches, and have the yoga instructor design a program you can follow daily at home to suit your individuality. Don't forget to stretch before and after your weight-training sessions, as discussed below. Begin with a warm-up of light aerobic exercise, then perform your stretching, followed by your weight-training routine, and end with more stretching during your cool-down period. Get into the habit of stretching each muscle group at the end of each set as you run through your routine. Most people begin to do this instinctively because it makes the fatigued muscles feel so much better, but the stretch will really help to keep the muscles limber, too. Now you can move on to the next body part.

If, after a few weeks of flexibility training, you find that you still have some hard and stiff muscles that are sore to the touch and do not readily soften when you firmly massage them with your fingers, you may need to invest in a professional therapeutic massage. These muscles are most likely in chronic spasm. A good massage therapist will work the muscles to relieve the tension and spasm and to release muscle adhesions that are locking your muscle fibers together. Give it time, however. While some people respond after a few sessions, others may have to

UPPER BODY STRETCHES

1. Front of Shoulder / Chest Stretch:

Standing perpendicular to the wall, raise one arm to the side and place your hand against the wall at shoulder level. Straighten your arm. Slowly turn body away from the wall feeling a stretch in the forearm, biceps, front shoulder, and chest. Repeat with the other arm.

2. Back of Shoulder Stretch:

Start with both hands grasped together behind the back, resting on the buttocks with elbows fully extended. From this position, raise both arms slowly as far as possible while maintaining a fully erect upright posture. If you can't get your hands to meet, try grasping a rolled-up towel behind your back.

3. Single Arm Shoulder Stretch:

Bring your arm in front of your chest, parallel with the floor, until you feel a stretch in the rear shoulder area. Repeat with the other arm.

4. Single Arm Overhead Shoulder Stretch:

Start by raising both arms above your head. Now bend your left elbow and grasp it with your right hand. Gently pull on your left upper arm so it is aligned straight up and down. Repeat with the other arm.

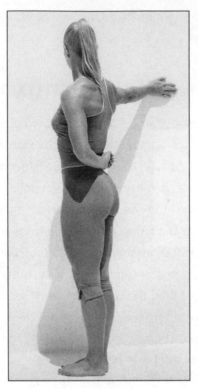
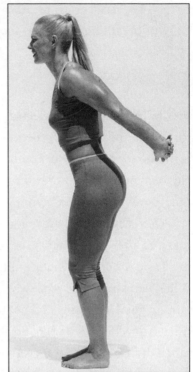

1.   2.

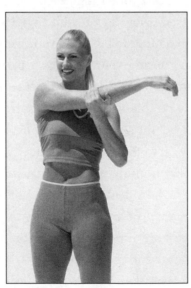
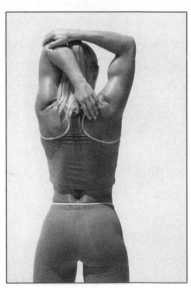

3.   4.

LOWER BODY STRETCHES

5, 6, 7. Calf Stretch:

Place your hands at shoulder height in front of you on a wall. Step back so that you are leaning forward as shown, keeping arms, back, and legs straight; you should feel a stretch in your calves. Then step forward with your right leg to increase the stretching in your left calf, keeping your left heel on the ground during the stretching movement. Repeat with the other leg.

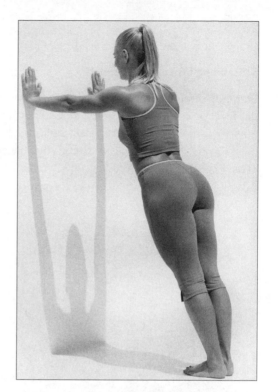

5.

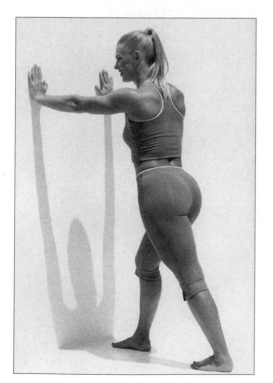

6.

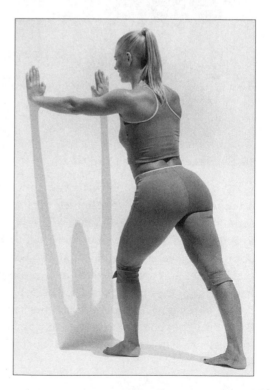

7.

LOWER BODY STRETCHES

8. Standing Quadriceps Stretch:

Standing straight, place your right hand about shoulder level on a wall. Lift your left foot so that you can grasp it with your left hand. Slowly pull your left foot back toward your buttocks to stretch the left quadriceps. Repeat with the other leg.

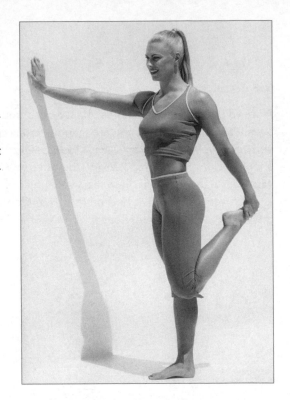

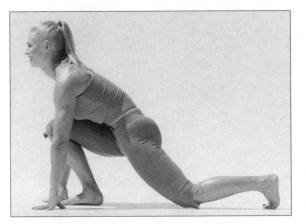

9. Hip Flexor Lunge Stretch:

Starting in a standing position, lunge forward with your right leg, keeping the left leg back with the knee bent. Lower the trunk of your body and position it as far forward as possible, resting your hands on the ground. You should feel the stretch in the groin area. Repeat with the other leg.

10. Single Leg Hamstring Stretch:

Start in the seated position with your right leg extended forward and your left leg bent with your left foot resting on your inner right thigh. Reach forward and grasp your right foot with both hands, keeping your leg straight. Slowly pull forward to create a stretch in your right hamstring. Grasp either your ankle, heel, or toes, depending on how flexible your hamstrings are. Bring the upper body as far forward as possible to stretch the hamstring. Repeat with your other leg.

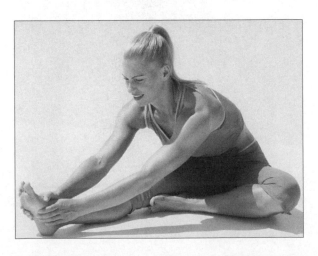

LOWER BODY STRETCHES

11, 12, 13, 14. Double Leg Hamstring Inner Groin Stretch:

Begin from a seated position on the floor with your legs spread apart and kept straight. Keep your arms shoulder length apart, resting in a U-shape as shown. Slide both hands down your legs, and lean forward. Then bring your arms and bend them on the floor in front of you and slide them forward, bringing your face to the floor.

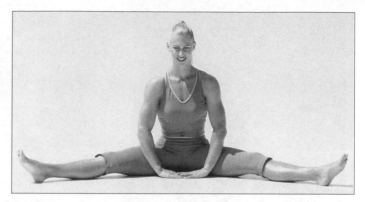

11.

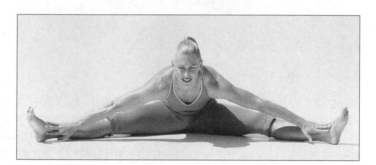

12.

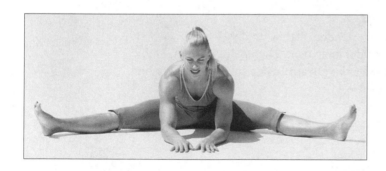

13.

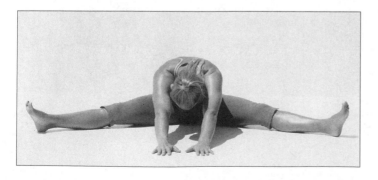

14.

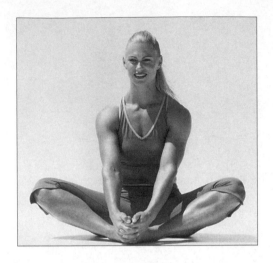

15.

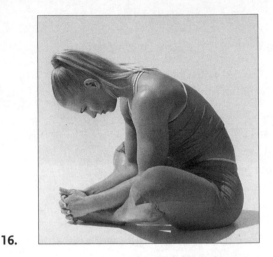

16.

LOWER BODY STRETCHES

15, 16. Groin Stretch:

Start by sitting on the floor with your knees bent toward your groin and the soles of your feet together, grasping both feet with your hands. Lean your upper body forward and rest both elbows on your lower legs. Continue to lean forward while pressing downward with your elbows on bent legs at the same time to create a stretch in the groin area.

17, 18. Spinal Twist:

Start in the sitting position with your legs fully extended. Place your right leg over your left leg, keeping your left leg straight and your right knee bent. Then place your left elbow against your right knee. Twist the spine toward your right arm, using your left arm to assist the twisting motion. Repeat on the opposite side.

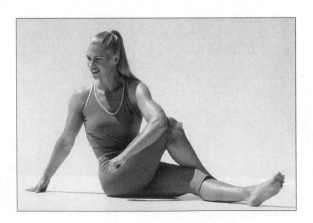

17.

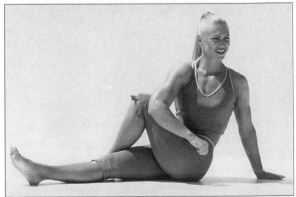

18.

LOWER BODY STRETCHES

19, 20. Lower Back Rotation Stretch:

Start by lying on your back. Bend your right leg and place it over the left leg so that it is perpendicular to your body, keeping your shoulders flat and your arms out to the side. You should feel a gentle stretch in your lower back. Increase the stretch by grasping your right leg with your left hand to pull your right knee toward the floor. Repeat with the other leg.

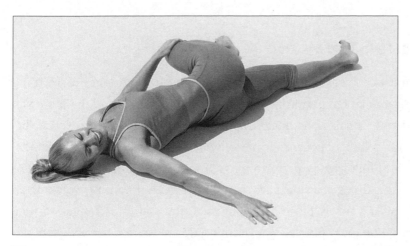

19.

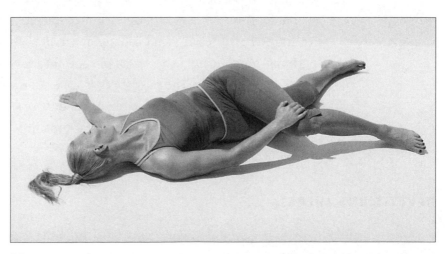

20.

make regular monthly visits to the massage therapist and see results develop more slowly. It all depends on how long the condition existed and what you do in your daily life that contributes to the condition.

The same is true for repetitive strain/muscle tension conditions such as carpal tunnel syndrome and tennis elbow. In most cases, after years of repeated motion in a limited range, if the muscles are not stretched or exercised to the full range of motion along with the other muscles, muscle tension syndrome sets in. Massage therapy can help relieve these muscle tension syndromes. The extra investment will be well worth it and just may keep you out of the doctor's office and operating room.

WARMING UP AND COOLING DOWN

If you are like most people, you were first taught about the importance of warming up way back in gym class in grammar school. The older you get and the more you advance in your athletic career, the more important warming up before exercise becomes. Warming up generally consists of doing some aerobic exercise, calisthenics, and stretching, followed by performing your weight training, sport event, or fitness activity a few times at a slow pace. If you are strength training or taking an aerobics class, start out slowly, picking up your pace after your muscles get warmed up and feel ready. The main purposes of warming up are to raise the body temperature, to limber up the muscles and connective tissues, and to get your blood flowing. Most warm-up periods take several to fifteen minutes before weight-training sessions, but for some athletes they can be much longer.

Most trainers also recommend cooling down after exercising. Cooling down consists simply of reducing the intensity of your physical activity gradually, as opposed to stopping abruptly. The purpose is to ease your breathing and heart rate back to their resting levels. This generally takes only several minutes and is well worth the time. This is a good time to perform some final stretching, focusing on the muscles that you just exercised.

REPETITIONS (REPS)

Every type of weight-training exercise consists of the execution of repetitions of muscle contractions. Each sequence of repetitions is called a set. The number of sets performed for a particular body part will depend on your level of fitness and your goals. In general, beginners can only tolerate a low number of sets. More is not better for the beginner. As your fitness level advances, you'll need to add more sets to stimulate greater improvements.

There is no fixed magic number of reps that will produce better results than another number. Everyone is different and you should use a combination of science, observation, and self-discovery to find out what works best for you. There are ranges of repetitions, related to the weight of the workload that will stimulate the specific muscle fibers to grow and develop. As you consult the Rep Zones table, you will notice that even high repetitions of lighter weights can be effective in building strength and muscle size. This will work up to a point—a point, incidentally, that most fitness exercisers will be pleased with. Then, as you advance in your weight training, you will need to increase the workloads and perform fewer repetitions to stimulate more fast-twitch muscle fibers, thereby building greater strength and gain in muscle size.

There are a few variables to consider. First, all of your muscle fibers have the capacity to increase in size from weight training, even slow-twitch muscle fibers. But remember that there are two primary types of fast-twitch muscle fibers that will respond to different workloads and repetition zones. The other major variable is you. While we can make generalizations that you can follow for tremendous results, you must also participate in the weight-training routine evaluation. You may genetically have more slow-twitch muscle fibers, and may find that your body responds to doing sets with higher repetitions, while your training partner may respond better to doing more sets with lower repetitions, using higher workloads.

Another variable is your current level of fitness. If you are an aerobically trained person, your body may respond more slowly than someone who is active in anaerobic sports or untrained. In the first case, this is because the anatomy and physiology of a person who has trained anaerobically is already in a muscle-building zone and, in the second case, because untrained individuals usually respond more quickly to weight training during the first few months. However, the Variable Weight-Training approach and weight-training routines take these differences into account. They are designed to stimulate growth and development in all of your muscle fibers to suit your performance and fitness goals. Guidelines are provided to enable you to customize the routines to best suit your individuality.

Aside from the number of repetitions to perform in a set, there are some dynamic aspects to the repetition itself. A repetition is composed of a positive resistance movement (concentric) when the muscle contracts, and a negative resistance movement (eccentric) when the muscle elongates. Research and experience shows that for maximum stimulation of muscle growth, emphasis on both the positive and negative movements of each repetition is important. As it turns out, the muscle can handle more weight on the negative movement. The classic bodybuilding repetition is slow and steady, using good form and technique as described in the next chapter. You must make sure to lower the weight slowly, over a count of two to three seconds. The positive or lifting movement should take one to two seconds.

As you advance, perhaps after weight training consistently for a few months, you can begin to mix up your routine somewhat by increasing the speed at which you perform reps and sets. Competitive athletes who do preseason weight training, as well as during the season, will most often benefit more from performing faster,

THE MECHANICS OF MUSCULAR CONTRACTION

To the naked eye, the external skeletal muscles appear grainy. This is due to the fact that they are made up of small fibers. These fibers are cylinderlike and may be several centimeters long. In length, they are divided into bands (striations), much like coins stacked in a pile. Each individual fiber is surrounded by a thin plasma membrane, the sarcolemma. Some 80 percent of the fiber's volume is filled with tiny fibrils, known as myofibrils—which may number from several hundred to several thousand per fiber. These fibrils are the structures that are directly involved in contraction of the muscle fiber. The remainder of the muscle fiber is filled with a jellylike intracellular fluid called sarcoplasm. The sarcoplasm contains many nuclei and other cell constituents, such as mitochondria, within which energy-producing biochemical reactions take place.

Further examination of the fibrils has revealed that they are made of two types of protein—actin and myosin—which are in the form of long filaments. The thick filaments consist of myosin, and the thin ones are made of actin. These filaments are able to interlock and slide over each other to accommodate the stretching of the muscle. During shortening (contraction), they slide into one another, and it appears that cross-links are made between the actin and myosin rhythmic repetitions, for improved functional strength. From time to time even intermediate and advanced fitness exercisers can benefit from lifting weights more rapidly, too. However, the amount of weight being used should be light enough to perform the repetitions easily. Even light weight will give you a very strenuous workout if you lift them quickly, and they can generate tremendous force on your joints. Increased force means increased risk of injury, so beginners should stick to using the slower-paced repetition movement and always concentrate on maintaining good technique and focusing on the particular muscles being exercised.

With the Rep Zones chart, you'll get a quick look at the different number of reps we recommend for a variety of strength-training goals. If you are a beginner, you should start with lighter rep zones. You will increase muscle size to a certain point by using this lower-intensity, longer-duration weight training. Then, as you become better trained, you'll move on to performing lower repetitions using heav-

THE MECHANICS OF MUSCULAR CONTRACTION

filaments. These cross-links are almost instantaneously broken, and new links are set up further along the filaments. The process of breaking these cross-links causes the two filaments to move toward one another, causing the muscle to shorten (contract).

The term "contraction" does not always refer to the shortening of a muscle. Technically, it refers to the development of tension within a muscle. There are two major contractions. A contraction in which the muscle develops tension but does not shorten is termed "isometric." A contraction in which the muscle shortens but retains constant tension is said to be "isotonic." For example, a person trying to curl a heavy barbell strains against the weight. The arm muscles develop tension but do not shorten because the amount of resistance generated by the heavy barbell is greater than the muscle's tension. But when the barbell is lightened by removing some plates, the working muscles shorten as they contract. This is an isotonic contraction. When muscles shorten by overcoming resistance to a load (weight), the isotonic contraction is said to be concentric. When the biceps lengthen while the barbell is let down but they maintain a constant tension during the lengthening movement, the isotonic contraction is termed "eccentric." The muscles lengthen as they act to maintain tension.

ier weight. However, it is still important to perform the high-repetition exercises at least once a week during your heavy-intensity weight-lifting sessions, and as a warm-up before all exercises.

ADVANCED WEIGHT-TRAINING TECHNIQUES— NEGATIVE FAILURE OR FORCED REPS

When you perform the second half of a rep (the negative or eccentric part), the muscle has the potential to resist higher workloads than it can lift during the first half. Some advanced body-builders use techniques called "negative failure" or "forced reps" to fully exhaust the muscle. We will bring these to your attention, but we do not recommend that you use these techniques until you've reached an advanced level. It's very possible that you'll come across them in your reading or at the gym, and we want you to understand that they may have a place in your weight training, but only when you are ready for them.

To do forced reps, you'll need to enlist the help of a training partner or "spotter." After you reach positive failure and cannot lift the weight any longer, your muscle still has the ability to lower the weight, so the spotter helps you bring the weight up a few more times while allowing you to bring it down during the negative phase. Continue this process until you can no longer control the speed at which you lower the weight. This is then called "negative failure."

Another way to utilize the muscles' ability to lift more weight during the negative phase of the rep is to have your spotter actually push down on the weight during the negative phase, fatiguing you more quickly. Negative-failure training may trigger a new growth spurt in your muscles.

It does this by producing more muscle-fiber damage, and will most likely result in more post-exercise muscle soreness that can last a few days. This technique is a double-edged sword. While it may help trigger new muscle growth and get you out of a slump, if used too often they can cause extreme muscle soreness, even damage to your joints. Because negative failure fatigues your muscles to the point where you cannot control the speed at which you lower the weights, it puts excessive pressure on your joints, and can result in injury or an accident if you are not closely monitored.

Also, in general, athletes should avoid going to negative failure, as this results in more damage to muscle fibers, and such damage may impair athletic performance. Individuals not looking for dramatic increases in muscle size should also avoid going to negative failure.

Rep Zones: Variable Weight-Training Approach			
Strength Training Objective	Explosive-Strength, Power-Strength, Speed-Strength Repetition Zone & Peak Muscle Mass	Speed-Strength Repetition Zone & Peak Muscle Mass	Stamina-Strength Repetition Zone & Moderate Muscle Mass	Endurance-Strength Repetition Zone & Minimum Muscle Mass
Training Level(s)	• Advanced • Competitive Athletes	• Advanced • Competitive Athletes • Intermediate	• Advanced • Competitive Athletes • Intermediate • Beginners	• Advanced • Competitive Athletes • Intermediate • Beginners
Intensity	Heavy	Medium	Medium Light	Light
Repetition Zone	3 to 6 reps	8 to 12 reps	15 to 24 reps	25 to 40 reps

Most people are looking to build strength and definition, and they should follow a program of lower repetitions with heavier workloads. Eight to 12 reps of moderately heavy weight is ideal for building strength and well-defined muscle mass. The heavier the weight you lift, the more strength and mass you will gain. Olympic weight lifters and powerlifters spend most of their time training with very heavy weights, performing fewer than six reps. Hence their greater strength. But keep in mind that with lifting heavier weights comes the greater risk of injury. So, while it is tempting to start showing off your new strength, we recommend that you avoid training with heavy weights for low repetitions until you develop to an advanced level, and only if your athletic performance will benefit from it.

Remember that you will also benefit from performing higher repetitions of lighter weights at least once a week to cross-train your anaerobic energy systems.

SETS

If you are untrained or new to weight lifting, you should perform one to two sets per exercise for the first few months. This should be sufficient to stimulate in-

---

THE COMPETITIVE EDGE FOR ENDURANCE JOCKS

Scientific studies yield mixed results about the usefulness of using low-repetition weight training during the competition season for endurance sports. Researchers report that while strength is improved, this may or may not translate into greater endurance. During the preseason, try using high-repetition weight training after your practice sessions to help increase your endurance. Do 25 to 40 repetitions, using weights that will make it challenging. In addition to building endurance strength, high reps will also help increase enzymes in your body that help clear lactic acid. It will also improve your ability to "sprint" at the end of your endurance event.

If you are considering weight training during your off-season, we recommend sticking to lighter weights and higher repetitions.

---

creases in strength and muscle size in most individuals. After a few months you will probably need to increase the number of sets for a particular body part to stimulate further improvements in strength and muscle mass.

The number of sets you eventually end up doing will depend on your personal goals. If you are a fitness exerciser, one to two sets may be all you ever need to do. If you are a competitive athlete lifting weights to augment your athletic performance, three to six sets per body part will work best. For some athletes, such as football players, more than 6 to 12 sets is usually required to build the strength and stamina needed to maintain explosive muscle contractions over and over during a game. If you aspire to be a weight-lifting athlete, you will surely need to eventually perform a high number of sets. For competitive athletes, there is no magic number of sets that can be applied to all individuals. That's why a good training log is of major importance so you can chart your progress and see how your strength increases in response to different workloads.

INCREASING THE WEIGHT—PROGRESSIVE OVERLOAD

One of the most common mistakes people make in weight training is to increase the workload too quickly. Don't let your eagerness determine when you are ready to increase the amount of weight you are using. Muscle tissue generally will increase in strength and size more quickly than the connective tissues that anchor them to your skeleton. A major benefit of weight training is that it builds a stronger body, so if you are a fitness exerciser you do not need to rush the process. Give yourself the time for complete body tissue growth.

This is especially true of beginners. It's hard enough to commit to an exercise program—the last thing you need is an injury that will prevent you from doing your workout and set you back several more weeks. So avoid packing on heavy weights to see how much you can lift for one repetition. Start using workloads that enable you to perform the recommended exercises within the target repetition range. Determining the exact workloads will take some trial and error. It is important to focus your initial efforts on establishing good weight-training technique and developing a good strength and muscle foundation.

With this in mind, evaluate potential increases in the weight you are lifting after your initiation period. Repeat this process about every three weeks. Use the repetition range as an indicator of when you should increase the weights, and even the number of sets. For example, if your repetition per set range is eight to 12 reps, you may be able to do 12 reps for the first set, then only 10 reps for the second, and barely eight reps for the third set. A good time to increase the weight would be when you can lift at least 12 reps to failure for all three sets, using the same workload. You can also opt to increase the number of sets at this point, if building stamina-strength is your goal. Generally, you should increase the weight by one- to

SPECIAL MESSAGE TO BEGINNERS AND EVERYONE ELSE

If you have never exercised with weights, or only have been doing so for a few months, keep the following in mind to maintain safety and derive maximum benefits. For the first three months, train only to near-positive failure and do not perform high-intensity workouts. Focus on your style, concentrating on good form. Do not overexert yourself and do not attempt to lift very heavy weights for one repetition. Always train with a spotter. If muscle soreness persists or injury occurs, immediately seek medical attention and stop exercising. Pace yourself and stick to realistic goals. Anyone engaged in an exercise program should get regular medical examinations and approval from their doctor to continue with their current exercise program or engage in a new one. This includes men and women of all ages, not just older adults—everybody!

ONE-REPETITION MAXIMUM

When you spend time in the gym and read the muscle-building magazines, you may encounter a system for determining your appropriate rep range called *one-repetition maximum* (1RM). This refers to maximum amount of weight you can lift one time. Let's say it's 100 pounds on the bench press. Then if you calculate a percentage of your 1RM, you will end up lifting a certain number of repetitions. For example, using 80% of your 1RM, 80 pounds, may result in performing six repetitions. For the purposes of this book, you do not need to be concerned with calculating your 1RM, except for the discussion on speed. Do not try to see how much you can lift for one repetition, unless required for your sport, as this can result in excessive muscle/joint strain.

2.5-pound increments for women and fitness exercisers, and 2.5- to 5-pound increments for male athletes.

REST BETWEEN SETS

If you are a beginner, take as much time as you need between sets to avoid feeling dizzy or overly fatigued, especially during the first three weeks. It takes your body some time to adjust to this new type of exercise. As your muscles develop and you

DON'T BE A CHATTY WEIGHTLIFTER

Look around the gym and you'll notice people sitting around too much during their weight-training routine. You have to approach your weight routine much as you would an hour of walking or running for exercise. Keep up a good pace with timed periods of rest, and stick to your plan. Don't get caught up in conversations and chit-chat during session. Stay focused and proceed through your routine with a passion. Concentrate on breathing correctly during your exercise. Take deep breaths, expanding your lower abdomen. Exhale when you lift the weights (contract your muscles), and inhale when you lower the weights (elongate your muscles). Breathing to full capacity is very important, as you need to provide your body with a maximum supply of oxygen and expel carbon dioxide with each breath you take. Save the conversation for after the workout.

advance to the intermediate level, start to keep track of the time spent resting between sets. Generally speaking, when exercising at a lower intensity, rest about one to two minutes between sets. If you're more advanced and are already lifting heavier workloads, a longer rest of two to four minutes between sets is recommended to allow lactic acid clearance and for your muscles' short-term energy system to be revived. If your goal is to increase muscle stamina-strength and endurance-strength, then rest periods should be short: 30 to 60 seconds.

An exception to this would be if you choose to engage in some type of circuit training, such as Universal or Nautilus. When circuit training, your rest between exercises is usually kept to a minimum to maximize cardiovascular benefits by keeping your heart pumping at an elevated rate. We recommend circuit training to maintain muscle tone and promote cardiovascular conditioning, but it is not the ideal way to build maximum strength and muscle mass. Additionally, if you are training for a sport that demands repetitive bursts of energy, such as basketball, football, or wrestling, try to keep your rest between sets to 40 to 60 seconds or less, to simulate the time it takes to recover between plays in the game. Remember, for athletes, weight training is meant to improve athletic performance first, and build a nice muscular body second. Focus on developing your energy level, specific muscle fibers, power, and stamina to best improve your athletic performance.

HIGH-INTENSITY/LOW-INTENSITY—THE VARIABLE WEIGHT TRAINING APPROACH

As the name implies, Variable Weight-Training approaches a variety of training intensities by employing different rep/set ranges. These in turn stimulate growth and development of different muscle fiber types, resulting in improvements to strength and muscle mass. Your training sessions should consist of different weight-training exercises for different body parts, which will be trained at different exercise intensities.

High-intensity training means training a particular muscle group using heavy weights, lifting them for a small number of reps, and performing the maximum number of recommended sets for your level of fitness. Low- and medium-intensity weight training means training a particular muscle group using lower workloads but performing higher repetitions per set.

Note, however, that on any weight-training day it is important to train with "high intensity of effort." This means that after your warm-up set(s), you need to train at least one of the work sets to complete failure, using all-out effort. Using high-intensity effort is important because it triggers the body to produce more of the hormones that stimulate muscle recovery and growth. If you don't feel some level of discomfort in the muscles during this set, then you are not working hard enough. While you should not feel sharp, intense pain, you will feel a burn and perhaps even begin to shake on the last reps of each set. You can make modest improvements by just going through the motions, but optimum improvements are only attained when you exercise with a high level of effort.

The sample weight-training programs alternate light-, medium-light-, and medium-intensity days. Never repeat high-intensity weight training for a particular muscle group two training sessions in a row. Your muscles need time to recover from high-intensity workouts. Eliminating rest days may actually be counterproductive. Follow hard days with moderate- to light-intensity weight-training sessions.

HOW MUCH TIME SHOULD I SPEND WEIGHT TRAINING?

This depends on how much time you have and what your strength and bodybuilding goals are. Ideally, after progressing from beginner to intermediate level, you should weight train each muscle at least twice a week, usually splitting your weight-training routines over four days per week. The time it takes for each weight-training session depends on your level of fitness and how many exercises and sets you are going to perform. For some dedicated people, quality training sessions can range from 30 to 60 minutes. If you are pressed for time, you can do a primary weight-training session at the gym, and another, shorter weight-training session at home. The key is to perform quality sessions. Have your plan ready before you begin. Perform the exercises with serious effort. Time your rest periods.

AEROBIC TRAINING

Most people should have an aerobic training session at least three times per week. If your goal is to maximize strength and develop a cut body, keep your aerobic exercise sessions at 20 to 30 minutes, but no more. Longer aerobic exercise stimulates your body to develop more slow-twitch muscle fibers and smaller muscles. This can be counterproductive to your bodybuilding. It's a delicate balancing act to choose the right amount of anaerobic and aerobic exercise. Many competitive strength athletes either use some form of short-duration aerobic exercise as a warm-up before weight training, or separate it completely from their weight training, so they can maximize their energy stores for high-effort weight-training sessions.

WHAT'S THE RIGHT AMOUNT OF REST BETWEEN WORKOUTS?

Quality periods of rest for recovery are just as important as quality weight-training sessions. Sometimes eager weight trainers who experience initial gains begin to train harder and longer, only to become frustrated when they stop seeing improvements. More is not always better, and sometimes more rest is required, not more weight training. Also, proper nutrition is absolutely necessary for optimum recovery. Chapters 7 and 8 contain complete nutrition plans. Sometimes a two-week break from weight lifting every three months can help prevent chronic overtraining.

The exact time it takes your muscles to fully recover from a weight-training session will depend on your genetics, sex, age, and level of fitness. In general men recover more quickly than women, and young people recover more quickly than people 35 and over. You usually need three to four days for a muscle group to recover after high-intensity weight training, and two to three days to recover after moderate and light weight-training sessions. These are general rules for strength and muscle-building programs. The rules may change for athletes in preseason and season training, depending on your sport.

WEIGHT-TRAINING PROGRAMS

Below are four examples of weight-training programs you can start using to build stronger and bigger muscles. These programs are based on the Variable Weight-Training method, and will result in comprehensive muscle-fiber development. We recommend that beginners and individuals with little weight-lifting experience begin by using Program A. This program is a total body workout, performed twice a week, using higher rep zones. For some people, this program may give you all the results you want, but for others, especially athletes, you will quickly proceed to Program B. The main difference between Programs A and B is the increased workout volume, from eight weight-training workouts per month in Program A, to ten workouts per month in Program B. Once you have completed the recommended cycle length, if you are pleased with the results, then you can repeat this program. Competitive athletes may also find that this level of weight training will be satisfactory to improve performance. If you still want more gains in strength and muscle size, then proceed to Programs C and D.

In Programs C and D the intensity and volume of workouts is cranked up to a new level. The number of sets per exercise is increased to three to six sets. The number of exercises is also increased for some muscles, and the frequency of workouts per month is increased. This higher volume of exercise demands a new approach to the total body workouts—the split workout. A split workout essentially means that you will divide your muscles into groups to accommodate the higher intensity and allow for improved quality of training on any given day. For example, Programs C and D divide training programs into upper body and lower body sections that are trained on different days, as well as abdominals, which are still trained on aerobic exercise days. Fitness exercisers should maintain a slow and steady movement when lifting, while athletes who wish to improve their speed should start executing faster, more rhythmic repetitions. Start slowly and selectively when implementing faster reps, as the extra speed increases the force on your muscles, connective tissues, joints, and bones. Focus on increasing speed during the concentric phase of the rep, while decreasing speed during the eccentric phase. Alternate repetition speeds from workout to workout—slow and steady with fast and rhythmic. See how your body responds and progress accordingly. Give yourself time to respond to the new gains generated by the faster reps.

WEIGHT-TRAINING PROGRAM A

LENGTH: SIX WEEKS

This weight-training program is a total body workout, repeated twice a week. Aerobic training should be performed on non-weight-training days two to three times per week. Abdominal exercises are performed on aerobic exercise days, after aerobic exercise. The training programs are presented in a weeklong schedule that you will repeat.

Make sure to perform a warm-up set, and only perform one working set for the first three weeks. Then perform two sets for each body part during weeks four to six.

Focus your attention on good form and weight-lifting technique. No jerking weights around. The last rep of each set should be difficult to complete within your rep zone—about one rep away from positive failure.

Choose workout days to best suit your personal schedule. If you are trying to lose excess body fat, then schedule workouts on the weekends (or your days off from work), as these tend to be the days most people with weight-control problems overeat. After six weeks take a week off from weight training.

Weight-Training Program A: Days 1–7

BODY PART	EXERCISES Choose one exercise for each body part or a set of exercises as indicated below.	Day 1 Workload: Medium-Light Intensity	Day 2 Aerobics Abdominals	Day 3 Rest	Day 4 Workload: Medium-Light Intensity	Day 5 Aerobics Abdominals	Days 6/7 Rest Aerobics Optional
Neck	Stretching/Manual Resistance	yes			yes		
Traps	Shoulder Shrug or Upright Row	15 to 24 reps			15 to 24 reps		
Shoulders	Military Press or Lateral Raise, Front Raise and Bent-over Lateral Raise	15 to 24 reps			15 to 24 reps		
Upper Back	Bent-over Barbell Rowing or Seated Cable Row or Lat Pulldown	15 to 24 reps			15 to 24 reps		
Lower Back	Back Extension	15 to 24 reps			15 to 24 reps		
Chest	Bench Press or Fly	15 to 24 reps			15 to 24 reps		

Note: If you are a long-distance (oxidative) athlete (see chapter 8), perform 24 to 40 reps per exercise.

The Strength and Bodybuilding Makeover: Exercise Programs

WEIGHT-TRAINING PROGRAM A: DAYS 1–7 (continued)

BODY PART	EXERCISES Choose one exercise for each body part or a set of exercises as indicated below.	Day 1 Workload: Medium-Light Intensity	Day 2 Aerobics Abdominals	Day 3 Rest	Day 4 Workload: Medium-Light Intensity	Day 5 Aerobics Abdominals	Days 6/7 Rest Aerobics Optional
Biceps	Standing Arm Curl or Preacher Curl or Incline Dumbell Curl	15 to 24 reps			15 to 24 reps		
Triceps	Lying Triceps Press or French Press or Triceps Kickback or Triceps Pressdown	15 to 24 reps			15 to 24 reps		
Forearms	Wrist Curl and Reverse Wrist Curl	15 to 24 reps			15 to 24 reps		
Abdominals (Abs)	Inclined Sit-up or Crunch and Reverse Crunch		as many as possible			as many as possible	
Obliques	Lying Side Oblique Crunch		as many as possible			as many as possible	
Buttocks, Hips, Legs	Leg Press or Lunge	15 to 24 reps			15 to 24 reps		

WEIGHT-TRAINING PROGRAM A: DAYS 1–7 *(continued)*

BODY PART	EXERCISES *Choose one exercise for each body part or a set of exercises as indicated below.*	Day 1 Workload: Medium-Light Intensity	Day 2 Aerobics Abdominals	Day 3 Rest	Day 4 Workload: Medium-Light Intensity	Day 5 Aerobics Abdominals	Days 6/7 Rest Aerobics Optional
Quadriceps	Leg Extension	15 to 24 reps			15 to 24 reps		
Hamstrings	Leg Curl	15 to 24 reps			15 to 24 reps		
Calves	Heel Raise or One-legged Standing Raise or Calf Machine	15 to 24 reps			15 to 24 reps		

WEIGHT-TRAINING PROGRAM B

LENGTH: EIGHT WEEKS

This weight-training program is a total body workout, repeated in cycles of three times a week and two times a week. This will increase the volume of weight training to 10 days per month. Aerobic training should be performed on non-weight-training days two to three times per week. Abdominal exercises are performed on aerobics days, after aerobic exercise. The training programs are presented in a two-week-long schedule, which you will repeat. Program B uses three rep zones to cross train your anaerobic energy systems and stimulate maximum muscle-fiber development.

Make sure to perform a warm-up set, and perform two to three working sets. Use this program for eight weeks, then proceed to Program C if you want additional improvements in strength and body build. Otherwise, use this program for maintenance, but introduce some new exercises for diversity.

Focus your attention on good form and weight-lifting technique. No jerking weights around.

Choose workout days to best suit your personal schedule. If you are trying to lose excess body fat, then schedule workouts on the weekends (or your days off from work) as these tend to be the days most people with weight-control problems overeat.

Choose exercise alternatives to work the muscles differently from workout to workout. After eight weeks, take a week off from weight training.

Weight-Training Program B: Days 1–7

BODY PART	EXERCISES Choose one exercise for each body part or a set of exercises as indicated below.	Day 1 Workload: Light Intensity	Day 2 Aerobics Abdominals	Day 3 Workload: Medium-Light Intensity	Day 4 Aerobics Abdominals	Day 5 Workload: Medium Intensity	Days 6/7 Rest Aerobics Optional
Neck	Stretching/Manual Resistance	yes		yes		yes	
Traps	Shoulder Shrug or Upright Row	25 to 40 reps		15 to 24 reps		8 to 12 reps	
Shoulders	Military Press or Lateral Raise, Front Raise, and Bent-over Lateral Raise	25 to 40 reps		15 to 24 reps		8 to 12 reps	
Upper Back	Bent-over Barbell Rowing or Seated Cable Row or Lat Pulldown	25 to 40 reps		15 to 24 reps		8 to 12 reps	
Lower Back	Back Extension	25 to 40 reps		15 to 24 reps		8 to 12 reps	
Chest	Bench Press	25 to 40 reps		15 to 24 reps		8 to 12 reps	
	Fly	25 to 40 reps		15 to 24 reps		8 to 12 reps	

WEIGHT-TRAINING PROGRAM B: DAYS 1–7 (continued)

BODY PART	EXERCISES Choose one exercise for each body part or a set of exercises as indicated below.	Day 1 Workload: Light Intensity	Day 2 Aerobics Abdominals	Day 3 Workload: Medium-Light Intensity	Day 4 Aerobics Abdominals	Day 5 Workload: Medium Intensity	Days 6/7 Rest Aerobics Optional
Biceps	Standing Arm Curl or Preacher Curl or Incline Dumbbell Curl	25 to 40 reps		15 to 24 reps		8 to 12 reps	
Triceps	Lying Triceps Press or Triceps Kickback or Triceps Pressdown	25 to 40 reps		15 to 24 reps		8 to 12 reps	
Forearms	Wrist Curl and Reverse Wrist Curl	25 to 40 reps		15 to 24 reps		8 to 12 reps	
Abdominals (Abs)	Inclined Sit-up or Crunch and Reverse Crunch		25 to 40 reps		15 to 24 reps		
Obliques	Weighted Side Bend or Lying Side Oblique Crunch		25 to 40 reps		15 to 24 reps		
Buttocks, Hips, Legs	Squat or Leg Press or Lunge	25 to 40 reps		15 to 24 reps		8 to 12 reps	
	Side Lunge	25 to 40 reps		15 to 24 reps		None	

WEIGHT-TRAINING PROGRAM B: DAYS 1–7 *(continued)*

BODY PART	EXERCISES *Choose one exercise for each body part or a set of exercises as indicated below.*	Day 1 *Workload:* Light Intensity	Day 2 Aerobics Abdominals	Day 3 *Workload:* Medium-Light Intensity	Day 4 Aerobics Abdominals	Day 5 *Workload:* Medium Intensity	Days 6/7 Rest Aerobics Optional
Quadriceps	Leg Extension	25 to 40 reps		15 to 24 reps		8 to 12 reps	
Hamstrings	Leg Curl	25 to 40 reps		15 to 24 reps		8 to 12 reps	
Calves	Heel Raise or One-legged Standing Raise or Calf Machine	25 to 40 reps		15 to 24 reps		8 to 12 reps	

WEIGHT-TRAINING PROGRAM B: DAYS 8–14 *(continued)*

BODY PART	EXERCISES *Choose one exercise for each body part or a set of exercises as indicated below.*	Day 8 Workload: Medium Intensity	Day 9 Aerobics Abdominals	Day 10 Rest	Day 11 Workload: Medium Intensity	Day 12 Aerobics Abdominals	Days 13/14 Rest Aerobics Optional Note: Repeat cycle from day 1
Neck	Stretching/Manual Resistance	yes			yes		
Traps	Shoulder Shrug or Upright Row	15 to 24 reps			8 to 12 reps		
Shoulders	Military Press or Lateral Raise, Front Raise and Bent-over Lateral Raise	15 to 24 reps			8 to 12 reps		
Upper Back	Bent-over Barbell Rowing or Seated Cable Row or Lat Pulldown	15 to 24 reps			8 to 12 reps		
Lower Back	Back Extension	15 to 24 reps			8 to 12 reps		

WEIGHT-TRAINING PROGRAM B: DAYS 8–14 (continued)

BODY PART	EXERCISES Choose one exercise for each body part or a set of exercises as indicated below	Day 8 Workload: Medium Intensity	Day 9 Aerobics Abdominals	Day 10 Rest	Day 11 Workload: Medium Intensity	Day 12 Aerobics Abdominals	Days 13/14 Rest Aerobics Optional
Chest	Bench Press	15 to 24 reps			8 to 12 reps		
	Fly	15 to 24 reps			8 to 12 reps		
Biceps	Standing Arm Curl or Preacher Curl or Incline Dumbbell Curl	15 to 24 reps			8 to 12 reps		
Triceps	Lying Triceps Press or Triceps Kickback or Triceps Pressdown	15 to 24 reps			8 to 12 reps		
Forearms	Wrist Curl and Reverse Wrist Curl	15 to 24 reps			8 to 12 reps		
Abdominals (Abs)	Inclined Sit-up or Crunch and Reverse Crunch		15 to 24 reps			8 to 12 reps	

WEIGHT-TRAINING PROGRAM B: DAYS 8–14 (continued)

BODY PART	EXERCISES Choose one exercise for each body part or a set of exercises as indicated below.	Day 8 Workload: Medium Intensity	Day 9 Aerobics Abdominals	Day 10 Rest	Day 11 Workload: Medium Intensity	Day 12 Aerobics Abdominals	Days 13/14 Rest Aerobics Optional
Obliques	Weighted Side Bend or Lying Side Oblique Crunch		15 to 24 reps			8 to 12 reps	
Buttocks, Hips, Legs	Leg Press or Squat or Lunge	15 to 24 reps			8 to 12 reps		
	Side Lunge	15 to 24 reps			None		
Quadriceps	Leg Extension	15 to 24 reps			8 to 12 reps		
Hamstrings	Leg Curl	15 to 24 reps			8 to 12 reps		
Calves	Heel Raise or One-legged Standing Raise or Calf Machine	15 to 24 reps			8 to 12 reps		

WEIGHT-TRAINING PROGRAM C SUMMARY

LENGTH: TWELVE WEEKS

From your progress in Programs A and B, you will be able to increase your working sets to three to six sets per exercise. This volume of weight training can make a total body workout impractical because it takes too much time and can be very exhausting. Therefore you'll need to follow a split workout: Upper Body, Lower Body, and abdominals and aerobics. The training programs are presented in a two-week-long schedule, which you will repeat.

Follow Program C for three months. Athletes involved in anaerobic sports that require immediate energy, and fitness exercisers who desire increased gains in muscle size and strength, should then advance to Program D. Program D is more intensive in terms of workouts per month. Also, more exercises for some body parts are included. This program should not be used by endurance (oxidative) athletes.

- Exercises: Choose one exercise per body part, unless otherwise indicated.

- More advanced exercises are added, such as the squat and dead lifts. Beginners should ease slowly into these exercises, focusing on good form and using weights light enough to perform them with ease.

After twelve weeks, take a week off from weight training.

WEIGHT-TRAINING PROGRAM C: DAYS 1–7

BODY PART	EXERCISES	Day 1 Upper Body Workload: Light	Day 2 Aerobics Abdominals	Day 3 Lower Body Workload: Light	Day 4 Aerobics Abdominals	Day 5 Upper Body Workload: Medium	Day 6 Optional Aerobics Abdominals	Day 7 Rest
Neck	Stretching	Yes				Yes		
Traps	Shoulder Shrug or Upright Row	25 to 40 reps				8 to 12 reps		
Shoulders	Military Press or Lateral Raise and Front Raise and Bent-over Lateral Raise	25 to 40 reps				8 to 12 reps		
Upper Back	Bent-over Barbell Row or Seated Cable Row or One-Arm Dumbbell Row	25 to 40 reps				8 to 12 reps		
Lower Back	Back Extension or Dead Lift	25 to 40 reps				8 to 12 reps		

WEIGHT-TRAINING PROGRAM C: DAYS 1–7 (continued)

BODY PART	EXERCISES	Day 1 Upper Body Workload: Light	Day 2 Aerobics Abdominals	Day 3 Lower Body Workload: Light	Day 4 Aerobics Abdominals	Day 5 Upper Body Workload: Medium	Day 6 Optional Aerobics Abdominals	Day 7 Rest
Chest	Bench Press or Incline/Decline Bench Press	25 to 40 reps				8 to 12 reps		
	Fly or Inclined Fly and Declined Fly	25 to 40 reps				8 to 12 reps		
Biceps	Standing Arm Curl or Preacher Curl or Incline Dumbbell Curl or Concentration Curl or Reverse Curl	25 to 40 reps				8 to 12 reps		
Triceps	Lying Triceps Press or French Press or Triceps Kickback or Triceps Pressdown or Dips	25 to 40 reps				8 to 12 reps		

WEIGHT-TRAINING PROGRAM C: DAYS 1–7 (continued)

BODY PART	EXERCISES	Day 1 Upper Body Workload: Light	Day 2 Aerobics Abdominals	Day 3 Lower Body Workload: Light	Day 4 Aerobics Abdominals	Day 5 Upper Body Workload: Medium	Day 6 Optional Aerobics Abdominals	Day 7 Rest
Forearms	Wrist Curl and Reverse Wrist Curl	25 to 40 reps				8 to 12 reps		
Abdominals (Abs)	Inclined Sit-up or Crunch and Reverse Crunch		25 to 40 reps				8 to 12 reps	
Obliques	Weighted Side Bend or Lying Side Oblique Crunch or Russian Twist		25 to 40 reps				8 to 12 reps	
Buttocks, Hips, Legs	Squat or Leg Press or Lunge			25 to 40 reps				
	Side Lunge			25 to 40 reps				
Quadriceps	Leg extension			25 to 40 reps				
Hamstrings	Leg Curl			25 to 40 reps				

WEIGHT-TRAINING PROGRAM C: DAYS 1–7 (continued)

BODY PART	EXERCISES	Day 1 Upper Body Workload: Light	Day 2 Aerobics Abdominals	Day 3 Lower Body Workload: Light	Day 4 Aerobics Abdominals	Day 5 Upper Body Workload: Medium	Day 6 Optional Aerobics Abdominals	Day 7 Rest
Calves	Heel Raise or One-legged or Standing Raise or Calf Machine			25 to 40 reps				

WEIGHT-TRAINING PROGRAM C: DAYS 8–14

BODY PART	EXERCISES	Day 8 Lower Body Workload: Medium	Day 9 Aerobics Abdominals	Day 10 Upper Body Workload: Medium-Light	Day 11 Aerobics Abdominals	Day 12 Lower Body Workload: Medium-Light	Day 13 Optional Aerobics Abdominals	Day 14 Rest Repeat 14-Day Cycle
Neck	Stretching			Yes				
Traps	Shoulder Shrug or Upright Row			15 to 24 reps				

Weight-Training Program C: Days 8–14 (continued)

BODY PART	EXERCISES	Day 8 Lower Body Workload: Medium	Day 9 Aerobics Abdominals	Day 10 Upper Body Workload: Medium Light	Day 11 Aerobics Abdominals	Day 12 Lower Body Workload: Medium Light	Day 13 Optional Aerobics Abdominals	Day 14 Rest Repeat 14-Day Cycle
Shoulders	Military Press or Lateral Raise and Front Raise and Bent-over Lateral Raise			15 to 24 reps				
Upper Back	Bent-over Barbell Row or Seated Cable Row or One-arm Dumbbell Row			15 to 24 reps				
Lower Back	Back Extension or Dead Lift			15 to 24 reps				
Chest	Bench Press or Incline/Decline Bench Press			15 to 24 reps				
	Fly or Inclined Fly or Declined Fly			15 to 24 reps				

Weight-Training Program C: Days 8–14 (continued)

BODY PART	EXERCISES	Day 8 Lower Body Workload: Medium	Day 9 Aerobics Abdominals	Day 10 Upper Body Workload: Medium-Light	Day 11 Aerobics Abdominals	Day 12 Lower Body Workload: Medium-Light	Day 13 Optional Aerobics Abdominals	Day 14 Rest Repeat 14-Day Cycle
Biceps	Standing Arm Curl or Preacher Curl or Incline Dumbbell Curl or Concentration Curl or Reverse Curl			15 to 24 reps				
Triceps	Lying Triceps Press or French Press or Triceps Kickback or Triceps Pressdown or Dips			15 to 24 reps				
Forearms	Wrist Curl and Reverse Wrist Curl			15 to 24 reps				

WEIGHT-TRAINING PROGRAM C: DAYS 8–14 (continued)

BODY PART	EXERCISES	Day 8 Lower Body Workload: Medium	Day 9 Aerobics Abdominals	Day 10 Upper Body Workload: Medium-Light	Day 11 Aerobics Abdominals	Day 12 Lower Body Workload: Medium-Light	Day 13 Optional Aerobics Abdominals	Day 14 Rest Repeat 14-Day Cycle
Abdominals (Abs)	Inclined Sit-up or Crunch and Reverse Crunch		8 to 12 reps		15 to 24 reps		15 to 24 reps	
Obliques	Weighted Side Bend or Lying Side Oblique Crunch or Russian Twist		8 to 12 reps		15 to 24 reps		15 to 24 reps	
Buttocks, Hips, Legs	Squat or Leg Press or Lunge	8 to 12 reps				15 to 24 reps		
	Side Lunge	None				15 to 24 reps		
Quadriceps	Leg Extension	8 to 12 reps				15 to 24 reps		
Hamstrings	Leg Curl	8 to 12 reps				15 to 24 reps		
Calves	Heel Raise or One-legged or Standing Raise or Calf Machine	8 to 12 reps				15 to 24 reps		

WEIGHT-TRAINING PROGRAM D

LENGTH: TWELVE WEEKS

Program D increases weight-training demands in three ways compared to Program C. First, you will be weight training 16 days a month, versus 12 days a month in Program C. Second, more exercises are performed. Third, the intensity levels are on the average heavier, and high-intensity rep zones are used once every two weeks. High-intensity reps are only performed for certain body parts. Program C is similar to Program D in its basic split workout format: Upper Body, Lower Body, and abdominals and aerobics. The training programs are presented in a two-week schedule, which you will repeat.

Follow Program D for three months. Program D is especially useful for athletes involved in sports that require explosive strength and speed-strength, such as athletes involved in strength sports (see chapter 8). The program will also benefit fitness exercisers who desire increased gains in muscle size and strength. Refer to the box on Super Speed for weight-lifting techniques to help increase muscle contraction speed. This program is not intended for endurance athletes.

Perform two to three warm-up sets per exercise to make sure the muscles are thoroughly warmed up.

If you find that on a particular workout day you are not up to performing at the recommended level of intensity, or can only seem to do one or two sets, your body may be displaying signs of overtraining because the intensity of weight lifting has increased too quickly. Ease up on the workout intensity for that day, and resume to the recommended intensity level specified in the next workout day. You don't need to try to make up for the "off-intensity" day. After twelve weeks take two weeks off from weight training.

Weight-Training Program D: Days 1–7

BODY PART	EXERCISES	Day 1 Upper Body Workload: Medium-Light	Day 2 Lower Body Workload: Medium-Light	Day 3 Aerobics Abdominals	Day 4 Upper Body Workload: Medium	Day 5 Lower Body Workload: Medium	Day 6 Aerobics Abdominals	Day 7 Rest
Neck	Stretching	Yes			Yes			
Traps	Power Clean	15 to 24 reps			8 to 12 reps			
Traps	Shoulder Shrug or Upright Row	15 to 24 reps			8 to 12 reps			
Shoulders	Military Press or Lateral Raise and Front Raise and Bent-over Lateral Raise	15 to 24 reps			8 to 12 reps			
Upper Back	Bent-over Barbell Row or Seated Cable Row or One-Arm Dumbbell Row	15 to 24 reps			8 to 12 reps			
Upper Back	Lat Pulldown	15 to 24 reps			8 to 12 reps			

WEIGHT-TRAINING PROGRAM D: DAYS 1–7 (continued)

BODY PART	EXERCISES	Day 1 Upper Body Workload: Medium-Light	Day 2 Lower Body Workload: Medium-Light	Day 3 Aerobics Abdominals	Day 4 Upper Body Workload: Medium	Day 5 Lower Body Workload: Medium	Day 6 Aerobics Abdominals	Day 7 Rest
Lower Back	Back Extension	15 to 24 reps			8 to 12 reps			
	Dead Lift	15 to 24 reps			8 to 12 reps			
Chest	Bench Press or Incline/Decline Bench Press	15 to 24 reps			8 to 12 reps			
	Fly or Inclined Fly and Declined Fly	15 to 24 reps			8 to 12 reps			
Biceps	Standing Arm Curl or Preacher Curl or Incline Dumbbell Curl or Concentration Curl or Reverse Curl	15 to 24 reps			8 to 12 reps			

WEIGHT-TRAINING PROGRAM D: DAYS 1–7 (continued)

BODY PART	EXERCISES	Day 1 Upper Body Workload: Medium-Light	Day 2 Lower Body Workload: Medium-Light	Day 3 Aerobics Abdominals	Day 4 Upper Body Workload: Medium	Day 5 Lower Body Workload: Medium	Day 6 Aerobics Abdominals	Day 7 Rest
Triceps	Lying Triceps Press or French Press or Triceps Kickback or Triceps Press-down or Dips	15 to 24 reps			8 to 12 reps			
Forearms	Wrist Curl	15 to 24 reps			8 to 12 reps			
	Reverse Wrist Curl	15 to 24 reps			8 to 12 reps			
Abdominals (Abs)	Inclined Sit-up or Crunch and Reverse Crunch			15 to 24 reps			8 to 12 reps	
Obliques	Weighted Side Bend or Lying Side Oblique Crunch or Russian Twist			15 to 24 reps			8 to 12 reps	

WEIGHT-TRAINING PROGRAM D: DAYS 1–7 (continued)

BODY PART	EXERCISES	Day 1 Upper Body Workload: Medium-Light	Day 2 Lower Body Workload: Medium-Light	Day 3 Aerobics Abdominals	Day 4 Upper Body Workload: Medium	Day 5 Lower Body Workload: Medium	Day 6 Aerobics Abdominals	Day 7 Rest
Buttocks, Hips, Legs	Squat or Leg Press		15 to 24 reps			8 to 12 reps		
	Lunge		15 to 24 reps			8 to 12 reps		
	Side Lunge		15 to 24 reps			8 to 12 reps		
Quadriceps	Leg Extension		15 to 24 reps			8 to 12 reps		
Hamstrings	Leg Curl		15 to 24 reps			8 to 12 reps		
Calves	Heel Raise or One-legged or Standing Raise or Calf Machine		15 to 24 reps			8 to 12 reps		

WEIGHT-TRAINING PROGRAM D: DAYS 8–14

BODY PART	EXERCISES	Day 8 Upper Body Workload: Medium-Light	Day 9 Lower Body Workload: Medium-Light	Day 10 Aerobics Abdominals	Day 11 Upper Body Workload: High	Day 12 Lower Body Workload: High	Day 13 Aerobics Abdominals	Day 14 Rest
Neck	Stretching	Yes			Yes			
Traps	Power Clean	15 to 24 reps			None			
	Shoulder Shrug or Upright Row	15 to 24 reps			3 to 6 reps			
Shoulders	Military Press or Lateral Raise and Front Raise and Bent-over Lateral Raise	15 to 24 reps			3 to 6 reps			
Upper Back	Bent-over Barbell Row or Seated Cable Row or One-Arm Dumbbell Row	15 to 24 reps			3 to 6 reps			
	Lat Pulldown	15 to 24 reps			3 to 6 reps			

WEIGHT-TRAINING PROGRAM D: DAYS 8–14 (continued)

BODY PART	EXERCISES	Day 8 Upper Body Workload: Medium-Light	Day 9 Lower Body Workload: Medium-Light	Day 10 Aerobics Abdominals	Day 11 Upper Body Workload: High	Day 12 Lower Body Workload: High	Day 13 Aerobics Abdominals	Day 14 Rest
Lower Back	Back Extension	15 to 24 reps			None			
	Dead Lift	15 to 24 reps			3 to 6 reps			
Chest	Bench Press or Incline/Decline Bench Press	15 to 24 reps			3 to 6 reps			
	Fly or Inclined Fly or Declined Fly	15 to 24 reps			None			
Biceps	Standing Arm Curl or Preacher Curl or Incline Dumbbell Curl or Concentration Curl or Reverse Curl	15 to 24 reps			None			

WEIGHT-TRAINING PROGRAM D: DAYS 8–14 (continued)

BODY PART	EXERCISES	Day 8 Upper Body Workload: Medium-Light	Day 9 Lower Body Workload: Medium-Light	Day 10 Aerobics Abdominals	Day 11 Upper Body Workload: High	Day 12 Lower Body Workload: High	Day 13 Aerobics Abdominals	Day 14 Rest
Triceps	Lying Triceps Press or French Press or Triceps Kickback or Triceps Pressdown or Dips	15 to 24 reps			None			
Forearms	Wrist Curl	15 to 24 reps			None			
	Reverse Wrist Curl	15 to 24 reps			None			
Abdominals (Abs)	Inclined Sit-up or Crunch and Reverse Crunch			15 to 24 reps			8 to 12 reps	
Obliques	Weighted Side Bend or Lying Side Oblique Crunch or Russian Twist			15 to 24 reps			8 to 12 reps	

WEIGHT-TRAINING PROGRAM D: DAYS 8–14 (continued)

BODY PART	EXERCISES	Day 8 Upper Body Workload: Medium-Light	Day 9 Lower Body Workload: Medium-Light	Day 10 Aerobics Abdominals	Day 11 Upper Body Workload: High	Day 12 Lower Body Workload: High	Day 13 Aerobics Abdominals	Day 14 Rest
Buttocks, Hips, Legs	Squat or Leg Press		15 to 24 reps			3 to 6 reps		
	Lunge		15 to 24 reps			None		
	Side Lunge		15 to 24 reps			None		
Quadriceps	Leg extension		15 to 24 reps			None		
Hamstrings	Leg Curl		15 to 24 reps			None		
Calves	Heel Raise or One-legged or Standing Raise or Calf Machine		15 to 24 reps			3 to 6 reps		

ADVANCING TO THE NEXT LEVEL

To maintain your strength and muscle-mass gains during the athletic season, weight training once to twice a week will usually be adequate. Remember to avoid lifting heavy or moderate workloads three days before your athletic event, as this may cause overtraining and not allow for full muscle recovery. Fitness exercisers who want to maintain their gains can return to Program A or B; if you like, you may keep following Programs C and D, but reduce the number of working sets to one to three.

For athletes or fitness exercisers who want to see continued gains in strength and muscle mass, try alternating Programs C and D. Make sure to take one- and two-week breaks between programs, and also take three to four weeks off per year. If you feel that you are overtraining, you can also cycle in a few weeks of Programs A and B. The bottom line is that for consistent improvements in strength and muscle mass, you have to expose your body to constant overload.

You can also turn to our monthly publications for additional weight-training programs, in particular, *Men's Fitness, Shape, Muscle & Fitness, Muscle & Fitness Hers,* and *Flex*. In addition to looking for new and exciting weight-training programs in our magazines, if you get the bodybuilding bug from following the weight-training programs in this book, you might try Joe Weider's Bodybuilding System (available via mail order from Weider Publications). This system provides weight-training routines that are more specifically designed for competitive bodybuilders.

GOT SPEED?

Once you start to develop bigger and stronger muscles, your athletic performance will begin to improve. Your muscles will be able to generate more powerful muscle contractions. Your total body training will give you the edge over athletes who do the bare minimum of traditional weight-training routines. Even so, developing maximum muscle speed-strength is of paramount importance for reaching peak athletic performance.

To develop optimal speed in combination with strength, you must focus on not only the workload you are weight training with, but also the speed and explosiveness with which you contract your muscle during a repetition. Of course, with increased speed in lifting comes more force and increased risk of injury to joints and muscles. To resolve this conflict sports scientists

GOT SPEED?

have spent a lot of time examining what workloads and rep ranges are effective in developing the muscles to get stronger and faster while reducing the risk of speed-training injury. What we and the exercise scientists have found is that while periodic use of heavy loads for a low number of reps is effective, most athletes develop greater speed-strength by lifting moderate workloads, but using explosive concentric movements. At this point we need to think in terms of the one-repetition maximum discussed earlier. The one-repetition maximum is the amount of weight you can lift in a particular exercise only one time. Based on our experience and taking into consideration a number of scientific studies, weight training with loads that are between 30 percent to 80 percent of the one-repetition maximum for a particular exercise is most effective in building optimum muscle contraction speed. Keep in mind that using workloads in this range will result in a wide variety of repetitions as already built into the weight-training programs. Begin a progressive speed-training program a few months before the competition season. Make sure to execute exercises using good form and under the supervision of your coach or qualified trainer. Start using lighter workloads, and progressively increase workloads during the several-week speed-building period. Do not progress too quickly. As a general rule, experts also caution that using speed-strength weight-lifting techniques with heavy workloads above the 50-percent one-repetition maximum range should be performed during the last weeks of a speed-strength training cycle, and only by advanced individuals under strict supervision. There will be exceptions to this general rule depending on your type of sport, such as in powerlifting. Be patient, and give the lighter speed-training workloads some time to produce an effect. Speed-strength training is not limited to the legs for the purpose of running faster. You can use this weight-training technique to build speed of muscle contractions in all muscles.

Also, think about your energetic zone—how long do you need to display this explosive speed-strength in your sport? Is it just a few seconds, as is the case for a football lineman? A split second that it takes for a shot-putter, Olympic weight lifter, powerlifter, or goalkeeper? Several seconds as for a 100-meter sprinter, football running back or end, or baseball player? Is it stop-and-go speed-strength, as for a tennis player or soccer fullback?

In addition to weight training, runners who want to maximize their speed should also perform sets of sprints. Experiment with training equipment that adds resistance while you are running, such as Speed Trainers, Saber Slave, Sled Sawg, and Power Fitness Chutes. Also try running up and down a road surface with a slight incline. All of these techniques can help improve running speed.

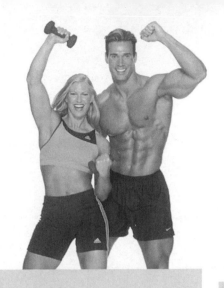

The Core Exercises

I n this chapter we include examples of many effective weight-training exercises and guidelines on how to perform them. Read the exercise descriptions carefully to make sure that you are executing them correctly. Be advised that there are limitations to conveying exercise instructions from a book. It is always best to consult a personal trainer at your gym to ensure that you are performing the exercises correctly. If you do not belong to a gym, you can have a personal trainer visit your home for private instructions. To keep costs down, ask a few of your friends to join in and negotiate a group rate with a personal trainer. In this way, you can get personalized expert advice for a modest investment. Athletes should consult with their coaches and trainers on proper weight-lifting technique.

WEIGHT-TRAINING EXERCISE EXAMPLES

This chapter focuses on the core strength and building exercises that work all the major muscle groups. These are the main exercises you need to do. Most of them can be performed in your home gym, using barbells and dumbbells. If you cannot perform one of the recommended exercises because you lack a spotter or equipment or have an injury, use the chart below to substitute exercises. Or if you feel you have reached a plateau in your gains, you can add different exercises from magazine articles found in Weider publications or from advice you may receive from a personal trainer. Always get a physical examination and get approval from your doctor before beginning a weight-training program.

THE EXERCISES			
Body Region	**Muscle Group**	**Exercises Included in this Chapter**	**Additional Exercises Not Included in this Chapter**
UPPER BODY	NECK	Stretching Manual Resistance	Nautilus Neck Machine Neck Bridging
	TRAPEZIUS	Shoulder Shrug Upright Row	Shoulder Shrug Machine
	SHOULDERS	Military Press Lateral Raise Front Raise Behind-the-Neck Presses	Lateral Arm Raise Machine Military Press Machine
	UPPER BACK	Lat Pull-down Bent-over Barbell Row Seated Cable Row One-arm Dumbbell Row	Seated Row Machine Pull-ups Chin-ups
	LOWER BACK	Dead Lift Back Extension	Back Extension Machine Reverse Back Raise Stiff-legged Dead Lift

	CHEST	Bench Press
		Incline / Decline
		   Bench Press
		Fly
		Incline / Decline Fly
			Pullover
			Seated Bench Press
			   Machine
			Seated Fly Machine
			Pushups

		THE EXERCISES (*continued*)	
Body Region	**Muscle Group**	**Exercises Included in this Chapter**	**Additional Exercises Not Included in this Chapter**
ARMS	BICEPS	Standing Arm Curl Preacher Curl Incline Dumbbell Curl Concentration Curl Reverse Curl	Seated Preacher Curl Machine
	TRICEPS	Seated Dumbbell Triceps Extension Lying Triceps Dumbbell Extension Triceps Kickback Triceps Pressdown Dips	Seated Triceps Extension Machine Lying Triceps Extension
	FOREARMS	Wrist Curl Reverse Wrist Curl	Supination-Pronation Wrist Roller Ulnar-Radial Flexion
MIDSECTION	ABDOMINALS (ABS)	Incline Sit-up Crunch Reverse Crunch	Abdominal Crunch Machine Hanging Leg Raise
	OBLIQUES	Weighted Side Bend Lying Side Oblique Crunch Russian Twist	Reverse Trunch Twist
LEGS	HIPS, BUTTOCKS, THIGHS	Squat Leg Press Leg Extension Lunge Side Lunge	Hip Joint Flexion Machine Hip Joint Extension Machine Hip Joint Adduction Machine Hip Joint Abduction Machine Good Morning

The Exercises *(continued)*			
Body Region	**Muscle Group**	**Exercises Included in this Chapter**	**Additional Exercises Not Included in this Chapter**
LEGS (continued)	QUADRICEPS	Leg Extension	
	HAMSTRINGS	Leg Curl	Stiff-legged Dead Lift
	CALVES	One-legged Standing Heel Raise Standing Calf Machine Seated Calf Machine	Heel Raise Toe Raise (for front of shin)
ADDITIONAL EXERCISE		Power Clean (for competitive athletes)	

FITNESS MODELS

In selecting athletes to demonstrate the weight-training exercises, we asked two of our world-class natural champions, Mike O'Hearn and Gea Johnson, to show you how to do them correctly.

More information about Mike and Gea can be found on page 379.

In most cases your neck muscles will naturally strengthen in response to general training, and specific neck weight-lifting exercises are not usually required. We do, however, recommend that you stretch the neck muscles as part of your warm-up by gently rolling your head in a circle, or turning your head from side to side. Roll your head around in a gentle, relaxed manner through all its available ranges of motion.

Some athletes, such as football players, wrestlers, and boxers, need to build tremendous neck strength. If you're actively involved in any of these sports (even on a weekend basis), you should add some neck-strengthening exercises. Below are some basic stretches for the neck.

Performing basic neck exercises. Start by sitting in an upright position with your hands pressed against your forehead. Slowly bend your head back as far as you can without forcing or overextending. Using your hands to supply firm but gentle resistance against the front of your forehead, bend or flex your head as far forward as possible. Go backward through the full range of motion, and repeat. Now tilt your head all the way to your left. Place the right hand up to the side of your head and bend all the way over to the right against the resistance of your arm and hand power. Now tilt your head to your right shoulder and, using your left hand against the side of your head, gently flex your head all the way to the right. You have now exercised your neck in flexion and side flexion. Now bend your head all the way forward and place your hands behind your head. Extend your head back through the full range of motion against the resistance supplied by your arms and hands. Repeat for the required repetitions.

As you become more advanced in neck work, you can use a towel instead of your hands to provide resistance. Using a towel is very effective for forward flexion and reverse extension, but not in sideways flexion. There are also some special machines specifically designed to exercise the neck.

TRAPS

SHOULDER SHRUG (Barbell or Dumbbells)

The barbell shoulder shrug is excellent for building up the trapezius muscles. It also exercises the deltoids, neck, and upper back muscles.

Performing the barbell shrug. Hold the barbell with an overhand grip, hands spaced about shoulder width, with your arms extended downward, as shown. Keep your arms at your sides and shrug your shoulders and shoulder girdle as high as possible, as if trying to touch them to your ears. Slowly lower the bar, returning to the starting position. This exercise can also be done with dumbbells.

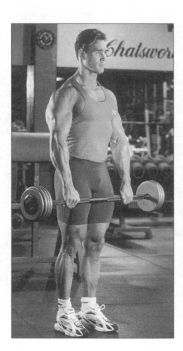
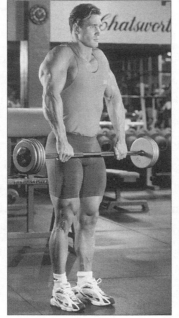
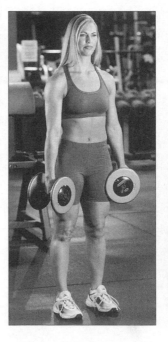
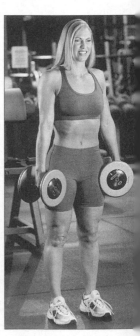

UPRIGHT ROW (Barbell)

The upright row is a great exercise that works both the trapezius and deltoids muscles, as well as the biceps and forearms. Perform this exercise on the alternate days you perform shrugs and other shoulder exercises.

Performing the barbell upright row. Hold the barbell with an overhand grip, with your arms extended downward as illustrated in the photo. Lift the barbell upward in line with your body, pulling your elbows up to keep them above the level of your

(continues on page 106)

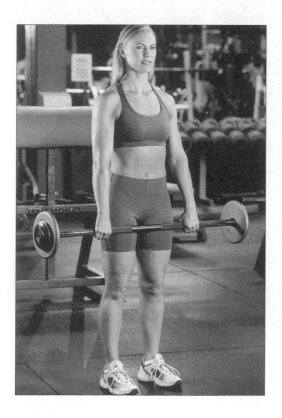
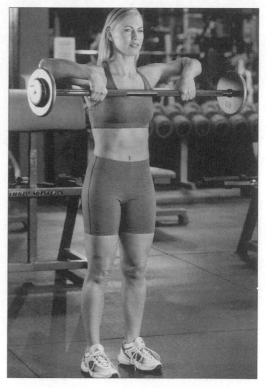

UPRIGHT ROW (Barbell) *(continued)*

hands at all times. Lift the bar to above your upper chest. Slowly lower the bar, returning to the starting position. This exercise can also be performed with a closer grip, but be careful of increased stress in the shoulders.

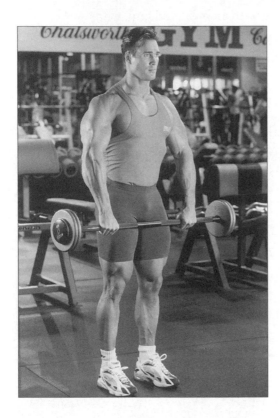
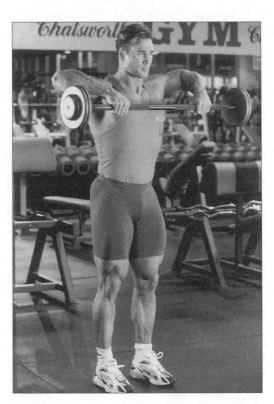

SHOULDERS

MILITARY PRESS (Barbell or Dumbbells)

The military press exercises the deltoids and triceps and other muscles of the upper body.

Performing the military press. Sitting with your back straight, hold the barbell so it is positioned at the top of your shoulders, using a grip that is wider than your shoulders as shown. Straighten your arms until the barbell is above your head. Slowly lower the bar, returning to the starting position. This exercise can also be performed using dumbbells, and in the sitting position.

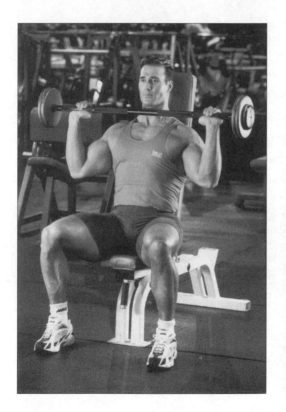

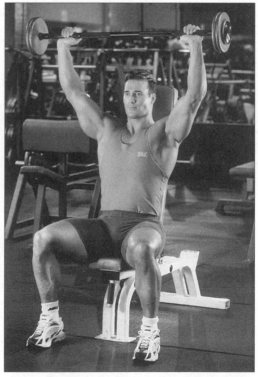

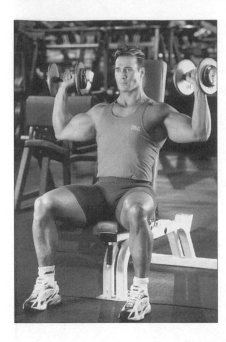
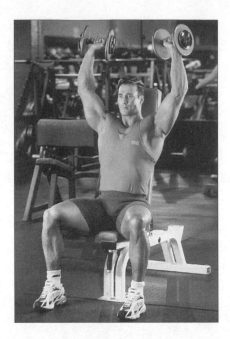

A variation of the military press is the **behind-the-neck press.** In this case, the barbell is positioned behind the neck. Keeping a wider-than-shoulder-width grip, press the bar up over your head to arm's length. Return slowly to your neck base. If you change the width of your grip periodically, you will stress the muscles slightly differently. Very wide grips work your deltoids to the max. Narrower grips shift more stress to your triceps muscles.

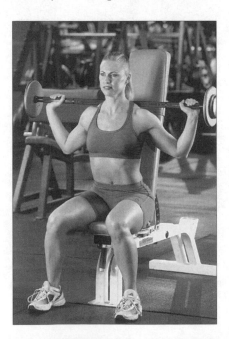
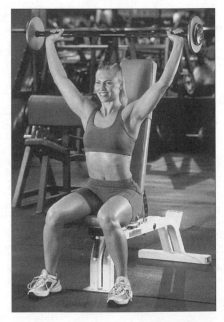

LATERAL RAISE (Dumbbells)

The lateral raise works the outside or lateral head of your deltoid muscles.

Performing the lateral raise. Stand erect, holding one dumbbell in each hand, elbows bent. Raise the dumbbells simultaneously away from the sides of your body until they are level with your shoulders. Lower the dumbbells under control to the starting position. If you always keep your elbows and wrists slightly bent, you will get a much better action on the lateral head of your deltoids. As you raise the dumbbells, rotate your hands so your little finger is higher than the thumb at the top of the movement. Reverse this twist as you lower the dumbbells.

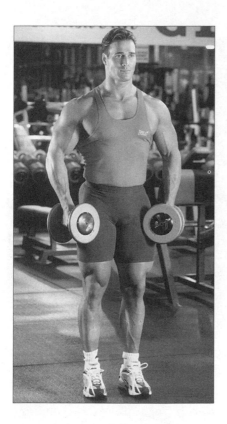
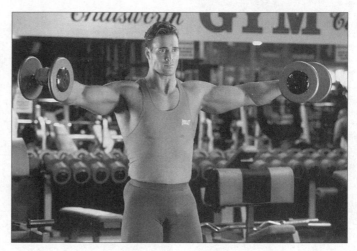

FRONT RAISE (Dumbbells or Barbell)

This front raise works the muscles of the front deltoid and upper chest.

Performing the front raise. Stand erect, holding dumbbells in each hand or a straight bar at arms' length across the middle of your thighs. Raise the dumbbells either one at a time or simultaneously with your elbows slightly bent until they are about eye level. Lower slowly to the starting position.

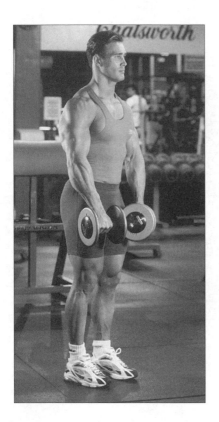

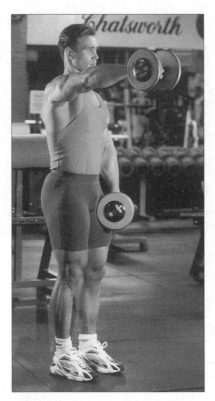

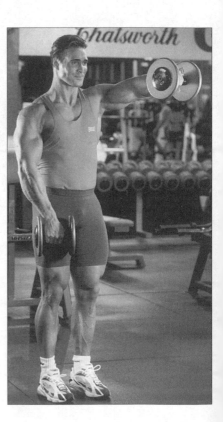

BENT-OVER LATERAL RAISE (Dumbbells)

The bent-over lateral raise works the posterior deltoids and upper-back muscles.

Performing the bent-over lateral raise. Hold one dumbbell in each hand. Lean over until your body is bent at a 90-degree angle. Bend your knees slightly to take the strain off your back. Raise the dumbbells together out laterally to the sides. After reaching the high point of the movement, lower the dumbbells, keeping the weight's motion under control. Keep your attention focused on the muscles being exercised. If you bend your elbows and wrists slightly, you can get more muscle contraction in the rear deltoid muscle.

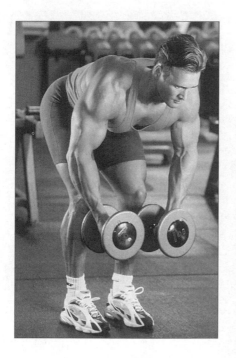

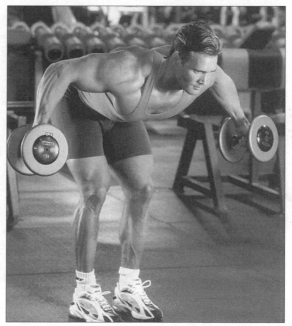

UPPER BACK

LAT PULL-DOWN

The lat pull-down is one of the most utilized exercises for the upper back muscles—the lats.

Performing the lat pull-down. Make the appropriate adjustments to the lat pull-down machine, grip the bar with a wide grip, hands facing away, and sit on the machine. Pull the bar down to your upper chest or behind your head, then return to the overhead position to complete the repetition.

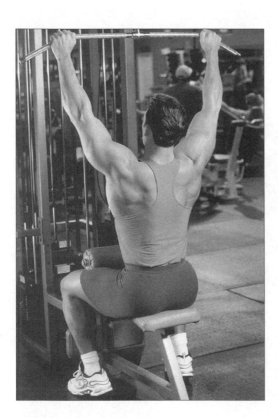 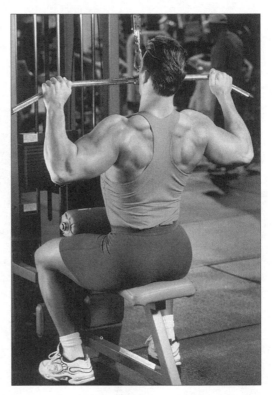

BENT-OVER BARBELL ROW

The bent-over barbell row primarily works the large latissimus (lat) muscles of your upper back, and also the trapezius, rhomboids, erector spinae, posterior deltoids, biceps, and forearms.

Performing the bent-over barbell row. With your feet about shoulder width apart, bend over until your torso is parallel to the floor. Bend your knees slightly to remove stress on your lower back and stabilize your stance. Hold the barbell with a shoulder-width grip, your palms facing your body. Your arms should be hanging straight down from your shoulders at the start of the movement. Making sure that your upper arms travel out to the sides, pull the barbell directly upward until it touches your upper abdominal, keeping your back flat during the exercise. Lower back to the starting position. For most barbell exercises, and particularly on the bent-rowing movement, you should periodically vary the width of your grip. This will put different degrees of stress on the muscles. The greater the number of grips, the greater the overall development.

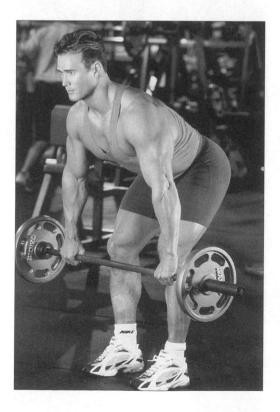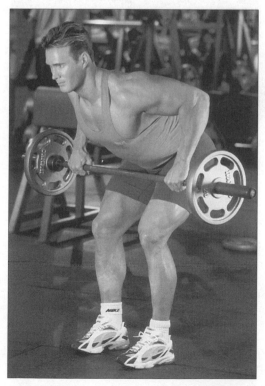

SEATED CABLE ROW

An alternative to the bent-over barbell row is the seated cable row.

Performing the seated cable row. Grasp the cable handle and sit upright on the bench. Keep your knees bent and place your feet on the footrest. Keep your back straight and perpendicular to the bench. Your arms should be extended forward. Now pull the cable handle into your upper abdominal area by bending your elbows and bringing them back past the plane of your body, while keeping your back straight and perpendicular to the bench. Hold the contraction for a second before slowly straightening your arms and lowering the weight until you feel a good stretch in your lats to complete the repetition.

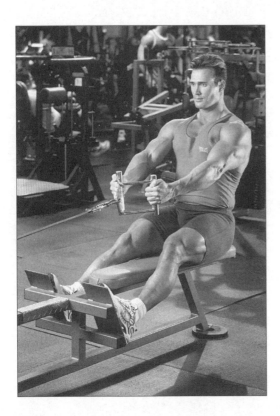
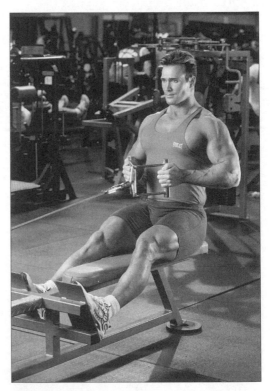

ONE-ARM DUMBBELL ROW

The one-arm dumbbell rowing exercise works the upper-back muscles, especially the lats, and muscles in your shoulders and arms.

Performing the one-arm dumbbell row. Bend forward, keeping one arm and one knee stabilized on the bench. Reach down with the other arm and pick up the dumbbell, holding it just off the floor, keeping your arm straight. Pull the dumbbell up to your ribcage, using your back muscles and keeping your back flat and abdominals tight. Twist your body a little as you pull the dumbbell up to create a greater range of motion. Then lower slowly back to the starting position, and stretch the back muscles for a moment.

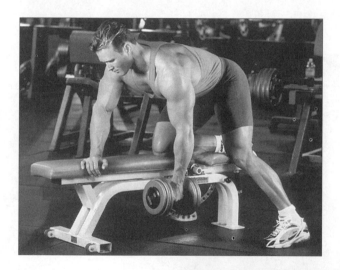

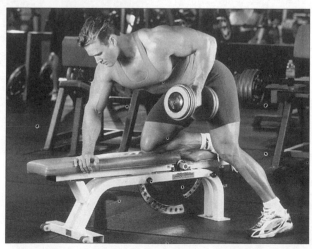

LOWER BACK

DEAD LIFT OR STIFF-LEGGED DEAD LIFT (Barbell or Dumbbells)

The dead lift is an exercise that works the muscles of your lower back, and also hip, middle back, hamstrings, and traps.

Performing dead lifts. Stand with your shins close to the barbell, bend down, and hold the bar with one hand facing forward and the other facing backward (alternate grip). The alternate grip increases your grip power. Then, stand erect using the power of your legs, hip, and back to perform the movement. Keep your arms straight and back as flat as possible as you lift the weight off the floor; avoid hunching the back. Keep the bar close to your body as you raise it to your thighs. Then slowly lower the bar.

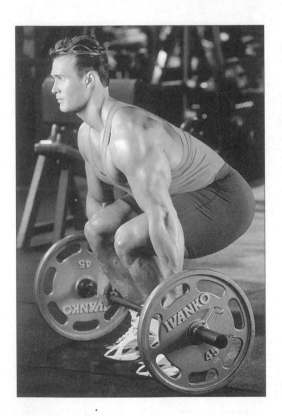
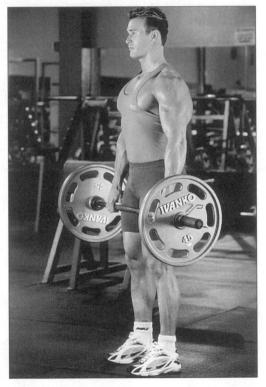

A modification of the dead lift, called the stiff-legged dead lift, isolates the lower back and also works your hamstrings. Use lighter weights for this advanced move, and focus on good form.

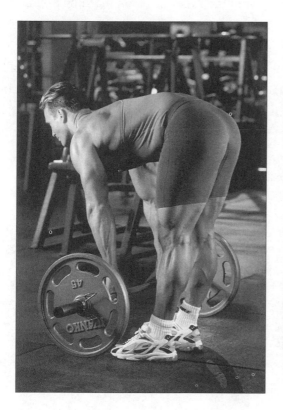 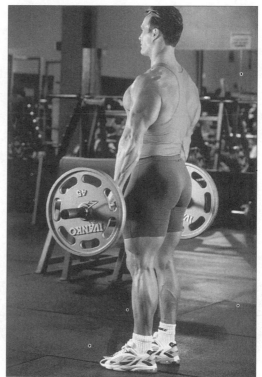

BACK EXTENSION (Back Raise)

The back extension is the primary exercise for working the lower back muscles through a full range of motion. In particular, it works the erector spinae muscle group and other muscles along the vertebrae that cause the spine to arch upward and maintain its natural curved posture.

Performing the back extension. Mount the back extension machine as illustrated, with your hips lined up on the pad. Do not extend your hip joint over the pad as this will take the focus off your lower back. Relax your back and assume the starting position with your back bent and head down, keeping your legs straight all the time. Your hands can be positioned across your chest (hold a weight if you are more advanced) or behind your neck. Straighten your spin slowly, raising your head and upper torso first, then your lower back in unison, until your upper body is about parallel with the floor. Hold this extended position for a second, then slowly return to the starting position.

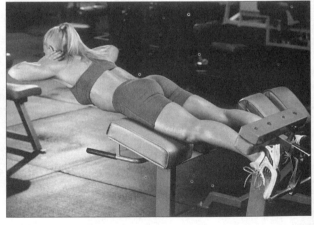

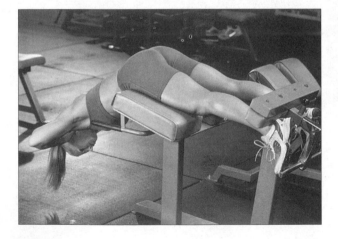

CHEST

BENCH PRESS (Barbell and Dumbbells)

The bench press is a classic exercise for building up the chest muscles. It also develops other upper-body and arm muscles.

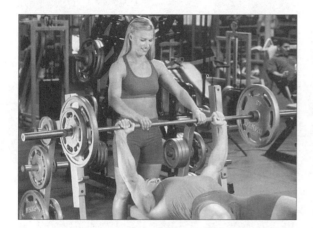
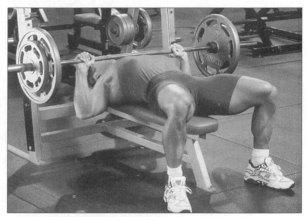

Performing the bench press. Lie on the bench, and grip the bar wider than shoulder width. With the help of a spotter, lift the barbell and extend your arms fully. As you lower the barbell to your chest, keep it just over the lower part of your chest muscles. Then begin pushing up, but bring the barbell slightly backward, so that the completion position is just over your neck. Return your arms to the fully extended position.

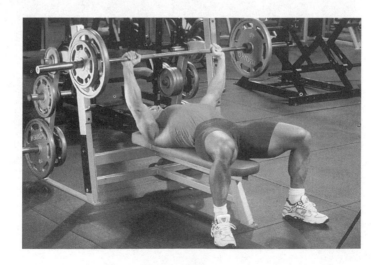

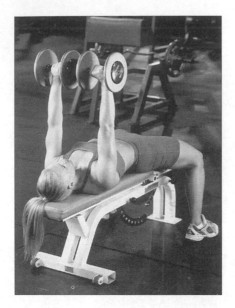

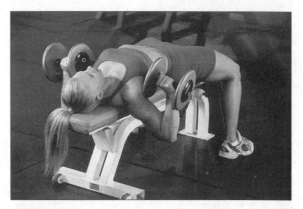

BENCH PRESS (Dumbbells) *(continued)*

INCLINE / DECLINE BENCH PRESS (Barbell and Dumbbells)

As the chest muscles work in a range of angular motion, performing the bench press at different angles will help evenly develop the upper, middle, and lower sections of the chest. Set the bench to either an incline (as shown) or a decline position to perform these variations of the bench press. Alternate among these three positions from workout to workout to fully develop your chest muscles.

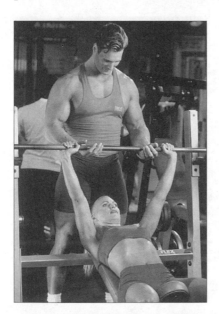

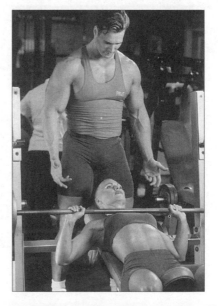

This fly exercise isolates the pectoral muscles of the chest, working them in a greater range of motion than in the bench press. It also works the deltoids.

Performing the fly.   Lie on your back on a flat bench, holding one dumbbell in each hand; you may want to have two spotters place the dumbbells into your hands. To begin, fully extend your arms above your chest as shown. Then lower the dumbbells horizontally, keeping your elbows just slightly bent, bringing the dumbbells out and away, down far enough until you feel a good stretch in your chest. Your upper arms should go below the line of your body. Be sure to take a very deep breath when lowering the dumbbells and exhale as you raise them back through the same arc to the top position. Focus on isolating the chest muscles during this exercise. To create a super-pump set, first perform flys to failure, then try to perform a few more repetitions using the dumbbell bench-press movement.

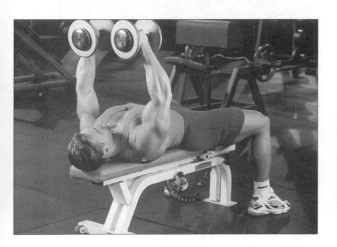

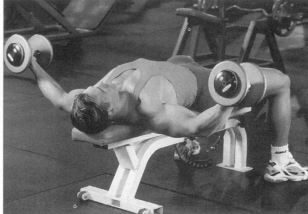

INCLINE FLY AND DECLINE FLY (Dumbbells)

Like the bench press, the fly can be performed in an incline (as shown) and decline position.

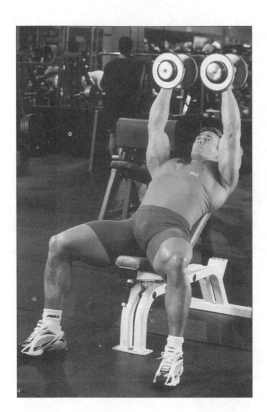
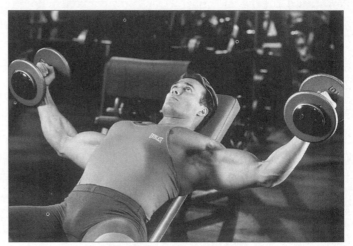

BICEPS

STANDING ARM CURL (Barbell or Dumbbells)

The standing arm curl builds the biceps and brachioradialis and the muscles of the forearms.

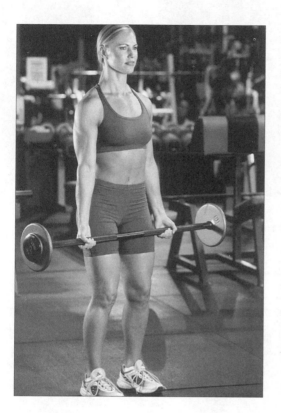 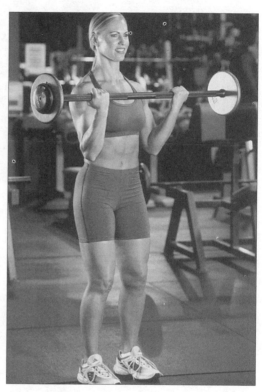

Performing the arm curl. Stand erect with your arms extended downward, grasping the barbell with an underhand grip, palms facing away from your body. Keep your elbows at your side and slowly curl the barbell to your chest. Then lower the weights to the starting position.

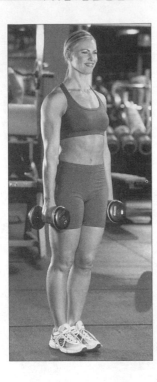
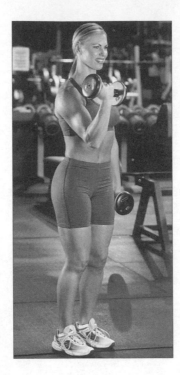
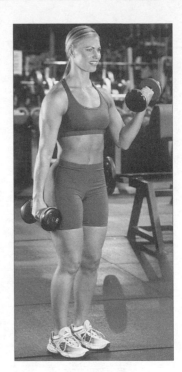

Arm curls can be performed using dumbbells, raising them at the same time or alternating left and right. You can also do curls from a seated position on a bench or standing using the cable machine, as illustrated.

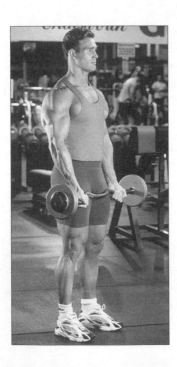
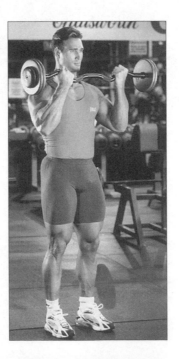
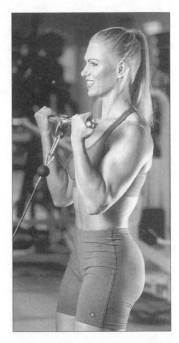

PREACHER CURL (Barbell and EZ-Curl Barbell)

The preacher curl is very effective for building the biceps and brachioradialis. It also exercises the forearm.

Performing the preacher curl. To begin, sit on the bench and rest your upper arm on the curl pad. Hold the barbell with an underhand grip and extend your arm. Slowly curl the barbell toward your chest, then lower the barbell to the starting position.

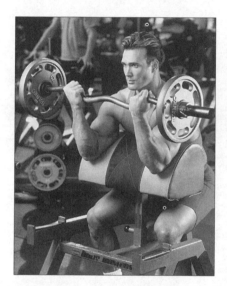
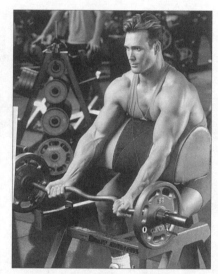

You can also do curls with an EZ-Curl barbell, varying the grip, narrow (as shown here) and wide.

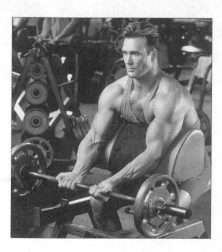
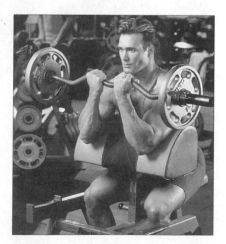

INCLINE DUMBBELL CURL (Dumbbells)

The inclined dumbbell curl works your upper-arm muscles, particularly your biceps and brachialis.

Performing the incline dumbbell curl. Holding two dumbbells, sit on the inclined bench. Keeping your body against the bench and your upper arms motionless, slowly curl the dumbbells from the down position up to your shoulders and then lower to the starting position. If you twist your hands from a fully pronated position (palms down with thumbs in) to a fully supinated position (palms up with thumbs out) at the top of your curl, you will get a better contraction. You can also alternate your arms while performing this movement.

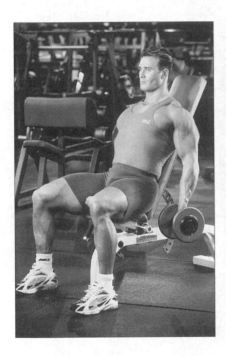 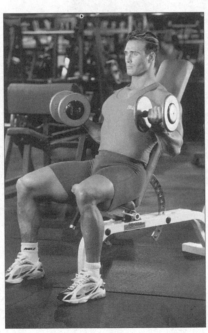 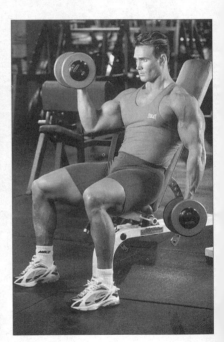

CONCENTRATION CURL (Dumbbells)

The concentration curl is another exercise that works your biceps.

Performing the concentration curl. Sit on a low bench with a dumbbell in hand, and bend forward from the waist with your arm braced against the inside of your thigh. Slowly curl the dumbbell up toward your chest, but keep your upper arm stationary, tucked in against your inner thigh. Keep your wrist straight during the upward movement. Hold and squeeze the contraction as hard as possible for a full two seconds, then lower slowly.

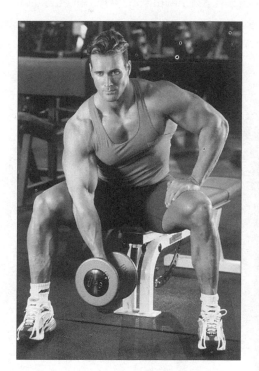
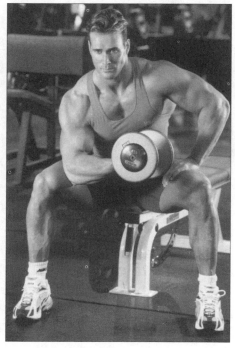

REVERSE CURL (Barbell or EZ-Curl Barbell)

The reverse curl works the large muscles at the top of your forearms, particularly the brachioradialis.

Performing the reverse curl. Stand, holding onto a barbell palms down with your arms down and extended in front of your thighs, the bar across your thighs. Keeping your elbows as fixed as possible, curl the weight up toward your shoulders slowly and evenly. Use a manageable workload that enables you to maintain good form, and focus on exercising the biceps. You can also use dumbbells to perform a slight variation of the reverse curl. Start with your arms extended and palms facing away from your body. As you curl the dumbbells, turn your palms inward.

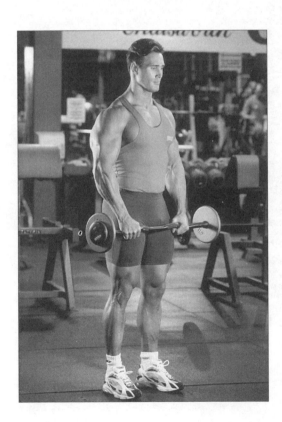
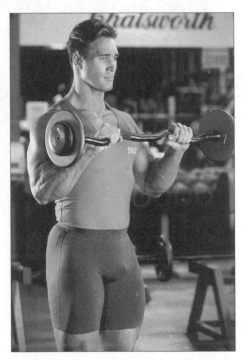

TRICEPS

LYING TRICEPS EXTENSION (Dumbbells)

The lying triceps extension isolates and works the triceps.

Performing the lying triceps extension. Take the same starting position as for the bench press. Start using a dumbbell in one hand, and lie on the bench as illustrated in the photo. Move your head slightly to the side opposite the arm lifting the dumbbell. Lift the weight up, and maintain good form by holding your elbow in place using your other hand. Lower the dumbbell slowly, making sure to keep your head out of the way.

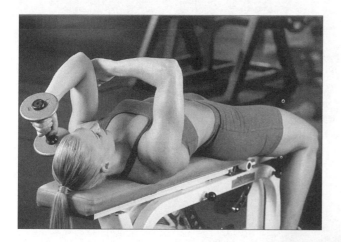

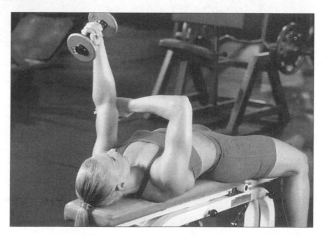

FRENCH PRESS (Seated Dumbbell Triceps Extension)

The Seated Dumbbell Triceps Extension and its variations places direct stress on the triceps muscles of the upper arm.

Performing the Seated Dumbbell Triceps Extension press. Grasp a light dumbbell in your left hand and sit on the end of a flat exercise bench. Place your right hand

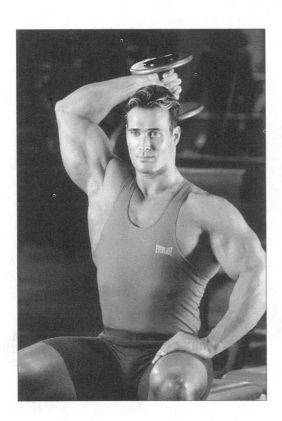

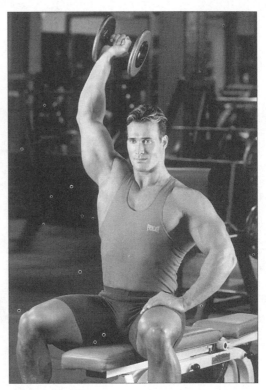

on your hip or thigh and extend your left arm straight upward from your shoulder, your palm facing forward throughout the movement. Keeping your upper arm motionless and elbow pointing upward, straighten the arm, then lower to the starting position. Seated triceps extensions can also be performed using a barbell or EZ-curl bar as illustrated in the photos.

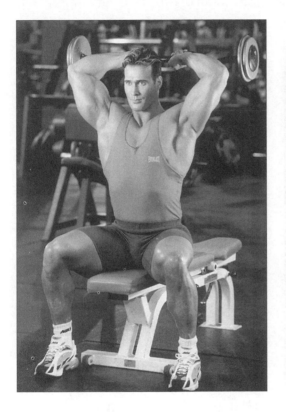 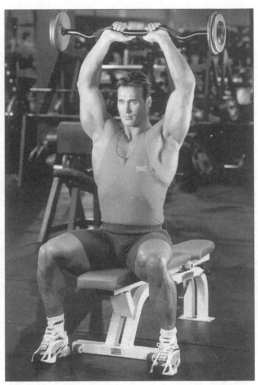

TRICEPS KICKBACK (Dumbbell)

The triceps kickback works the triceps muscles.

Performing the triceps kickback.   Lean over, with one hand stabilizing the body on the end of a bench and the other hand holding a dumbbell as illustrated. Keeping your upper arm parallel to the floor, straighten out the forearm and kick the dumbbell back and slightly upward, moving only the forearm. Contract your triceps very hard at the end of the movement for a count of two before lowering back down, for maximum effectiveness.

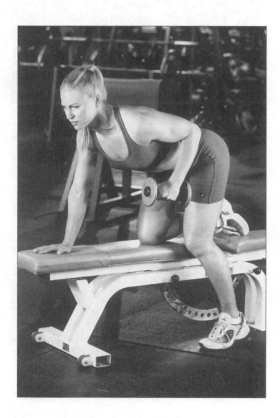

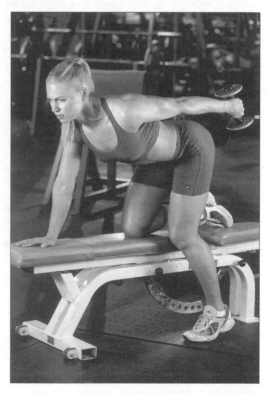

TRICEPS PRESSDOWN (PUSHDOWN) (Cable Machine)

The triceps pressdown is ideal for exercising the triceps, while maximizing safety.

Performing the triceps pressdown. Standing with your feet about shoulder-width apart, grasp the bar of the machine with palms facing down. The bar should be about chest height for the starting position. Lean slightly forward and, keeping the upper arms stationary, push the bar down only moving the forearms, then return to the starting position. Avoid using weights that are too heavy, as this causes bad technique. Isolating the triceps and maintaining good form is key to this exercise.

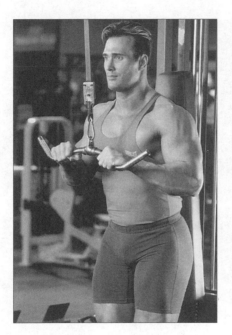 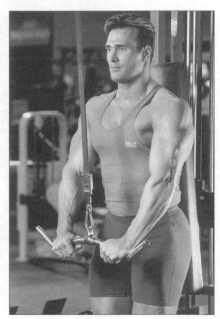

DIPS

While the dip works the triceps, it also exercises the chest, back, and shoulders. This makes it a good combination exercise that can be done on days when your workout time is limited and you want to work a few muscles at a time. It also builds good functional strength. Athletes should especially include dips in their regular training programs.

Performing the dip. The dip is best performed using a machine designed for this exercise. To begin the dip, grasp the bars and straighten your arms to the up posi-

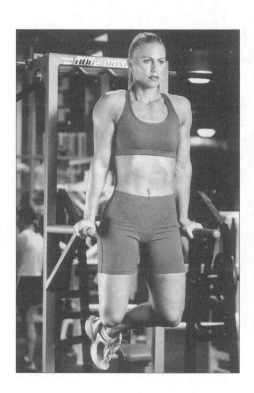

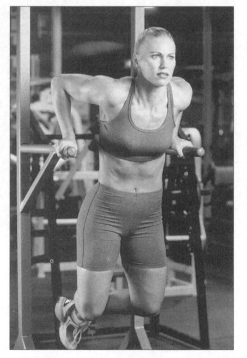

tion. Then lower your body, as shown, until you feel a stretch in your shoulder joints. Then return to the starting position. Focus on maintaining good form and working the muscles through their full range of motion. Advanced individuals can also increase training resistance by adding weights as shown. If you cannot support your body weight, place a sturdy box or low step under your feet, and assist the movement by using your legs to partially support the weight of your body.

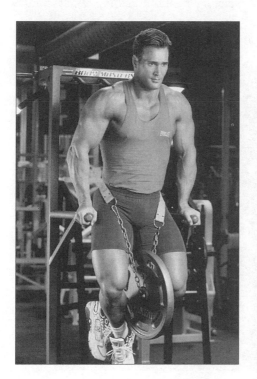

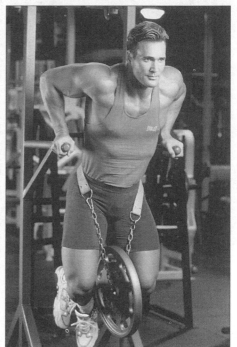

FOREARMS

WRIST CURL (Barbell or Dumbbells)

The wrist curl strongly exercises the muscles of your forearms.

Performing the wrist curl. Sit at the end of a flat exercise bench with your fore-arms resting on your thighs so your wrists are hanging over your knees. Grip the barbell with your palms up. Flex your forearms, curling the barbell upward as high as you can. Return to the starting position. Doing wrist curls with palms up stresses the flexor muscles on the insides of the forearms.

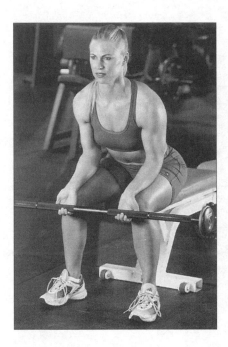 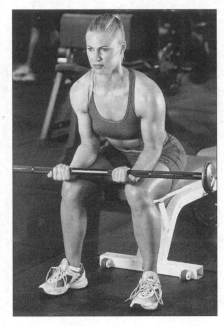

REVERSE WRIST CURL (Barbell or Dumbbells)

The reverse wrist curl exercises the extensor muscles of your forearms. These muscles are often underdeveloped, so weight training will help build and strengthen them and develop forearm muscle balance.

Performing the reverse wrist curl. Sit at the end of a flat exercise bench with your forearms resting on your thighs so your wrists are hanging over your knees. Grip the barbell with your palms facing down, and assume the starting position with your knuckles aimed at the floor. Flex your forearm extensor muscles, curling the barbell upward as high as you can, with your knuckles aimed up to the ceiling. Return to the starting position to complete one repetition.

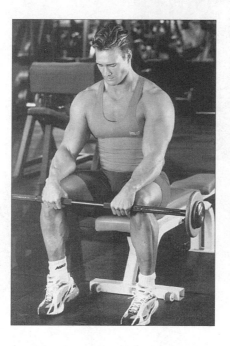 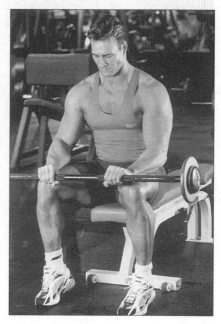

ABDOMINALS

INCLINE SIT-UP

The incline sit-up exercises the abdominal muscle.

Performing the incline sit-up. Start by lying down with your hands crossing your chest or behind your neck as shown. Tighten the abdominal muscle and raise your torso as illustrated. Return to the starting position to complete one repetition.

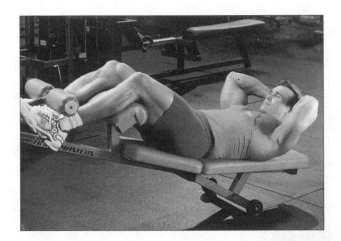

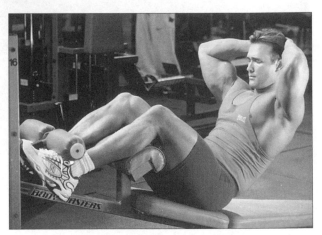

CRUNCH

The crunch exercises your abdominal muscle.

Performing the crunch.   Lie on the floor, with your arms across your chest or your hands lightly clasped behind your head. You can keep your feet on the floor or raise them as shown in the photos. Tighten your abdominal muscle and slowly curl your shoulders up off the floor and toward your knees until your shoulder blades come one to two inches off the floor. Hold this position for a second before slowly returning to the starting position.

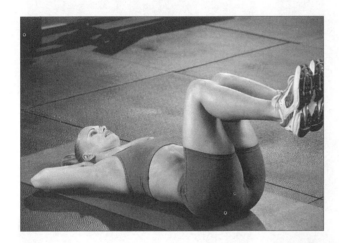

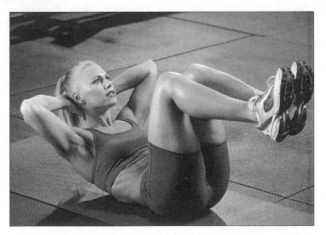

REVERSE CRUNCH

The reverse crunch exercises the lower abdominal muscle.

Performing the reverse crunch. The reverse crunch can be performed lying down on the floor or using the inclined sit-up board as shown in the photos. Starting with your legs bent, lift your feet a few inches from the board, then flex your abdominal muscle and raise your knees toward your chest. Return your legs to the starting position.

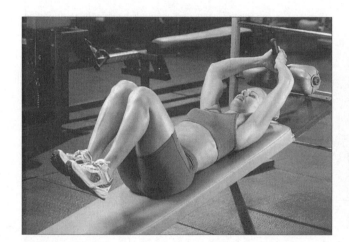

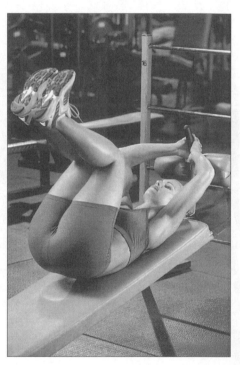

OBLIQUES

WEIGHTED SIDE BEND

The weighted side bend exercises your obliques in an alternating sequence.

Performing the weighted side bend. Start this exercise by performing some side bends without holding weights to warm your muscles. Grab a dumbbell in one hand and stand straight, with your other hand placed on the oblique you will be exercising. Bend to the side you are holding the weight on, keeping the hips straight. Then contract your oblique on the side opposite the one you are holding the dumbbell on, and hold the contraction for a second before returning slowly to the starting position. Perform this exercise with caution, as most people are unaccustomed to moving side to side in this way.

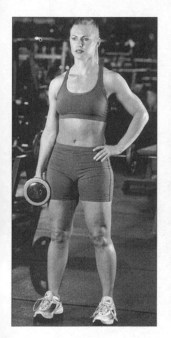
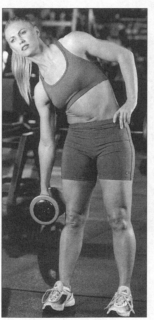
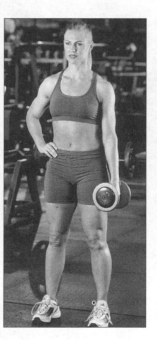
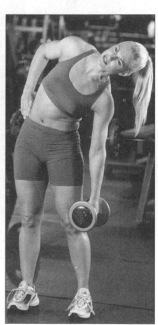

LYING SIDE OBLIQUE CRUNCH

The lying side oblique crunch is another exercise that can be used to exercise the obliques.

Performing the lying side oblique crunch. Lying on your side as shown in the photo, place your hands behind your neck. To initiate the motion of this exercise, contract your oblique and lift your shoulders toward your hip, in a short range of motion. Relax your oblique, and return to the starting position. After performing the desired number of repetitions, lie on the other side to exercise your other oblique.

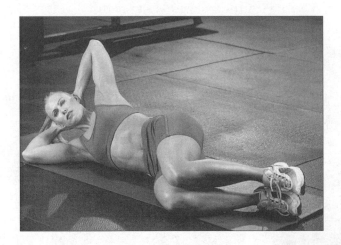

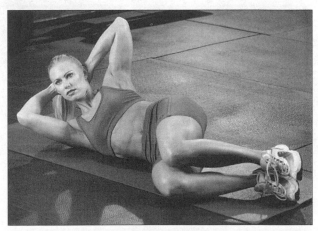

The Russian twist is considered an advanced exercise for the midsection, and should only be performed by competitive athletes who need to build strength and speed for twisting their torso.

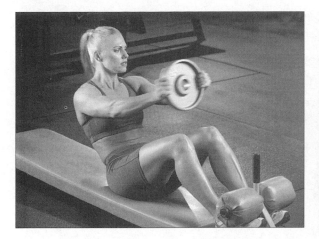 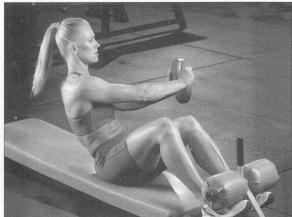

Performing the Russian twist. Using a sit-up board, assume a bent knee sit-up position with your torso tilted backward as illustrated in the photo. Holding your hands out (or holding a weight), start to twist your torso from one side to the other over and over again.

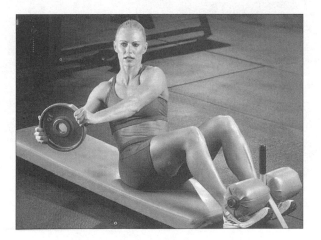

BUTTOCKS, HIPS, THIGHS

SQUAT (Barbell)

The squat is a good all-around exercise for the buttocks, hips, and quadriceps.

Performing the squat. Two spotters should be used when performing the barbell squat, as well as a safety squat apparatus or smith machine. Stand with your legs about shoulder width, or slightly wider, with toes pointed straight or slightly outward, and rest the barbell on your upper back, using some type of padding if desired. Keep your spine straight through the exercise. Try tilting your head up, and look at the ceiling during the repetition movement, as this helps keep the back

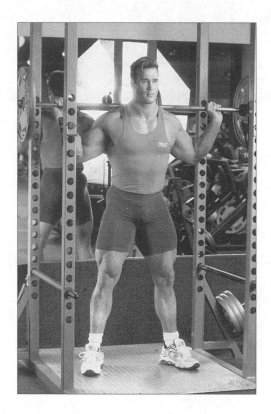

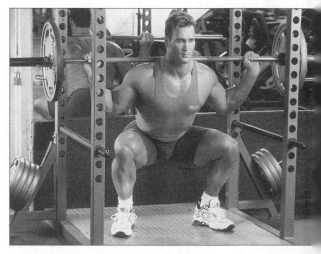

straight. Slowly bend your legs as shown, and lower you buttocks until your thighs are parallel to the floor. You may lean slightly forward during this downward motion. Then return to the starting position.

Using a lighter weight, you can also hold the barbell in front of your chest as shown (front squat). Begin with light weights and focus your efforts on developing good form when doing the squat. Most people will want to perform higher repetitions for general fitness conditioning.

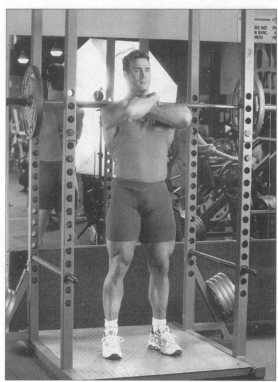

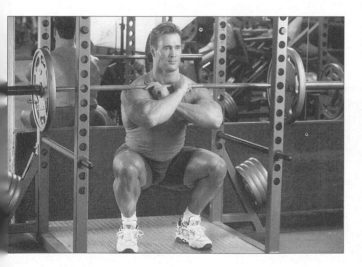

LEG PRESS

The leg press exercises the buttocks, hips, and upper legs in a way similar to the squat, while reducing pressure on the spine.

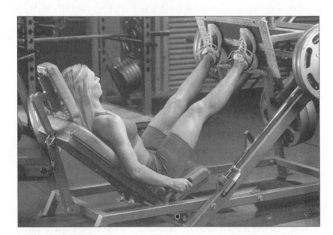 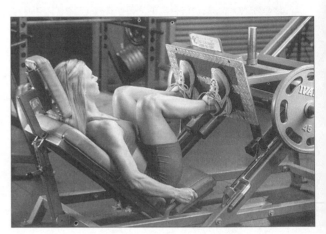

Performing the leg press. Sit on the machine and position your feet about six to 12 inches apart. Straighten your legs to the starting position, then lower them slowly. Straighten to the starting position.

You can also perform calf exercises using the leg-press machine as shown.

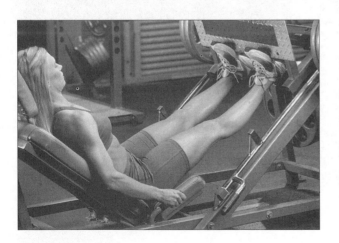 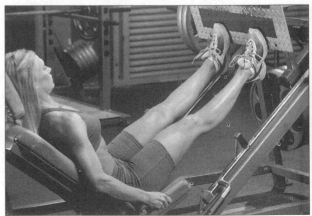

LEG EXTENSION (Machine)

The leg extension isolates and exercises the quadriceps (thighs).

Performing the leg extension. Sit on the bench or leg extension machine, with your feet under the lower pads of the foot support. Flex your quads and lift your legs as shown until they are straight, and hold for a second. Return slowly to the starting position.

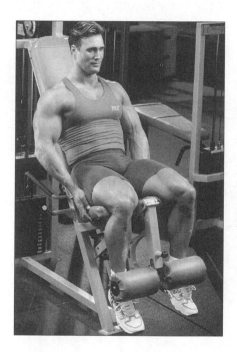
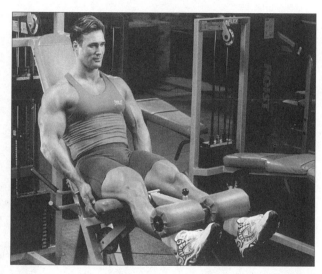

LUNGE (Barbell or Dumbbells)

The lunge, like the squat, exercises the buttocks, hips, and upper legs, as well as the calves. It can be performed with or without weights, and is a great exercise for athletes and fitness exercisers.

Performing the lunge.   Stand straight and hold the dumbbells at your sides. Keep your back straight. Step forward with one leg, bending your knees as shown, resulting with the lower leg perpendicular to the floor. Return to the starting position, and alternate legs with each repetition. Advanced individuals can perform the lunge using a barbell. Another popular variation of the lunge is the walking lunge.

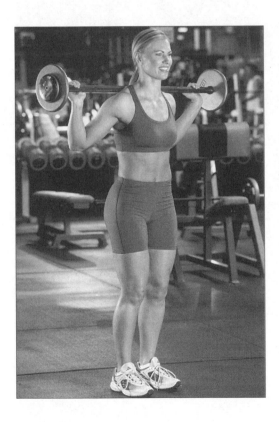
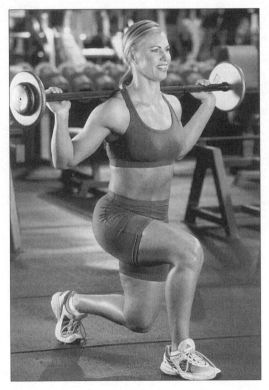

SIDE LUNGE

The side lunge is a useful exercise, especially for runners. It also works the buttocks, hips, quadriceps, and calves, as well as the hip abductors and adductors, and helps develop greater flexibility in the inner thigh and groin regions.

Performing the side lunge. Stand straight with your feet just slightly wider than your shoulders. Step out to one side with your right leg. As the right foot lands,

(continues on page 150)

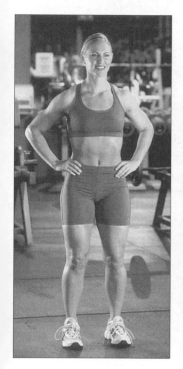

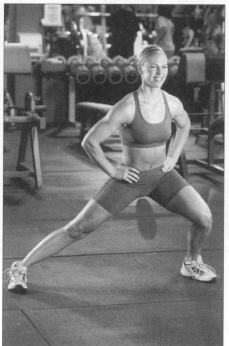

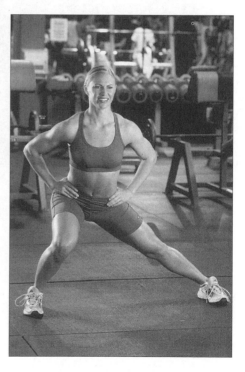

SIDE LUNGE *(continued)*

turn it outward, and assume the squat position with your right leg. Keep your torso erect and facing forward. Then push back to the starting position, and repeat this movement with your left leg. As you progress in this exercise, you can add weights.

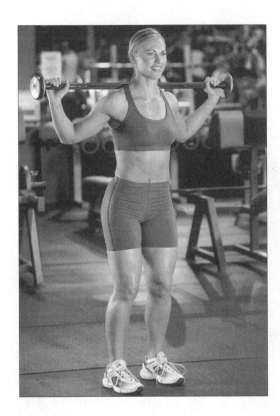 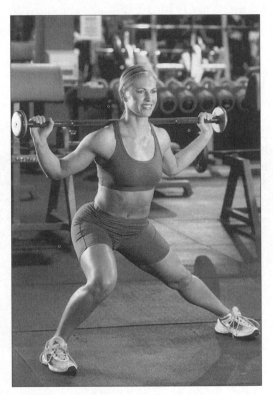

HAMSTRINGS

LEG CURL (Machine)

The leg curl is the primary exercise for the hamstring muscles.

Performing the leg curl. Lie prone (face downward) on the bench, with your ankles under the upper pads of the leg lever and kneecaps just off the bench, as shown. Curl your feet toward your buttocks and hold for a second. Return to the starting position. Maintain smooth, rhythmic movement in the knee joint, and avoid jerking your body. Keep your hips flat on the bench during the repetitions.

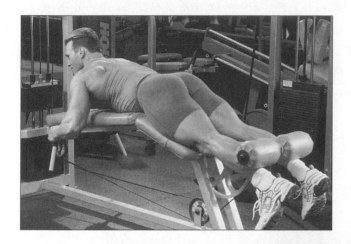

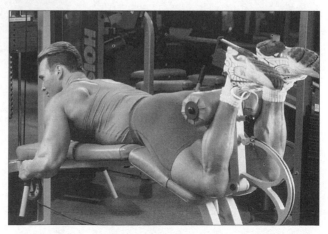

CALVES

ONE-LEGGED STANDING HEEL RAISE (Dumbbells)

This exercise is excellent for working your calves.

Performing the one-legged standing heel raise. Stand with your toes and the balls of your feet on a 4 × 4-inch or 2 × 4-inch block of wood (toes pointed directly ahead). Shift all your weight to one foot and bring the other off the block by bending your knee and letting it dangle behind you. Keeping your leg straight, rise up as high as possible on your toes. Lower slowly back to the starting point and repeat. You can also do this while holding dumbbells in your hands. You might find it difficult to balance yourself, but if you rise up slowly you should be able to manage. Large gyms have a special calf machine that eliminates the balance problem.

On your second set of calf raises, point your toes outward at 45-degree angles. On your third set, point them inward at 45-degree angles. Each foot position stresses the calves somewhat differently.

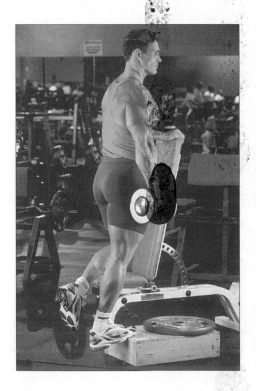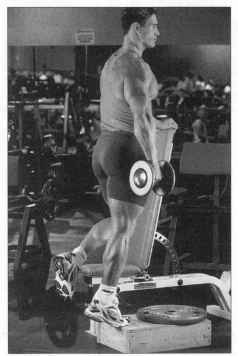

CALF MACHINE

The seated and standing calf exercise machines train the calves with heavy loads. The seated calf machine is the best choice for using the heaviest load, as it eliminates pressure on the lower back.

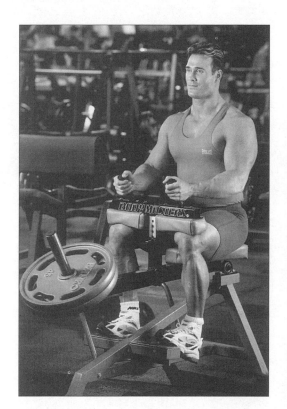
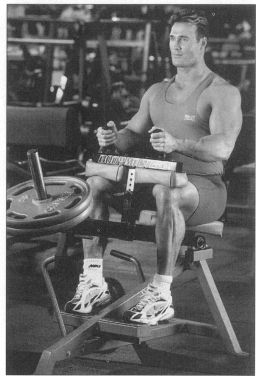

Performing the seated or standing calf exercise machines. Assume the appropriate position on the machine. Start by lowering your heels. Then stand up on your toes as high as possible, while maintaining good position as you contract the calf muscles. Lower your heels to the starting position.

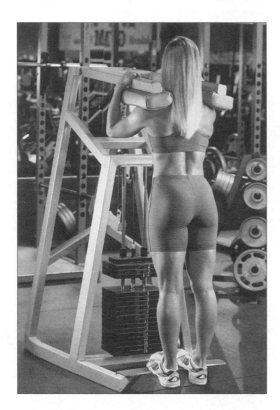

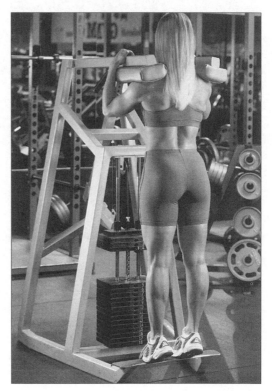

ADDITIONAL EXERCISE—ADVANCED ATHLETES

POWER CLEAN (Barbell)

The power clean is an advanced exercise for athletes who wish to build explosive strength in their legs, hips, and upper body. It combines the dead lift, shrug, squat, and reverse curl performed in a sequence of rapid movements. This is an exercise for advanced-level individuals only. If you are unaccustomed to performing this exercise, use light weights until you perfect the technique.

Performing the power clean. With the barbell in front of your shins, bend down, keeping your back flat, and grip the barbell with an overhand grip. Use a shoulder-width or slightly wider grip. Pull the barbell up rapidly to your shoulders as illus-

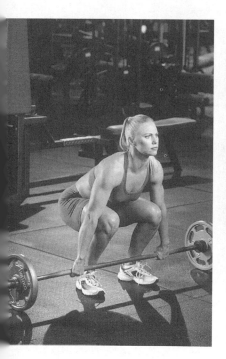 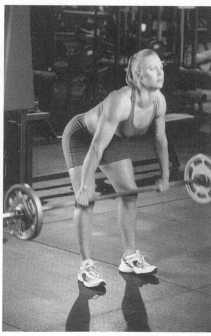 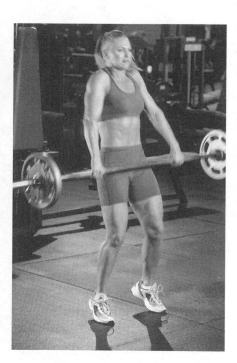

trated in the photos. Return the barbell to the floor and assume that starting position for another repetition. The trick to performing the power clean is to let your legs and back do most of the work in the beginning of the movement. The upper body then snaps the barbell up, while your legs squat down to shorten the height you need to lift the barbell to the chest position. Then with the barbell held at your chest, straighten your legs to complete the upward motion of the sequence.

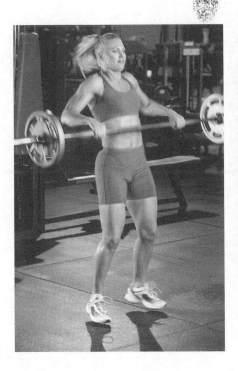
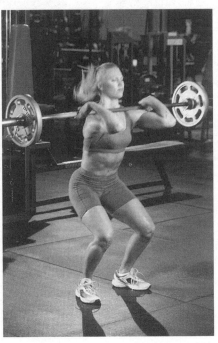
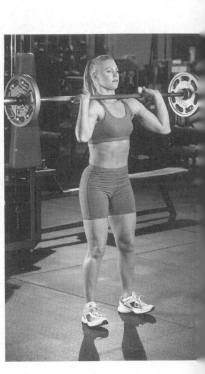

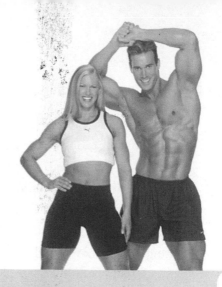

Dynatrition—The New Commandments of Nutrition

6

Energy from optimal nutrition is the base of the Weider Triangle Method. Without the right food to fuel your workouts, you may survive, but you'll never thrive. You may be surprised to learn that most people follow nutrition plans that scarcely provide the bare essentials; even professional athletes succumb to diet fads in an effort to tweak gains. Adequate nutrition is a science—something that should be adhered to every day. If you work out on a regular basis and have performance goals, it's even more essential to follow a sophisticated meal program, one that maximizes the performance of your entire body. This is why we developed Dynatrition, to distinguish regular nutrition from high-powered, performance-based sports and fitness nutrition.

Dynatrition takes your individual needs into account, whether they are sport-specific or issue-specific. For example, you may need to lose weight, build muscle, or boost energy levels. Gender and age are also considerations. Dynatrition emphasizes the role of dietary supplements in your daily eating plan, based on cutting-edge research that shows what really works. Our newly updated Commandments of Performance Nutrition give you the easy to follow Dynatrition eating guidelines, complete with supplement guidelines and sports-specific meal plans.

FIVE PRINCIPLES OF SPORTS NUTRITION

Athletes have special needs that cannot be easily met by the typical American diet. Even if you don't consider yourself an "athlete," there are some very simple but important changes you can make to your daily diet that will have a significant effect on your performance and fitness. So what is optimum nutrition? Is it three square meals a day from the five food groups, as some books suggest?

The problem with finding the answers to these questions is the mass of conflicting information found in books, magazines, and on the Internet. Scientific organizations also publish various guidelines. But these allowances are based on average food needs for the nation at large—average, sedentary people. In fact, the RDA committee states emphatically in their handbook that guidelines should not be confused with requirements for specific individuals. Despite this clear statement, the RDAs are constantly misused to estimate requirements for individual athletes. This is a big mistake, and the most recent research on sports nutrition confirms this.

These days, it's almost impossible to avoid processed foods, most of which are loaded with fat, salt, and sugar. Eating junk food while training leads to permanent injury to muscles and bones, because they are insufficiently supplied with enough nutrients to combat the strain of the intense exercise. What's worse, poor dietary habits contribute to the development of degenerative and deadly diseases, such as cardiovascular disease, diabetes, obesity, and cancer.

We're going to show you how to devise a healthy eating program that will take all the guesswork away. Make these important principles of performance-nutrition— Individuality, Synergy, Complete Nutrition, Evolution, and Consistency—part of your thinking, and we guarantee you the fastest and best results in your physical development and health.

1. INDIVIDUALITY

Each person is biologically unique and has different nutrient requirements. From the hair on your head to the bottom of your feet, these differences are what make us unique and special. Your perfectly normal stomach may vary in size from what is considered normal, and the digestive juices your stomach uses may be a hundred times stronger or weaker than those of the next person. Compared to the textbook average, you may have inherited low or high blood pressure, poor or 20/20 eyesight, high or low levels of sex hormones, sluggish or explosive gland function. The unique combinations are endless. And while there are obviously many similarities among the nutritional requirements of the masses, there are many requirements that are unique to you, based on your activities and performance goals. While your training partner may swear that peanut butter and jelly sandwiches helped build his abs, it doesn't mean it will work for you if weight loss is your number-one priority. Use your science sense. For optimum performance and health you need a blend of nutrients to suit your specific needs, activity level, metabolism, size, etc. Nutritional individuality is the first principle of Dynatrition.

2. SYNERGY

It is the interaction of vitamins, minerals, and other nutrients, not their individual actions, which is the basis of their biological functions. Medical science has only recently begun to understand the delicate interplay among the hundreds of nutrients our bodies need—many of which we must get from the food we eat. There is rarely a deficiency or inadequacy of only one vitamin, mineral, or amino acid. In fact, it is the multiple interactions of these essential substances that result in healing, muscle repair, bone growth, and the hundreds of other bodily functions that occur daily. How well your body performs depends on a balance of nutrients being supplied to the body in the same mixtures and concentrations that occur in nature, but geared to your specific demands of training. Rarely will eating just a few types of food, or supplementation with one nutrient, do any real good.

There is controversy over the use of supplements, mainly because scientists have relied on evidence from single-nutrient studies. These studies sometimes fail to show positive results because complementary nutrients are not sufficiently available in the diet. For example, the power of vitamin C to stop colds depends as much on other nutrients in the diet as on the supplemental vitamin C. If the diet is deficient in nutrients that interact with vitamin C in promoting resistance to colds, it is impossible for the body to use the vitamin C supplement. You also need adequate amounts of B_6, B_{12}, zinc, folic acid, choline, etc. Similarly, there is a well-known interplay between calcium and vitamin D—you need both for healthy bones. Every nutrient and essential element operates by multiple interactions. This is the second principle of Dynatrition.

3. COMPLETE NUTRITION

The principle of synergy leads to the rule of complete nutrition. As said above, arbitrary supplementation of the diet with large amounts of any single nutrient produces imbalances in overall nutrition and is damaging to peak performance and health. Athletes require different proportions of protein, carbohydrates, fats, vitamins, and minerals to meet the various demands of training.

Focus on complete nutrition. You need to make sure that your diet contains the full spectrum of nutrients from foods and high-quality sports supplements designed to provide you with precise performance nutrient combinations. This is the third principle of Dynatrition.

4. EVOLUTIONARY DYNAMICS

Amino acids, sugars, starches, fatty acids, vitamins, and minerals are some of the essential components that are absolutely essential to life. It is certain that the current list of essential nutrients is incomplete. Many elements and other substances under intense study are bound to yield discovery of new essential nutrients. For example, chromium was once thought to be appropriate only for car bumpers, but we now know that chromium is essential for proper metabolism. For performance-fitness nutrition, we must ensure that our diet contains all nutrients we know are essential. This is the fourth principle of Dynatrition.

5. NUTRITIONAL CONSISTENCY

The action of nutrients in building and in rebuilding the body is slow, safe, and enduring. It is fairly common to hear of athletes going on a good diet for six weeks or so to get ready for competition. Champions don't do that. Champions are careful of their diet year round. Bodybuilding greats like Lou Ferrigno, Frank Zane, Arnold Schwarzenegger, Lee Haney, Dorian Yates, and Ronnie Coleman believe that year-round attention to diet is the difference between winning and losing, and they're right. Long-term maintenance of good nutrition is crucial for so many reasons. For example, did you know that your blood cells live for only 60 to 140 days before they are renewed? Each year your blood is completely renewed about four times. All the cells of your muscles are also renewed during your life. The rebuilding of this new tissue depends on what you eat. You really are what you eat. You can be of great service to yourself and others by emphasizing physiological dynamics and the necessity of year-round attention to nutrition for optimum body growth, performance, and health. This is the fifth principle of Dynatrition.

COMMANDMENTS OF PERFORMANCE-FITNESS NUTRITION

Okay, we're done with the science behind eating, and hopefully you understand why these five principles are so important. Now here are the absolute Commandments of Sports Nutrition. They apply to athletes, fitness exercisers, and everyone else. When we first developed these guidelines, we called them the Commandments of Sports Nutrition and they turned out to be way ahead of their time. It took the medical community two decades to realize their truth. Follow them, and you will be rewarded with improved performance, a healthy body, and longer life. Make copies of this page, post it in your kitchen, and take it with you when you shop or

TAKE A DAILY MULTIVITAMIN SUPPLEMENT

Despite high calorie intake, athletes are frequently deficient in many nutrients. In a comprehensive four-year study of university athletes, researchers found that for athletes with high calorie intakes, fat comprised more than 50% of their diets. Vitamin A and potassium were deficient, and the women's teams showed low iron, despite high-protein and high caloric intake. The situation is worse in sports that demand a very low level of body fat such as bodybuilding, wrestling, weightlifting, martial arts, boxing, gymnastics, dance, and ballet. One noteworthy study of college wrestlers found that many of the participants did not meet even two-thirds of the RDA for protein, vitamin A, vitamin C, vitamin B_2, vitamin B_6, magnesium, iron, and zinc. In such cases supplementation with vitamins, minerals, and amino acids is essential to maintain good health. If you are on a reduced calorie diet to lose weight, it is vital that you supplement your limited food intake to reduce the risk of nutritional deficiencies.

eat out. It makes pefect sense to always eat a healthy and performance-enhancing diet. Memorize the commandments and practice them daily.

THE NEW COMMANDMENTS OF SPORTS NUTRITION

> Commandment 1: Drink clean water.
>
> Commandment 2: Eat foods that are high in complex carbohydrates and fiber.
>
> Commandment 3: Eat protein in moderation.
>
> Commandment 4: Eat a diet low in saturated fats and cholesterol.
>
> Commandment 5: Eat essential fatty acids.
>
> Commandment 6: Eat a diet low in processed sugar.
>
> Commandment 7: Eat salt in moderation.
>
> Commandment 8: Eat a variety of healthy foods.
>
> Commandment 9: Take a daily nutritional supplement.
>
> Commandment 10: Eliminate junk foods.

When you think of it, what you put into your mouth is one of the few things in life over which you have total control. So why not eat with purpose? Before consuming something, ask yourself, "Is this healthy for me?" "Will eating this food or drinking this beverage help me reach my goals?"

Watch for the pitfalls of travel, when your healthy choices may be limited and you can easily overeat or eat the wrong foods. It's much harder to eat clean when you're at a restaurant, so make an extra effort to avoid dishes laden with sauces and fat. But even then, there are plenty of choices that won't kill your whole plan. Be smart and avoid the cream sauces and fried items.

If you have cookies and potato chips in your house, you're going to eat them, so clean your cupboards.

Let's look at the Commandments a bit more closely.

Commandment 1: Drink Clean Water.

Our bodies are more than two-thirds water, and so good clean water is the most important starting point. Some athletes training long, intensive hours can perspire and excrete over two gallons of water a day. When you are on a weight-loss diet, you increase your risk of becoming dehydrated. The body can make some water from metabolic processes, but not much. You have to replace it constantly. You must maintain a regular intake of pure water to maintain adequate hydration.

Even a tiny, temporary shortage of water can disrupt your body's functions. If your muscles become dehydrated only 3%, you lose 10% of contractile strength and 8% of speed. Water balance is the most important variable in peak performance and maintenance of good health.

The quality of your muscles reflects the quality of the water you drink. But clean water is becoming a rare commodity. Tap water is treated only to minimum standards, and chemicals are sometimes added to keep it germ-free. Even low levels of contaminants can ruin your performance. Make sure the water you drink is pure. Start by checking with the company that supplies your water. Ask to get a copy of the tests. Then have your water tested by an independent testing service to verify the results. If your water is too high in contaminants, then get a water-filtering device installed to correct the problem. Turning to bottled water is also an option. Select a brand you like that is convenient and economical. Then contact the company and request a copy of their water quality test to confirm that the product you are purchasing is indeed as pure as you expect. If the company resists, then contact other companies until you get the information you want and are satisfied.

Commandment 2: Eat Foods That Are High
in Complex Carbohydrates and Fiber.

Carbohydrates are an essential energy source for both strength and stamina, and when your body is depleted of carbohydrates, physical and mental performance is compromised. Make sure 55 to 60 percent of the daily calories you eat come from high-quality complex carbohydrates, such as vegetables, whole grains, and fruit. Increase carbohydrate intake even more on the day of competition to 70–90 percent, or for the meal before your exercise sessions.

But not all carbohydrates are created equal. A diet high in simple carbohydrates or sugar can disrupt your metabolism of fat. In both animal and human studies, excess sugar raises both cholesterol and triglycerides levels in your blood. The more processed a grain or vegetable, the more deficient in nutrients it is, especially in fiber. Some foods high in carbohydrates are better than others. Champion athletes need the champion carbohydrates, especially for stability of blood sugar and for maintenance of glycogen (energy) stores.

The key to eating carbohydrates is to choose ones that are low-fat, made from whole grains or whole foods (like potatoes), and contain fiber and protein. Be careful not to overindulge in carbohydrates. Because your body can easily digest them, you can easily overeat them. Chapter 7 includes a list of the best carbohydrate foods from which to choose. Make carbohydrates part of all of your meals and snacks for super energy and peak performance.

Commandment 3: Eat Protein in Moderation.

Maintain intake of high-quality protein foods and supplements. Athletic people need more protein than non-athletes and the RDA standard. Depending on your sport, aim for a diet of 15 to 30 percent protein.

Protein is most often recognized as the key "muscle food." The more muscle you develop, and the more you exercise, the more protein your body needs to repair and maintain muscle tissues. In particular, the more fast-twitch muscle fibers you develop, the greater your need for protein becomes, because fast-twitch muscle fiber is more fragile than slow-twitch muscle fiber. So the more you strength train and the bigger your muscles get, the more protein you need. But even a lean marathon runner, whose muscles are high in slow-twitch muscle fibers, needs about double the protein of a sedentary person. Chapter 7 includes a detailed discussion of why athletes need more protein.

Amino Acids There is another side to protein that is often overlooked by nutritionists. Proteins are made up of amino acids. In addition to making muscle-tissue proteins, amino acids have other functions. They are part of many enzymes that are needed to make your body run correctly. Amino acids are also used to make neurochemicals that are used in your brain and nervous system. Since your nervous system controls your muscles, keeping it well nourished will fuel performance. It is interesting to note that in all studies where people are given protein supplements, their health improves, their body composition improves, and their performance improves. In a recent study, scientists discovered that whey protein supplements actually reduced feelings of stress and anxiety. We can all benefit from this, especially athletes.

Commandment 4: Eat a Diet Low in Saturated Fats and Cholesterol.

Most sensible athletes try to keep fats low in their diets but it's easy to fail because of all the hidden fats found in processed foods. Let us set the record straight on fats. There are good fats and bad fats. Saturated fats should be minimized at all costs. Saturated simply means that all the carbon atoms of the fat are filled with hydrogen atoms. Most saturated fats are solid at room temperature like the fat you see around steak. Most foods high in saturated fat are low in essential fats and high in cholesterol. Because saturated fats are not essential to your body, they tend to be easily stored as body fat and make you unhealthy.

Foods that are higher in unsaturated and polyunsaturated fatty acids (oils) can lower body cholesterol levels and reduce the risk of heart disease. They tend to be high in the essential fatty acids that are used to build your cells, as well as high in other important substances your body needs to thrive. Plant oils tend to be high in unsaturated fats, as do fish oils.

But beware that food processing can make a good fat into a bad one. For example, some cooking oils, margarines, and spreads are prime examples of how the food industry can screw up Mother Nature. Most of the oils in these products are hydrogenated during processing to improve shelf life, taste, and smell. That is, hydrogen atoms are added, making the unsaturated vegetable oils nearly as saturated as beef drippings. Margarine is the prime example. You might as well use butter. It tastes better, too. Also, don't believe the advertisements showing how liquid some oils are, therefore presumably less saturated. Coconut oil can be liquid, yet is primarily composed of saturated fat.

Commandment 5: Eat Essential Fatty Acids.

Some classes of fatty acids are essential to health and beneficial to athletes. In addition to plant oils and oils in nuts, fish oil is extremely beneficial. Eating fish just two to three times a week makes for a healthier cardiovascular system. Recent studies have shown this level of dietary intake can prevent and even stop the progression of cardiovascular diseases. Additional benefits include reducing joint pain and inflammation and muscle soreness. Long-term health benefits include preventing development of arthritis, cardiovascular disease, and cancer. In the last few years, controlled scientific studies have shown that it is likely the "omega-3" fatty acids in fish oils are the protective agents.

Almost everyone develops some degree of arthritis as they age. But until recently, there was no scientific evidence for the idea that joints, tendons, and membranes "dry" with aging, resulting in pain and stiffness, and that fish oils help offset this deterioration. Now some evidence is in. Dr. Joel Kramer and colleagues at Albany Medical College and New York University gave rheumatoid arthritis patients 1.8 g of an omega-3 called eicosapentaenoic acid (EPA) daily for 12 weeks, and compared their responses with rheumatoid arthritis patients given placebo capsules. The group receiving the EPA showed significant decrease in tender joints and in pain. When the EPA was withdrawn, the patients deteriorated again, showing clear increases in pain and stiffness. New research confirms the results of these earlier studies.

Numerous studies have shown benefits to fish oil ingestion in the prevention and treatment of heart disease as well. Dr. J. Singer and colleagues showed that a high-EPA diet (mackerel fillets) lowered systolic blood pressure significantly in both hypertensive and normal subjects. As rising blood pressure with age is one of the main causes of heart attacks, any food that lowers it is important. For athletes it is especially important to keep blood pressure below 120/80. The average athlete needs only a gram or so of fish oils daily, about equivalent to one serving of sardines, salmon, or mackerel. Fish is also a healthy source of protein. Start eating more fish. But stick to grilled or baked fish, prepared without added oils or butter.

In addition to the healthy omega-3 fatty acids, there are numerous medical studies that report on the benefits from supplementing the diet with linoleic and linolenic acids, the essential fatty acids from which the body makes all other fatty acids. The published research runs the gamut from lowering cholesterol and blood pressure to improving intelligence. And women will be pleased to know that a diet low in saturated fatty acids and adequate in essential fatty acids is associated with a reduction of symptoms of premenstrual syndrome.

Commandment 6: Eat a Diet Low in Processed Sugar.

While it is true that your body will digest complex carbohydrates into the same glucose molecule that is found in sugar, there are some good reasons to reduce your consumption of sugar and high-fructose corn syrup. Sugar is composed of glucose and fructose. Because it is refined and removed from other nutrients and fiber, which would slow down its digestion, refined sugar gets into the bloodstream very quickly and causes a rapid rise in insulin. Drinking too many high-sugar drinks and eating too many high-sugar foods can cause problems with maintenance of blood sugar levels and insulin production. High-sugar diets are also linked to diabetes and can ruin your teeth.

The fructose content of many foods has also become a problem. Fructose tends to be used at a slower rate by your muscles than glucose for energy. Your liver can convert fructose to energy or fat more quickly than your muscles, but new evidence reveals that the liver can be overloaded by too much fructose. Years ago fructose was touted as a healthy sugar, because it causes a slower rise in insulin and blood-sugar levels than glucose. However, new research indicates that too much fructose can make you fat and cause your liver to increase fatty deposits, leading to a malfunctioning metabolism.

We think that applying some common sense will do you better than reviewing all the scientific details. The problem with refined sugars and flour is that fiber and nutrients have been removed. Fiber is Mother Nature's regulator of proper digestion. It slows down digestion to a healthy rate. When your diet is higher in refined sugar, it is lower in fiber and essential nutrients. This is not healthy. The other downside to eating too much sugar is that because it surges through your body rapidly, it gets broken down into molecules that have been associated with accelerating the aging process. This is why eating complex carbohydrates from whole foods and whole grains is important. They don't rush through your system and overwhelm it. They are digested at a healthy rate, and contain essential nutrients beneficial to your health.

We will review in chapter 7 some instances where ingesting sports drinks containing glucose or special glucose polymer drinks can benefit your exercise sessions and athletic performance. But as a general rule, reduce your dietary consumption of foods that contain added sugar and refined flour.

Commandment 7: Eat a Diet Moderate in Salt.

Salt is an essential nutrient, but it's a double-edged sword. If you don't get enough, your health and athletic performance are compromised; if you get too much, your heath is compromised. Realistically, most diets are too high in salt (sodium chloride), so cutting back on adding salt to your food and reducing the consumption of packaged foods that are usually high in salt will automatically adjust your salt intake to where it should be.

Of course, as with any essential nutrient, the higher your activity, the more you need. When it comes to salt it is also important to consider your potassium intake. Your body works best when you have achieved total nutrient balance. Eating a lot of packaged foods high in salt and adding salt to your foods upsets your body's balance of salt and potassium. Too much salt can upset your body's water balance and slow you down. When you starting eating whole foods, they restore a naturally healthy balance of these nutrients. So keep aware of your salt intake and don't overdo it.

Commandment 8: Eat a Variety of Healthy Foods.

If variety is the spice of life, then let a variety of healthy foods be the spice in your life. By eating a variety of foods, especially vegetables, you are more likely to get an adequate supply of essential nutrients.

When traveling in Asia, it is typical to encounter meals that consist of a wide variety of foods, especially vegetables. In Japan, the population is preoccupied with eating healthy foods that promote health and prevent diseases. The importance of eating a variety of foods is so important to the Japanese that the Japanese Ministry of Health and Welfare has officially recommended eating a varied diet of at least thirty foods daily. So when you are planning your next meal, think of the health-savvy Japanese.

Commandment 9: Use Nutritional Supplements Daily.

The use of nutritional or dietary supplements is mandatory for athletes and fitness enthusiasts. The research is clear and proven in more than 50,000 medical studies: When athletes take supplements, their performance improves. When non-athletes take supplements, their general health improves. People on weight-loss diets can benefit by taking supplements to ensure they are getting the essential nutrients they need while reducing calories.

The research is so impressive that during the 1990s, special regulations were implemented for dietary supplements here in the United States, in order to make them more available and to allow more claims on labels to educate the public about their many health benefits. The National Institutes of Health even established the Office of Dietary Supplements to fund research and maintains a database on existing research.

The benefits of taking dietary supplements are so vast that we have included an entire reference chapter explaining the best dietary supplements for different purposes. Use it as a guide to help evaluate and construct a personalized nutritional supplement plan that suits your performance-fitness needs.

Commandment 10: Eliminate Junk Foods.

This should be obvious by now. Junk foods often contain the very ingredients that the other commandments are aimed at avoiding, such as too much sugar, saturated fats, cholesterol, and salt. Most fast foods offer little in the way of healthy complex carbohydrates, protein, fiber, essential fatty acids, vitamins, minerals, and other healthy substances.

Avoiding junk food is the single most important factor that will make you healthier and more productive. When we work with athletes and fitness enthusiasts, if we can get them to master just this one commandment, in days we observe beneficial improvements in their physical and mental performance and physique.

When these commandments become ingrained in your thinking, they will act to filter out the foods you should avoid. Think of it this way: You follow rules and programs for your weight training, so why not be equally disciplined to feed your body the healthy nutrients it needs for optimum performance and health? The next chapter presents Dynatrition daily menu guidelines to help you create an eating plan worthy of a champion.

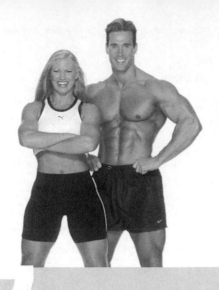

Putting Dynatrition into Practice

B y now you know that one size does not fit all when it comes to weight training and fitness, and the same is certainly true for meal plans and nutrition. For example, your individual metabolism and activity level determine your total caloric needs, as well as the amount of protein, carbohydrates, and fat you should consume. In the pages that follow, we teach you how to synthesize and use your new nutrition knowledge about Dynatrition, developed with our coauthor, sports nutrition, fitness, and dietary supplement expert Daniel Gastelu.

Why so many diets?

Why are there so many different theories on nutrition? This is probably the question we answer most frequently in our magazines and in our lectures. It's likely that you've come across hundreds of nutrition plans and tips in your reading, so let's take a look at what may or may not be based on meaningful science. (We cover nutrition for weight loss in chapter 9, so here we refer to overall nutrition for health and performance.)

NUTRITION FOR STRENGTH AND BODYBUILDING

If your goal is to increase muscle mass and strength, you need special nutrition that includes supplementation. Eating more may not be enough, especially if you are not eating a proper diet in the first place. You need specific nutrients to help muscles attain maximum growth. Your specific athletic conditioning determines which foods and supplements work best for you. Of course, everyone needs to follow the general rules of healthy eating, but you can modify your intake of certain nutrients to help you achieve maximum performance. This chapter covers the basics of sports nutrition and will help provide the essential information you need to benefit the most from the information in this book.

While it's important to eat a balanced diet containing adequate amounts of all of the essential nutrients, scientific research has shown that a balanced diet alone does not provide sufficient nutrition to individuals doing strenuous physical activities.

What are macronutrients and micronutrients?

Optimal nutrition for peak performance means more than just the food groups you learned about in school. Sports nutrition refers to several categories of nutrients from a variety of sources. *Macronutrients* are those nutrients needed in large amounts, such as protein, carbohydrates, fats, and water. *Micronutrients* are those nutrients required in smaller amounts, particularly vitamins and minerals. Micronutrients are measured in milligrams (mg) and micrograms (mcg) and macronutrients are measured in grams (g).

MACRONUTIENTS

PROTEIN AND AMINO ACIDS

Under certain circumstances protein is used for energy, especially during exercise. Adequate protein will ensure you don't draw upon valuable stores of muscle for energy. Like carbohydrates, protein can be converted to fat if you eat too much or if your total daily caloric intake is too high. Eat a moderate amount of protein that meets your body size and exercise demands for optimum performance and muscle growth.

Protein comes from both animal and plant food sources, as well as from special protein supplement formulations. Animal protein tends to be more complete than plants because it contains all the amino acids your body needs. However, animal protein is also high in saturated fat and cholesterol. Be sure your protein source is low in saturated fats and cholesterol. Good choices include egg whites (or whole eggs if eaten sparingly), chicken, turkey, shellfish, and lean fish. Minimize fatty cuts of beef, pork, and lamb, and always trim excess fat and skin.

When it comes to designing an eating plan for athletes, there are different protein requirements for different levels of conditioning. Later in this chapter we will determine what amount of protein is adequate for your specific sport and level of conditioning. We'll also introduce you to some of the amino acids that have been shown to enhance athletic performance.

Protein is an essential nutrient, which means that you must take in adequate amounts of it through your diet for continued health. In fact, it is the basic component of all living cells and can be found in virtually every part of your body, including your muscle tissue.

Protein provides your body with the raw material it needs—in the form of amino acids—for tissue growth, repair, and maintenance. Protein is also vital to the creation of biomolecules, such as hormones and deoxyribonucleic acid (DNA)—the molecule that stores your genetic code. Also referred to as polypeptides, proteins contain anywhere from less than a dozen to over a hundred amino-acid molecules. Amino acids are the building blocks of proteins. They are linked together by a chemical bond, known as a peptide bond. Although many amino acids exist in nature, twenty-two are considered biologically significant.

Some amino acids play important metabolic roles as precursors, or starting materials, of other molecules and act as intermediates, or go-betweens, in some metabolic pathways. (A pathway is a sequence of metabolic reactions.) For example, some amino acids are important in the urea cycle, which is the pathway responsible for clearing nitrogen waste from the body. Other amino acids are important precursors of some neurotransmitters—chemical substances that help transmit nerve impulses throughout the body.

Your body needs amino acids for the formation of enzymes—catalysts, or starters, of different biochemical reactions, such as energy production. Researchers estimate that as much as 10 percent of an athlete's energy production can come from amino acids. Apparently, as your muscles become better conditioned, and you undergo one to several hours of physical training each day, your body will use more amino acids for energy production during exercise and even at rest.

What are the different types of amino acids?

The essential amino acids—the amino acids that your body cannot manufacture and therefore need to be ingested—are valine, lysine, threonine, leucine, isoleucine, tryptophan, phenylalanine, methionine, and histidine. Nonessential amino acids are amino acids that the body can manufacture on its own. However, it's still important to ingest nonessential amino acids from dietary sources and spare the supply of essential amino acids for other functions. Some of the nutritionally important nonessential amino acids are glycine, alanine, serine, cystine, tyrosine, aspartic acid, proline, hydroxyproline, citrulline, arginine, ornithine, hydroxyglutamic acid, glutamine, and glutamic acid.

Are there certain amino acids that my body is more likely to use as energy?

The branched-chain amino acids, including isoleucine, leucine, and valine—which also happen to be essential amino acids—are the preferred group of amino acids for energy use. Scientific research has concluded that the body uses all three of these branched-chain amino acids for energy during exercise as well as during rest, but uses leucine most often.

When selecting your protein and amino acid supplements, make sure they supply a plentiful amount of the branched-chain amino acids, as well as the other essential and nonessential amino acids. Some products will provide a complete listing of the amino acid profile per serving. Shopping around for a protein/amino acid supplement that suits your particular needs and budget may take a while; however, when you find the product that works best with your metabolism, you will be rewarded with many beneficial health and performance effects.

*What do the letters D and L mean when they appear
before the name of an amino acid?*

Most amino acids occur in two forms, which are mirror images of each other. Chemists refer to them as isomers. The letters D and L distinguish between these mirror image forms. In general, the L form of an amino acid is more compatible with human biochemistry and is usually the only form that should be ingested. The D form should be avoided except in a few instances. For example, the D and L forms of the amino acids phenylalanine and methionine are biologically active, meaning that they can be used by the body. Finally, it's interesting to note that one common amino acid—glycine—does not have an isomer form. Thus, you will never see an L or D listed before its name.

How is adequate protein intake determined?

In addition to the molecules of carbon and hydrogen that are common to all organic molecules, amino acids contain nitrogen as part of their molecular structure. Researchers can determine if protein intake is adequate by looking at how different diet compositions of the macronutrients affect nitrogen balance in your body. (Nitrogen balance refers to the condition in which the amount of dietary nitrogen taken in is equal to the amount of nitrogen excreted.) In order to achieve a positive nitrogen balance, you must take in more nitrogen than your body excretes.

There is a home testing system, created by Robert Fritz and marketed under the name NitroStix, that measures nitrogen balance to determine if your protein intake is sufficient. Use of these diagnostic sticks can also help you determine how other factors—training intensity and duration, and carbohydrate, lipid, and calorie intake—affect your nitrogen balance. A positive nitrogen balance indicates potential growth of body tissues. A negative balance may indicate that your protein intake is inadequate and that your body is experiencing a net loss of muscle tissue.

How can you tell if a protein is high quality or low quality?

Nutritionists have developed a few techniques and rating systems that are helpful in determining the quality of a particular protein. Whether a protein can be turned into tissue for growth and development is the most basic criteria of quality. When researchers discovered that some amino acids are essential and some are non-essential, they tried applying this concept to the different dietary proteins. Hence, the earliest protein rating system rates a protein on whether or not it is complete or incomplete. A complete protein has adequate amounts of all the essential amino acids needed for normal growth and development. An incomplete protein may be deficient in one or more of the essential amino acids. An essential amino acid deficiency in the body can result in abnormal growth and development.

There are other rating systems that attempt to more accurately rate how much of a protein's amino acids are absorbed and turned into tissue and biomolecules. These include the protein efficiency ratio (PER), biological value (BV), and the protein digestibility-corrected amino acid score (PDCAAS). An important point to keep in mind with all of these protein-quality rating systems is that they are derived using animal models. This does not mean that these tests are useless, but they do not tell the whole story as far as human nutrition is concerned.

What proteins are considered high quality?

All of the protein quality-rating systems demonstrate that whey isolates and concentrates, casein, and egg-white protein are high quality. (Whey and casein are both produced from milk.) Soy protein, which used to be considered incomplete by some rating systems, has recently been reevaluated using the PDCAAS system. (Soy protein will be covered in the next question.) Casein and egg proteins are high-quality proteins with a long track record of use in foods and supplements, but whey protein supplements are among the most popular protein supplements. Whey protein has been reported to increase the production of protein and glutathione—the body's primary antioxidant enzyme. It has also been reported to enhance the immune system. Whey protein is high in the beneficial branched-chain amino acids and may stimulate the anabolic hormone, insulin, which is involved in muscle growth and maintenance.

What are the benefits of soy protein?

The consumption of soy protein products has been shown to benefit gastrointestinal health and help maintain healthy blood cholesterol and triglyceride levels. A benefit of reducing blood cholesterol levels is better circulation. This is important for general health, but also for the efficient exchange of oxygen and nutrients to exercising muscle tissue and the clearance of metabolic waste products. Other health benefits reported from soy protein intake include reduction of heart disease, reduced risk of developing certain cancers, reduced incidence of osteoporosis, and improved kidney function. For women, soy protein can help manage menopausal symptoms, as well as the symptoms of premenstrual syndrome (PMS). However, even if you include soy protein in your diet, these health benefits can only be achieved if you also maintain a diet low in saturated fats and cholesterol and high in fiber, vegetables, and fruit.

In addition to the above health benefits, research suggests that soy protein offers athletes some distinctive health benefits. For example, a research study using a special isolated soy protein called Supro was conducted in 1992 by researcher I. Dragan and coworkers. They performed a clinical study on 45 male and 21 female Romanian endurance athletes engaged in Olympic rowing events to examine the biological effects of soy protein on certain physical and biochemical characteristics. In addition to their daily diet, the athletes were given Supro at the rate of 1.5 g per 2.2 pounds of body weight per day for eight weeks. The control group did not receive any soy protein supplement. At the conclusion of the 12-week study, the athletes taking Supro every day showed an increase in their lean body mass and reduced body-fat levels. In addition, the soy protein group had more hemoglobin in their blood—meaning there was an increased ability for the blood to carry oxygen to the cells. The soy group also experienced a decrease in fatigue after training sessions. There was also a decline in the urine excretion of certain proteins that in higher levels can indicate kidney stress. Moreover, no adverse effects or side effects were noted and Supro was well tolerated. Other studies using soy protein on different groups of athletes have reported similar results.

What are good sources of high-quality protein?

Good sources of high-quality protein include whole eggs or egg whites, poultry, lean cuts of meat, fish, seafood, low-fat dairy products, high-protein nutrition supplement bars, and protein supplement drinks. Choose products that have anywhere from 15 to 35 g of protein per serving. Look for either sole source or a combination of the high-quality proteins and clinically tested soy protein isolates, such as Supro.

Another thing to remember when selecting a protein product is that it is a good idea to ingest some lipids (fats and oils) along with the protein. The reason for this is that lipids help with the digestion of amino acids. Therefore, eating pure fat-free protein like egg whites or fat-free and carbohydrate-free protein supplements may not be the most efficient way to ingest your protein sources.

Are there any particular amino acid
supplements for strength athletes?

Some studies indicate that certain growth-hormone-stimulating amino acids can benefit strength athletes. Most of these studies report that taking a dose of 1 to 3 g per day of both L-arginine and L-ornithine will stimulate higher growth hormone levels. For example, to test the benefits of these amino acids on strength athletes, a group of researchers examined the short-term effects of arginine and ornithine administration. The results of this study were reported in *The Journal of Sports Medicine and Physical Fitness.* Twenty-two adult males participated in a five-week progressive strength-training program. Half of the subjects received 1 g each of L-arginine and L-ornithine daily, and the other half received a placebo, an inert substance. The strength-training sessions lasted approximately one hour and were undertaken three times per week. At the beginning and at the end of the five-week program, each subject was measured for total strength and lean body mass. The researchers found that the group taking the amino acids produced more significant increases in total strength and lean body mass than the placebo group did.

What effect does the amino acid glutamine
have on athletic performance?

Because of its beneficial effects on athletic performance, healing, and the immune system, L-glutamine—one of the major amino acids found in the body—is among the most studied amino acids. One interesting role attributed to glutamine is its anti-catabolic effect, which protects muscle breakdown during times of exercise-induced stress. Glutamine does this by suppressing the rise in the hormone cortisol, which can contribute to breaking down muscle tissue and other body components. Therefore, glutamine plays a dual role in muscle building: in protein synthesis, and in decreasing protein breakdown in skeletal muscle.

Glutamine is also vital to immune-system function and is required for cellular replication of immune-system components. In addition, a recent article published in the *American Journal of Clinical Nutrition* reports that a study using 2 g of L-glutamine increased the levels of growth hormone in study subjects within thirty minutes and elevated the level of plasma bicarbonate, which increased the buffering capacity of the body fluids. All athletes, especially strength and power athletes, can benefit from these additional effects of L-glutamine supplements. The best recommendation at this time would be to keep glutamine intake from the free-form glutamine supplements to around 1 to 3 g per day. Higher dosages—over 3 g and sometimes 5 to 10 g per day—should be used during periods of high-intensity training that usually occur in the preseason and athletic season. There is more on glutamine in chapter 11.

What are the benefits of taking gelatin supplements?

Although gelatin is considered an incomplete protein, it does contain high amounts of two amino acids, proline and hydroxyproline, that are important to the formation, maintenance, and repair of connective tissues. There are some recent studies showing that taking hydrolyzed gelatin products, high in these two amino acids, can increase the growth and size of connective tissues. A recent study was conducted on athletes in Spain who were taking 10 g per day of a special hydrolyzed gelatin made by Protein Products, Inc., in addition to micronutrients, such as magnesium and B vitamins. The results showed an increase in connective tissue mass. This could be of significance to athletes because it is probable that athletic training, especially with weights, stimulates the skeletal muscle system to increase in size and strength more quickly than connective tissues do. This disproportionate development could lead to the muscles overpowering the very connective tissues that anchor them together. If you are prone to connective tissue injuries, or if you are recovering from one, including a hydrolyzed gelatin supplement in your sports-nutrition program can have beneficial effects.

Are there any amino acids that can help
with injury repair and pain relief?

The amino acid phenylalanine is an essential amino acid that has many functions in the body. For example, phenylalanine is a precursor, or starting material, of several important metabolites such as the skin pigment melanin and several catecholamine neurotransmitters, including epinephrine and norepinephrine. Catecholamine neurotransmitters are important in memory, learning, locomotion, sex drive, tissue growth and repair, immune system function, and appetite control. Supplements containing both the D- and L-phenylalanine forms have been used successfully to help control pain. This could be of interest to athletes who suffer from acute or chronic pain from injuries. The dosage of phenylalanine that has been shown to be effective for pain management ranges from 500 to 1,500 mg per day.

Scientists believe that DL phenylalanine can help protect endorphins—the body's pain-control substances—from destruction, thereby allowing them to distribute pain relief for longer periods. These naturally occurring endorphins are a thousand times more powerful than morphine, a potent analgesic. This means that a very small amount of endorphins can go a long way in pain control. A word of caution: When taking DL phenylalanine or any isolated or individual amino acid formula, it is best not to take very large doses (over 6 g), especially if you are undergoing weight loss, training strenuously, or using phenylalanine for injury recovery. In these instances, you should use amino acids only under the supervision of a medical doctor. An additional word of caution: People with a condition known as phenylketonuria (PKU) should not take any supplements containing DL phenylalanine because they have problems metabolizing this amino acid. Refer to chapter 12 for more information on natural pain control and healing methods.

CARBOHYDRATES

The second macronutrient group is carbohydrates, which are a major source of fuel for athletically fit people and an essential part of the diet for everyone. Recent research has shown that the different varieties of carbohydrates—depending on when they are ingested—can either enhance or hinder performance. Knowing which carbohydrates work best can mean the difference between winning and los-ing. This chapter will help you determine how to use carbohydrates to enhance your performance.

What types of carbohydrates should you include in your diet?

The primary carbohydrates to include in your diet are the complex carbohy-drates—starches and fiber. Starchy complex carbohydrates are chains of glucose (sugar) that are freed up during digestion to be used for energy. Fibrous complex carbohydrates are not digested well by humans, but provide necesary bulk and have other beneficial characteristics, making them quite important to health. Stick with food sources that are wholesome and unprocessed, such as whole-grain rice, whole-grain flour pastas, whole-grain breads, and potatoes. These foods will pro-vide you with fiber, which is important for proper digestion, and will keep the complex carbohydrates from digesting too rapidly. Note, however, that just because a carbohydrate source is complex doesn't mean that it won't cause a rapid rise in your blood-sugar levels. On the other hand, just because a carbohydrate source like glucose or fructose is simple doesn't mean that it won't produce a lesser rise in blood-sugar levels.

How can you tell how a carbohydrate will act in your body?

To determine the effect a certain carbohydrate will have on the body, nutritionists have developed the glycemic index. This is a method for determining the response of blood-sugar levels to various carbohydrate-rich foods. As a general rule of eating, foods with lower glycemic index values can help you maintain a more stable blood-sugar level. In addition, these foods help prevent the overproduction of the hor-mone insulin, which is often associated with a rapid decrease in blood-sugar levels followed by a feeling of physical or mental fatigue. The glycemic index rating sys-tem is important for athletes for two main reasons. First, it indicates the metabolic consequences that different foods can have on the body. And second, it helps to de-termine which foods should be consumed in relation to exercise sessions.

The table on page 181 lists some common foods and their glycemic index values.

GLYCEMIC INDEXES OF SELECTED COMMON FOODS

GLYCEMIC INDEX	FOOD
Rapid Inducers of Insulin Secretion	
100 percent	Glucose
80–90 percent	Corn flakes, carrots*, parsnips*, potatoes (instant mashed), maltose, honey
70–79 percent	Bread (whole-grain), millet, rice (white), Weetabix cereal, broad beans (fresh)*, potatoes (new), rutabaga*
Moderate Inducers of Insulin Secretion	
60–69 percent	Bread (white), rice (brown), muesli, Shredded Wheat cereal, Ryvita crispbreads, water biscuits, beetroot*, bananas, raisins, Mars Bars
50–59 percent	Buckwheat, spaghetti (bleached), sweet corn, All Bran cereal, digestive biscuits, oatmeal biscuits, Rich Tea biscuits, peas (frozen), yams, sucrose, potato chips
40–49 percent	Spaghetti (whole-wheat), oatmeal, potatoes (sweet), beans (canned navy), peas (dried), oranges, orange juice
Slow Inducers of Insulin Secretion	
30–39 percent	Butter beans, haricot beans, black-eyed peas, chickpeas, apples (Golden Delicious), ice cream, milk (skim), milk (whole), yogurt, tomato soup
20–29 percent	Kidney beans, lentils, fructose
10–19 percent	Soybeans, soybeans (canned), peanuts

* This food item was tested in portions containing 25 grams of carbohydrates.

The above table is reprinted with permission from Diabetes Care, Vol. 5, 1982 Copyright 1982 by the American Diabetes Association, Inc.

When should you eat carbohydrate-rich foods?

Much of the research on how carbohydrates affect athletic performance has been conducted on athletes during endurance events, such as marathon running and long-distance cycling. What these studies have found is that it is important to maintain your body's glycogen (stored glucose) levels. This can be accomplished by taking in plentiful amounts of carbohydrates throughout the day, ranging anywhere from 55 to 60 percent of your total daily calories.

It's best to consume a high-carbohydrate, moderate-protein, low-fat meal two to three hours prior to your training session to fuel your energy system. Including complex carbohydrates in your meal tends to help your body load up with a good

---

EATING BEFORE, DURING, AND AFTER EXERCISE

You've probably heard of runners and cyclists who consume huge plates of pasta the night before a big race. Is there any benefit to this carbo-loading? In a word, yes (especially for marathon events), but depending on your workout, you may need carbs before, during, and after you exercise. We now have a vast array of carbohydrate beverages available that are much more efficient than heaping plates of noodles. We recommend eating two to three hours before your event. Your meal should be low in fat (1 to 10 percent), moderate in protein (10 to 20 percent), and high in carbohydrates (70 to 90 percent).

If you find that drinking a carbohydrate beverage before or during training gives you an upset stomach, then make sure you take in extra carbohydrates during your pretraining meal and directly after training. Keep well hydrated during your practice sessions by drinking water instead of a carbohydrate drink.

If you are involved in sports like sprinting, wrestling, high jump, and martial arts, which require short bursts of explosive energy, you should get in the habit of drinking a carbohydrate sports drink during practice, since your energy stores will become depleted quickly. When this happens, fatigue sets in and athletic performance will suffer. Some athletes refer to this as "bonking," meaning your body simply runs out of gas.

Make sure that your body's carbohydrate supply is replenished the day before, along with a

> ## EATING BEFORE, DURING, AND AFTER EXERCISE *(continued)*
>
> high-carbohydrate pregame meal. However, your performance in longer-duration sports (generally more than an hour long) will benefit from carbohydrate ingestion before and during the events. During practice it is important to maintain carbohydrate beverage intake to maintain glycogen stores, as most training sessions last more than two hours.
>
> Experiment with different brands of drinks and different caloric amounts to discover which one is best for your digestion. Generally, carbohydrate solutions of pure glucose (about 50 calories per eight ounces) are the easiest to digest. As the amounts of carbohydrates, electrolytes, and other nutrients increase in the solution, the rate at which your stomach empties may slow down, and you may feel bloated. Again, it may take some experimentation on your part to discover which product works best for your system. Don't wait until right before a competition to figure out what pregame meal/drink works best for you. Start testing now.
>
> Some carbohydrate ready-to-drink sports beverages we like are American Body Building's Carbo Force and Turbo Tea. For post training/recovery drinks, try American Body Building's Pure Pro Protein Formula, Pure Pro Shake, Lean Protein, Mass Recovery, White Lightning, Kick Some Mass, Blue Thunder, Extreme XXL and Super Shake, Weider Sports Meal drinks and nutrition bars, and American Body Building's Extreme Body Nutrition Bars.

supply of glucose and recharge your body's glycogen system. This is recommended for precompetition meals, too. More important, foods high in complex carbohydrates do not usually cause a rapid rise in insulin levels, which is preferred for optimum physical performance. If insulin levels are too high during exercise, they will conflict with the hormone glucagon, which rises during exercise to release energy from your tissues.

Should you refuel with carbs after a workout? That depends on your sport. In the world of bodybuilding and powerlifting, athletes want to maintain muscle mass, and therefore they time meals around the growth hormone surges and potential insulin surges that occur right after high-intensity workouts. Eating a meal containing high-glycemic-index carbohydrates approximately half an hour to an hour after a workout helps the body to restore its glycogen more quickly.

If you are primarily involved in long-distance aerobic workouts, you should eat a meal plentiful in low-glycemic-index carbohydrates about an hour to an hour and a half after major events and practice to replenish your glycogen stores. You should also try to eat properly throughout the day and drink a carbohydrate beverage during and after exercise sessions, especially if your activity lasts more than an hour. If you don't follow this rule, your hard practice may actually cause you to deplete glycogen levels, overtrain, and not perform your best at competition time.

Is it a good idea to drink carbohydrate beverages before a workout or competition?

Sports nutrition research has determined that in endurance sports and training sessions that are going to be an hour or more in duration, ingestion of a high-glycemic-index beverage just before exercise will allow carbohydrates into the bloodstream quickly, providing exercising muscles with a readily available supply of energy. Once you start to exercise, your muscles display what is called an insulin-independent uptake of nutrients. This means that exercising muscles can use glucose directly from the bloodstream, independent of insulin. This is important because during exercise, if there is a high amount of insulin released, it can cause the body to try to store glucose. This process conflicts with the function of glucagon, which rises during exercise to release glucose from the glycogen stores of the muscles to be used as energy. Thus, if your pre-exercise eating is not right, high blood levels of insulin may result. In competitive athletes, high blood levels of insulin have been shown to cause reduced athletic performance. Therefore, when consuming a carbohydrate beverage prior to training or an event, start drinking it about fifteen minutes beforehand, so that your exercising muscles will offset the need for insulin increases.

What happens to the glucose that your body doesn't use right away for energy?

Glucose that is not immediately used for energy is converted into a storage molecule called glycogen. Excess glucose can also be stored as fat and serves as a building block for other compounds and tissue formation. Glucose is also used by the body to make glucosamine, which is needed for the synthesis of connective tissues. (Note, however, that excess glucose consumption does not result in extra connective-tissue formation.) Glucose, which can be used by all of the body's cells, is taken up at a much higher rate by muscle cells and will therefore be used very quickly to meet the energy demands of exercising muscle. Fructose, a simple sugar, on the other hand, has a higher affinity to replenish liver glycogen and does not replenish muscle glycogen as well as glucose does. Giving athletes glucose drinks, fructose drinks, placebo drinks, or complex carbohydrate drinks during exercise has shown that glucose has a significant performance-enhancing effect during oxidative sports. Furthermore, ingested glucose has a greater muscle-glycogen-sparing effect (which means there is more muscle energy to exercise or compete longer) than fructose does. This is because the enzymes necessary to metabolize fructose and glucose in the muscles favor glucose.

How can you keep your glycogen supplies
well replenished for peak performance?

A dietary technique called carbohydrate loading—also called carbohydrate super-compensation—can super-load your muscle glycogen stores. Researchers found that this could be accomplished in a few ways. Using the traditional technique, carbohydrate consumption is reduced for a few days, which actually depletes glycogen stores. Timing is important; this glycogen-depletion phase should be done five to six days before an important event. A two- to three-day glycogen-depletion phase would include reducing carbohydrate levels to about 10 percent of your total daily calories. Obviously, during that period, exercise performance will be impaired. This period of glycogen depletion is then followed by a high-carbohydrate diet—up to 90 percent carbohydrates—for three days to build up glycogen levels to much higher levels than would normally be attained. However, many athletes find it difficult to follow this six-day traditional method of glycogen depletion and don't wish to experience reduced performance during the glycogen-depletion phase. To compensate for this, researchers have come up with other ways to effectively deplete and load the glycogen system by modifying the diet less drastically than the traditional method.

One of these modified methods of glycogen loading recommends keeping training levels high, while maintaining a macronutrient intake over five or six meals at approximately 15 percent fat, 30 percent protein, and 55 percent carbohydrates for four days. After four days of this phase, two days before your competition, begin glycogen loading by ingesting a plentiful amount of carbohydrates. The diet you should follow during this phase should provide 15 percent fat, 15 percent protein, and 70 percent carbohydrates. Stress the intake of carbohydrates that have low to medium glycemic indexes up to a rating of 49 percent, and restrict the intake of high-glycemic-index carbohydrate beverages to immediately before, during, and after exercise.

Are there any side effects to carbohydrate loading?

Some athletes may experience some minor side effects from carbohydrate loading. These include muscle stiffness, which may result in muscle cramping and premature fatigue. During the depletion phase of the traditional carbohydrate-loading technique, some individuals experience fatigue and dizziness. Therefore, you should not perform any exercise that can result in injury during traditional glycogen depletion.

Athletes interested in using carbohydrate loading should do so a month before a major event to see how their body responds to it. It is interesting to note that every gram of glycogen in the body is stored with about 4 g of water. This explains the mystery behind many of the fast weight-loss diets, which are low in calories and low in carbohydrates. Individuals will lose several pounds of water weight as they deplete their glycogen system. Note that it is important to pay extra attention to being properly hydrated when using carbohydrate loading. Finally, scientists have determined that the body becomes nonresponsive if you try to carbohydrate load too many times during the season. Restrict it to three or four or maybe up to five times during any particular athletic season. This means you should use carbohydrate loading strategically to boost your endurance performance for special competitions.

Are there dietary supplements that help
with carbohydrate loading?

Taking extra amounts of vitamins B_3 and B_6 a couple of days before you begin the glycogen-depletion phase, and then on the first day of the glycogen-depletion phase, can help stimulate the rate at which glycogen is depleted from your body. Then, during the glycogen-loading phase, take in extra chromium (up to 600 mcg a day) and double your normal amounts of vitamin C and beta-carotene to help increase the rate at with the muscles store glycogen. Utilizing carbohydrate sports drinks can help maximize your body's glycogen content. Choose drinks that contain only glucose for use before, during, and after exercise for best results. In addition, there is some indication that ingestion of 1 to 3 g per day of the amino acid L-glutamine can help with the glycogen-loading phase. It's also important to ingest a complex carbohydrate food or beverage that contains approximately 400 to 600 calories per serving in the morning and an hour before bedtime to prevent muscle glycogen depletion. It can also contain protein, but should be low in fat content. Keep in mind that carbohydrate loading is no panacea or magic bullet. However, as part of a total sports-nutrition program, it can help give you a competitive edge.

LIPIDS (FATS AND OILS)

The third major macronutrient group is lipids (fats and oils). Lipids have many vital body functions and are an essential part of every cell. In the diet, lipids are found with important essential fat-soluble vitamins, such as vitamins A, D, E, and K. They are also a source of essential fatty acids (EFAs), such as linoleic acid and alpha-linolenic acid, which have both a structural role and various metabolic roles in the body, including the production of neurotransmitters and steroid hormones. Lipids also make foods taste better—one of the characteristics that often leads to their overconsumption. New research on athletes has shown that in addition to maintaining the proper daily intake of lipids for health, there are certain lipid supplements that can help boost performance.

What is the difference between fats and lipids?

Lipids is the scientific term used to describe a diverse group of biomolecules that vary considerably in composition and structure; contain carbon, hydrogen, and oxygen; and are insoluble in water. Fats and oils are therefore subcategories of lipids. Fats are solid at room temperature, and oils are liquid at room temperature. Fats and oils consist mainly of triglyceride molecules. Other lipids include cholesterol and phospholipids.

What are the main functions of lipids in the body?

> Lipids provide the body with fuel, aid in the absorption of fat-soluble vitamins, act as energy storehouses within cells, and supply the essential fatty acids important to growth, development, and health maintenance. In addition, lipids provide protective padding for body structures and organs, supply building blocks for other molecules, serve as building blocks for all cell membranes and other cell structures, and provide the body with insulation from cold.

What are essential fatty acids?

> The two primary essential fatty acids are linoleic acid and alpha-linolenic acid. These two fatty acids cannot be made in any significant amount by the body; therefore, it is essential that they are taken in on a daily basis from the diet. Under certain circumstances, a third fatty acid called arachadonic acid, which the body makes from linoleic acid, becomes essential if dietary intake of linoleic acid is deficient. Linoleic acid and alpha-linolenic acid are both unsaturated fatty acids that are 18 carbon atoms long. In addition to their structural roles in the body and their roles as precursors of important biomolecules and hormones, these two fatty acids are also used for energy.

How do eicosapentaenoic acid (EPA) and
docosahexaenoic acid (DHA) fit into the lipid picture?

> These two fatty acids were plunged into the media limelight in the 1980s when scientists examining the traditional diet of Eskimos in Greenland—high in fats and animal proteins—discovered that these people experienced a very low rate of cardiovascular diseases. Researchers discovered on further examination that one of the health-contributing factors was the cholesterol-lowering effect of EPA and DHA—also referred to as omega-3 fatty acids. There are studies documenting the improvement of athletic performance using anywhere from 2,000 mg to 4,000 mg per day of EPA and DHA from eating fish and taking EPA/DHA dietary supplements. Researchers have observed improvements in strength and aerobic performance as well. On the athletes tested, these improvements included increased strength in the bench press, faster running times, reduced muscular inflamma-

tion, and greater jumping distances. Scientists speculate that these effects are due to the beneficial functions of EPA and DHA. These functions include growth hormone production, anti-inflammatory action, enhanced oxygen metabolism, and lowered blood viscosity (blood-thinning effects). The latter leads to better oxygen and nutrient delivery to the muscles and improved recovery after rigorous bouts of exercise and training. In addition to getting EPA and DHA through supplements, these fatty acids are found in high amounts in cold-water fish, such as cod, salmon, sardines, trout, and mackerel, and in lower amounts in tuna fish—an economical source of low-fat protein.

What other lipids have beneficial effects on athletes?

Recently, attention has turned to a special phosphate lipid called phosphatidylserine (PS). PS is derived from the lipid lecithin. Lucas Meyer, Inc., a manufacturer of phosphatidylserine, has performed many clinical studies on the biological effects of PS. The original research focused on PS's ability to improve memory, concentration, and learning. More recently, researchers have found that PS can protect the body from tissue breakdown caused by the catabolic hormone cortisol, which is produced by the body during exercise and periods of mental stress and plays a role in molecular breakdown. A recent study conducted on athletes who were using PS discovered that there was a reduction of muscle soreness and an improvement in tissue buildup and muscle formation. Moreover, an overall sense of well-being was observed by the athletes taking PS. Therefore, PS may give you the mental edge that is important to any athlete who is undergoing the rigors of intensive training.

Researchers believe that the group of athletes taking PS probably experienced less muscle soreness because the amount of cortisol in the body was reduced, which in turn reduced the amount of muscle breakdown and tissue damage.

How can I maintain a dietary intake of healthy lipids without overdoing it?

For starters, avoid adding fats to your foods. This is one of the biggest sources of fat in the diet. Added dietary fats include oils and butter used in cooking and high-fat dips and spreads. Also, stay on the lookout for high-fat foods, such as baked goods, breads, and cream cheese. Additionally, it is wise to keep your total fat intake to below 30 percent of your total daily calories, or as low as 15 percent depending upon your specific sport requirements. You should minimize your intake of saturated fatty acids and cholesterol, which occur mostly in animal products. You should also include a high-quality supplement in your nutrition program that contains the essential fatty acids—especially in the preseason and during your athletic season. Trimming visible fats from beef and pork and removing the skin from poultry are good nutritional habits.

Another guiding rule is never to overeat at any particular meal. Every time you overeat, the excess calories are stored as body fat. It is always a sound practice to avoid having excess fat on your body. This only creates dead weight that will slow you down and impair your performance. As you develop your sport nutrition skills and focus on the proper protein and carbohydrate intake, the fat-management part of your diet will automatically fall into place. Don't reprimand yourself if you occasionally have the urge to spread some mayonnaise on a sandwich or to use high-fat salad dressing, just as long as it doesn't become the norm. And always remember that it is extremely important not to lose control of your eating habits around an important competition.

MICRONUTRIENTS

The main micronutrients include vitamins, minerals, and vitaminlike nutrients. There are bout 26 that have been identified as essential for human health, and more will probably be identified in the future. Micronutrients are involved in every biochemical process. For example, it was recently determined that the trace mineral chromium is an essential cofactor for insulin functioning. This is important because when you eat, nutrients pour into your bloodstream and need the proper stimulus to let them into the cells. As it turns out, insulin is the hormone that performs this function. Think of insulin as being the hand that opens the door to let in food. However, insulin needs a key to open the door, which is chromium. This means that if chromium levels are low, insulin cannot work efficiently and the nutrients circulating in your bloodstream, notably glucose and amino acids, may not be used efficiently and may in fact end up being converted to fat. This example of chromium is only one of many important micronutrients that can be provided by supplements. See chapter 11 for the Nutritional Supplement Review.

THE ROLE OF ESSENTIAL NUTRIENTS		
Nutrient	**Major Function(s)**	**Food Sources**
Protein	Builds and repairs tissues. Contains amino acids, vital to many body structures and functions.	Egg whites, eggs, lean meats, such as chicken, fish, turkey, and lean cuts of beef and lamb.
Carbohydrates	Provide energy.	Whole grains, pasta, rice, bread, cereal, beans, and potatoes.
Unsaturated Fat	Part of every cell membrane, used in making important biochemicals, carries fat-soluble vitamins, important source of energy.	Plant oils, such as flaxseed oil, borage oil, hemp oil, peanut oil, soy oil, walnut oil, olive oil, corn oil, and fish oils.
Essential micro-nutrients (vitamins and minerals)	Regulate body functions, make up body structures.	All whole foods.
Water	Vital to health and peak performance.	Pure water, other beverages, foods with high water content such as fruits and vegetables.

WHOLE FOOD VERSUS SUPPLEMENTS

While whole foods provide a diversity of both micronutrients and macronutrients, research has shown that food alone is not a reliable source of fixed amounts of micronutrients. Quantity varies greatly. Additionally, micronutrients are commonly destroyed in the cooking process, and their bioavailability is unpredictable.

In addition to supplying you with a pure, high-quality nutrient source, supplements are specially blended to have the exact amounts of nutrients in each tablet. Daily supplementation is a guaranteed way of optimal nutrition. Sports supplements are often good sources of both macro- and micronutrients. Other substances found in sports supplements include metabolites (products of metabolism, such as creatine, carnitine, and CoQ_{10}) and semiessential nutrients, such as bioflavonoids (plant compounds with antioxidant and other health-promoting properties).

What sports supplements should you consider taking?

From the start, you should keep in mind that the foods and supplements you need will be dictated by the physical activity you are undertaking. In general, however, your sports supplements should include a good multi-vitamin and -mineral formula that contains all of the antioxidants, such as vitamin C, beta-carotene, and bioflavonoids. And because many studies show that a large percentage of athletes do not take in adequate amounts of dietary protein, a protein supplement is also recommended. Carbohydrate drinks have been shown to act as potent performance beverages and are particularly useful directly before, during, and after exercise. You'll also benefit by including an essential fatty-acid supplement in your regimen. Each of these supplements will be discussed individually in chapter 11.

FORGET ABOUT THREE SQUARE MEALS A DAY

We have found that it is much better to spread your food intake over five to seven meals per day, including snacks, than it is to lump your meals into three sittings per day. The reason is very simple. Depending on your body size, activity level, and metabolism, your body can only use a fixed number of calories per meal. If you eat too much at any one meal, the excess calories usually end up getting converted to fat and the valuable proteins and other nutrients are wasted.

YOU ARE WHAT YOU EAT

This old adage is more appropriate today than ever. A diet high in fat makes you fat. Studies show that when people eat the same amount of calories per day, but one group eats a diet high in fat and the other eats a diet low in fat, the people on the low-fat diet tend not to gain weight. Furthermore, depending on the amount of calories eaten, they can lose weight faster. There are other benefits of eating a low-fat diet—namely, you can eat more. Fat contains more than twice the calories as protein or carbohydrates per unit weight:

Fat	9 calories per gram
Protein	4 calories per gram
Carbohydrate	4 calories per gram

This means that for every ounce of fat you reduce in your diet, you can replace this with twice the amount of protein or carbohydrates. Also, note that alcohol has about seven calories per gram.

We all need some fat in our diet, but the type of fat you eat makes a huge difference. Fats contain fatty acids, which are part of every cell in your body. This means that the types of fat you consume determine what your body is composed of. Eating too much fat, especially saturated fatty acids, has negative effects on health. When eaten in moderation, unsaturated fatty acids are a healthier form of fat because they contain certain essential fatty acids your body needs to survive. These essential fatty acids are used to make cells and compounds in your body, and are less likely to become stored as excess body fat. Eating these healthy fats and reducing your consumption of unhealthy saturated fats will also result in a better-functioning circulatory system, which translates into better blood flow and improved performance.

These are very important nutrition considerations if you want to increase strength and muscle mass. Resistance training exercise tends to burn calories from stored muscle carbohydrates and does not burn much body fat. This means that while you may be burning 600 or more calories per workout, you're not burning many fat calories. That's why it's so important to keep fat intake low. The lower your fat intake, the less you'll store.

HOW MANY CALORIES DO I NEED, AND IN WHAT PROPORTIONS?

It is now well established that athletic people need to consume more calories and protein than nonathletic people. To help guide your efforts for determining optimal protein intake, follow the table on page 196. Because this table recognizes that people of different sizes need different amounts of protein, it is more useful than food labels, which provide one fixed number for the entire adult population. Note that the protein estimates are based on your lean body mass. It is your lean body mass that utilizes most of the protein, not your body fat stores. Looking at protein intake on a lean body mass basis also makes this table suitable for men and women. The government's standardized calorie and nutrient intake guidelines for men and women are only different in that they take into account women being smaller on average, and having more body fat on average than men. When this data is examined from a lean body mass—pound for pound muscle basis—the differences become less significant.

Another feature you will find in the table is the activity factors columns. As an individual becomes more active, his or her protein intake increases, as well as total caloric and nutrient intake. Also note that regardless of sport, heavy weight training increases protein intake the most. This has to do with your lessons learned in the earlier chapter on muscle fibers. Strength athletes have more muscle mass that is composed of the type II fast-twitch muscle fibers, which tend to break down more than type I slow-twitch muscle fibers. More protein is therefore required to help rebuild and maintain the larger, fragile type II fast-twitch muscle fibers. This table will suit most individuals. As you become more sophisticated in your sports-nutrition skills, a detailed nutrition analysis by a trained health professional is recommended to confirm your exact needs. The Dynatrition Sport-Specific Plans in chapter 8 have this variable protein requirement built in. The generalized nutrition plan which follows in this chapter is based on a 60 percent carbohydrate, 20 percent protein, and 20 percent fat macronutrient composition, which is a good basic nutrition plan for athletes and fitness enthusiasts to get started with and follow most of the year, and fine tune as indicated in chapter 8, during the competition season based on your sport. In clinical studies the 60-20-20 plan has also been shown to reverse cardiovascular disease. So, it is a great performance-enhancing diet, as well as a health-promoting and healing diet.

ESTIMATING YOUR DAILY PROTEIN REQUIREMENT

Too often, athletes eat either too much or too little protein. The following method was developed by Dr. Hatfield as an easy way to estimate your daily protein requirement. It will help you determine approximately how much protein you should consume from food and supplement sources on a daily basis.

Your estimated protein requirement is determined using your lean body mass and activity factor. Your lean body mass is all of your body's bones, muscles, organs, blood, and water—all of your bodily tissues apart from your body fat. Your activity factor is the average intensity of a normal day's activities. If you are more active on a particular day, or during your athletic season, you will need to up your protein intake to meet your increased requirement. If you are less active, you should lower it, since your demand is reduced.

To estimate your daily protein requirement:

1. Calculate your lean body mass (in pounds).

2. Determine your activity factor using the Activity Factors Table below.

3. Determine your daily protein requirement (in grams) using the Daily Protein Requirement Table on page 196. First, find the lean body mass closest to your own from step 1 in the Lean Body Mass column. Then, read across the row until you find your activity factor from step 2. The answer is the grams of protein you should consume from food and supplement sources on an average day. For example, if your lean body mass is 173 pounds and you train with heavy weights every day, you would find the 170-pound row and read across to the .9 column. Your daily protein requirement would be 153 grams.

ACTIVITY FACTORS TABLE	
Activity Factor	**General Daily Activity**
.5	Sedentary; no sports participation or fitness exercising.
.6	Jogging or light fitness exercising.
.7	Sports participation or moderate fitness exercising three times a week.
.8	Moderate weight training or aerobic training daily.
.9	Heavy weight training daily.
1.0	Heavy weight training plus sports training daily ("two-a-day" training).

Reprinted from *Dynamic Nutrition for Maximum Performance*. Avery, 1997.

DAILY PROTEIN REQUIREMENT TABLE

Lean Body Mass in Pounds	Activity Factor (Columns represent Daily Protein Requirements in Grams)					
	.5	.6	.7	.8	.9	1.0
90	45	54	63	72	81	90
100	50	60	70	80	90	100
110	55	66	77	88	99	110
120	60	72	84	96	108	120
130	65	78	91	104	117	130
140	70	84	98	112	126	140
150	75	90	105	120	135	150
160	80	96	112	128	144	160
170	85	102	119	136	153	170
180	90	108	126	144	162	180
190	95	114	133	152	171	190
200	100	120	140	160	180	200
210	105	126	147	168	189	210
220	110	132	154	176	198	220
230	115	138	161	184	207	230
240	120	144	168	192	216	240

KEEPING FATS LOW

If you really want results, you must keep calories from fat at or below 20 percent of your total daily intake. A good rule of thumb is to avoid food that has more than 2 grams of fat per 100 calories. Because most protein sources contain more than 20 percent fat calories, you will need to make an extra effort to watch the fat content of the other foods you eat.

TOTAL DAILY CALORIE REQUIREMENTS

Scientists have developed a number of ways to estimate total caloric energy needs—perhaps too many. For our purposes here, we will present some general guidelines, and examples of nutrition plans that provide 2,600 to 3,400 calories per day. People on weight-loss diets can refer to chapter 9 for guidelines on body-fat reduction.

To determine your total daily caloric needs, it is first important to eat a healthy diet with adequate macronutrients and micronutrients. This means eating no excess fat, getting the right amount of protein, eating high quality, complex carbohydrate foods, fruits, and vegetables, taking your supplements, and drinking plenty of pure water. In terms of estimating how many calories you need to meet the demands of your activity level, the requirement for most nonathletic adults is 1,800 to 3,000 calories per day. As your activity level increases, so does your need for more calories. Depending on your size and daily activity level, your caloric intake needs may be quite varied. On a lazy day, you may only need 2,600 calories or less. For active days you may require 3,400 calories or more. Some long-distance endurance athletes require more than 6,000 calories per day. But the general range of daily caloric intake for the majority of men and women will be between 2,600 and 3,400 calories per day.

Two nutrition plans are included here to give menu examples that supply about 2,600 calories and 3,400 calories per day. Active people of normal body composition weighing less than 160 pounds should start with the 2,600-calorie-per-day eating plan. Active people over 160 pounds can use the 3,400-calorie-per-day plan. See how your body responds. If your weight and body fat start to increase, then cut back 10 percent on the total daily calories. If your weight starts to decrease too much, then increase your total daily caloric intake by 10 percent (unless weight loss is your goal). It will take a few weeks to fine-tune your performance-fitness eating plan, so be patient and allow for some experimentation. Balancing your food intake to meet your caloric needs is a daily task. Keeping track of your body weight and body composition will help you to perfect your performance-fitness and weight-maintenance sports-nutrition plan.

USING THE DYNATRITION FOOD CHOICE GUIDE

If you're confused about making healthy food selections when you shop or eat away from home, you're certainly not alone. Most people get confused with all the choices available, and deceptive food labels don't make it any easier. To assist you, we provide some serving suggestions and meal plans that fit within the Dynatrition guidelines.

The serving suggestion chart that follows includes each food group and a range of caloric intake from 2,600 to 3,400 calories per day. Aim to eat a variety of servings from each food group. You'll notice that the chart offers a range in the number of servings (11 to 14 servings of carbs, for example). Aim to eat a variety of servings from each food group. The lower number of suggested servings is for a diet of approximately 2,600 calories per day. The higher number of servings will provide about 3,400 calories per day. These diets are designed to provide a total daily calorie intake consisting of the following macronutrient percentages: 20 percent protein, 60 percent carbohydrates, and 20 percent fat, which will suit the needs of most fitness exercisers and athletes in their off season training. If you are a competitive athlete, chapter 8 provides specific nutrition guidelines based on your particular sport activity, to further fine-tune your diet during the competition season. The table starting on page 199 contains a shopping list that will help you choose healthy and performance-enhancing foods and supplements.

Many people who weight train make the mistake of significantly increasing their daily calorie intakes and end up gaining a lot of body fat. Remember to balance your food intake with activity. The Dynatrition guidelines will steer you away from high-fat foods. Remember to spread out food intake over a combination of three or four meals per day, and one to three snacks, eating about every three to four hours. Grazing like this maintains a constant flow of nutrients to your muscles, spreads the caloric intake out over several meals, and prevents conversion of food to body fat. It may take you a week or two to fine-tune your food intake. Take a look at the examples of daily menus for 2,600- and 3,400-calorie-per-day nutrition programs to get some ideas.

Keep these general guidelines in mind:

Minimize consumption of saturated fats and sweets.

Avoid consumption of alcoholic beverages.

Minimize salt intake.

DYNATRITION FOOD AND SUPPLEMENT SHOPPING LIST

Photocopy this list and use it regularly to help choose nutrient-rich, healthy foods. Add some of your favorite healthy foods to this list.

FRUIT

Apples	Nectarines	Tangerines	Pineapples
Bananas	Peaches	Persimmon	Figs
Cantaloupe	Oranges	Mango	_____
Pears	Grapefruit	Honeydew melon	_____
Plums	Guava	Star Fruit	_____
Grapes	Watermelon	Blueberries	_____
Kiwi	Blackberries	Cherries	_____
Apricots	Raspberries	Limes	_____

VEGETABLES

Asparagus	Eggplant	Cucumbers	Endive
Artichokes	Peas	Onions	Avocados
Broccoli	Green beans	Green onions	Beets
Cauliflower	Lettuce	Potatoes	Radishes
Red peppers	Cabbage	Sweet potatoes	_____
Green peppers	Collard greens	Zucchini and other	_____
Brussels sprouts	Salad mix	squash	_____
Carrots	Spinach	Garlic	_____
Celery	Tomatoes	Swiss chard	_____
Corn	Mushrooms	Snow peas	_____

BEANS

Pinto beans	Navy beans	White beans	_____
Soybeans	Fava beans	Lima beans	_____
Lentils	Green beans	Mung beans	_____
Black-eyed peas	Kidney beans	_____	_____

BREADS

Bagels
English muffins
Pizza crust
Rolls
Sourdough bread

Tortillas (low-fat)   _____
Whole-wheat bread   _____
Whole-wheat pita   _____
Whole-grain breads   _____
_____   _____

RICE

Brown rice   _____
Wild rice   _____

_____   _____
_____   _____

DAIRY PRODUCTS/EGGS
(choose low-fat or nonfat only)

Cheese   Egg substitute   Sour cream   _____
Cottage cheese   Egg whites   Tofu   _____
Ricotta cheese   Light margarine   Yogurt   _____
Eggs*   Milk   _____   _____

*Eggs aren't low-fat, but you can use whites only for nonfat protein. For healthy, active people, whole eggs are permitted.

MEAT/POULTRY/FISH

Chicken breast   Fresh fish, such as: pollock   Venison
Precooked chicken   bass   red snapper   Canadian-style bacon
   strips   catfish   roughy, orange   Leg of lamb
Beef pot roast   cod   salmon   Lean whole cut deli
Round steak   flounder   shark   meats
Sirloin steak   grouper   snapper
Pork tenderloin   haddock   sole   _____
Lean ground beef   halibut   trout   _____
Lean ground turkey   mackerel   tuna   _____
Turkey-breast fillets   perch   Scallops   _____
                                                                      _____

CEREALS
(choose any variety with at least 3 grams of fiber per serving and minimum sugar content)

Cheerios	Quaker Shredded	General Mills Fiber	Kellogg's All-Bran
Oatmeal	Wheat	One	Extra Fiber
Post Shredded	Quaker Oat Bran	Shredded	Other whole-grain
Wheat'n Bran	Kellogg's Raisin	wheat	cereals
Raisin bran	Bran	Wheat Chex	_____

CANNED FOODS

Tuna	Green beans	Broth	Tomato sauce
Salmon	Peas	Pineapple	_____
Black beans	Spinach	Peaches	_____
Kidney beans	Tomatoes	Pears	_____
Lima beans	Soup (low-fat,	Applesauce	_____
Garbanzo beans	low sodium)	(unsweetened)	_____

FROZEN FOODS

Strawberries	Fruit juice bars	Other vegetables	Healthy frozen
Blueberries	Asparagus	Cooked frozen	dinners
Peaches	Broccoli	shrimp	_____
Orange juice	Soybeans	Packaged meals	_____

CONDIMENTS

Honey	Mustard	_____
Horseradish	Nonfat mayonnaise	_____
Low-fat salad	Salsa	_____
dressings	Vinegars	_____

PASTA AND SAUCE

Spaghetti	Noodles	High-protein pastas	_____
Macaroni	Whole-grain pastas	Nonfat pasta sauce	_____

SNACKS AND STAPLES

Peanut butter	Cajun spices	Raisins/dried fruit	Sherbet
Almonds	Mexican spices	Flaxseeds	Nuts
Walnuts	Spices and	Pretzels	_____
Flour	flavorings	Low-fat chips	_____
Bulgur	Vanilla flavoring	Popcorn	_____
Couscous	Canola oil	Rice cakes	_____
Wheat germ	Olive oil	Whole-wheat	_____
Garlic powder	Cooking spray	crackers	_____

BEVERAGES

Bottled water	grapefruit	Black tea	_____
(primary beverage)	Tomato juice	Green tea (with every	_____
100% fruit juices:	Diet soda	meal)	_____
orange	(occasional)	_____	_____
apple	Coffee	_____	_____

SUPPLEMENTS

Weider Sports Nutri-	Creatine	Super Mega Mass	Phencal
tion Products	Soy products	Creatine ATP	Ultra AC Fat Burner
Schiff Vitamins	Diet aids	Complete RX	Mega Ripped Cap-
American Bodybuild-	Sports Meal Bars	Dynamic Muscle	sules
ing Products	Sports Meal Powder	Builder	_____
Nutrition bars	Sports Meal RTD	Tiger's Milk Bars	_____
Protein powders	Ultra Whey Pro	Fi-Bar	_____
Vitamins/minerals	Lean Pro	Metaform	_____
Glutamine	Mass 1000	Fat Burners	_____

DYNATRITION BASIC FOOD CHOICES		
Food Group	**Suggested Servings Per Day**	**Example of Serving Size**
High-Protein Foods: meat, poultry, fish, eggs, dry beans, and peas.	3 to 4 servings. Choose lean cuts of meat, skinless chicken and turkey, fish 5 or more times a week. Count protein drinks and high-protein nutrition bars as one serving.	Amounts per serving should be about 4 to 6 ounces of cooked lean meat, poultry, or fish. Count 1 egg, or 1/2 cup cooked beans as 1 ounce of meat.
High-Carbohydrate Foods: bread, cereal, and other whole-grain products. Choose low-fat when possible and avoid white processed flour.	11 to 14 servings. Include several servings of whole-grain products.	1 slice of whole-grain bread 1/2 hamburger bun or English muffin. A small roll, biscuit, or muffin 3 to 4 whole-grain crackers 1/2 cup cooked cereal (oats), wild rice, or whole-grain pasta 1 ounce of whole-grain breakfast cereal
Vegetables	5 to 8 servings. Include all types; use raw chopped vegetables, leafy green vegetables.	1/2 cup of cooked vegetables 1/2 cup of chopped raw vegetables 1 cup of leafy raw vegetables
Fruit	4 to 6 servings.	1 piece of whole fruit, such as an apple, banana, or orange 1 grapefruit half 1 melon wedge 3/4 cup of juice 1/2 cup of berries 1/2 cup cooked or canned fruit (no sugar added) 1/4 cup dried fruit
High-Carbohydrate/ Moderate Protein Foods: dairy: milk, cheese, and yogurt.	1 to 3 servings. Choose low-fat or fat-free dairy products whenever possible to reduce your fat intake, yet provide moderate protein and high carbohydrates.	1 cup of low-fat or nonfat milk. 8 ounces of low-fat yogurt or cottage cheese 1 1/2 ounces of natural cheese

Watch out for high-fat snacks, like chips, cake, and ice cream.

Choose fresh whole foods and whole-grain foods when possible.

Drink at least 8 to 10 eight-ounce glasses of water per day.

Take your dietary supplements every day.

Divide food intake over three or four small meals and one to three snacks per day.

DYNATRITION DAILY MENU EXAMPLES

The sample daily menus beginning on page 205 will give you some guidance as to what you should be eating every day, and how to spread out the calories over several meals and snacks. When you eat the right foods (low in fat, high in complex carbohydrates and fiber, and moderate in quality protein), you can eat an awful lot, while still keeping the calories down where they should be.

DYNATRITION GUIDELINES FOR SELECTING YOUR DAILY ESSENTIAL DIETARY SUPPLEMENTS

Now that you have a feel for planning daily meals, let's take a look at dietary supplements you should consider using, and what dosages might be right for your core dietary supplement program. Use the Dynatrition Dietary Supplement chart on page 209 as a guide. This chart integrates years of research and the findings of numerous scientific studies and guidelines published by both government and independent dietary supplement organizations.

When selecting and choosing supplements to meet your dietary requirements, keep a few points in mind. First of all, no matter how well you eat, most nutritionists have determined that many dietary needs cannot be attained by food alone. Dietary supplements meet a real need. They don't just give you expensive urine, although it is true that when you increase the dosage of nutrients, you will excrete them at a higher rate. Scientific research proves you do benefit from the extra amounts. There are trillions of cells, with thousands of biochemical reactions happening each day in your body. Taking supplemental amounts of essential nutrients ensures that each of these cells will be properly nourished.

2,600-Calorie-Per-Day Menu

Breakfast

1/3 medium cantaloupe
2 medium bran muffins (about 100 to 120 calories each)
2 teaspoons low-fat spread
2 teaspoons jelly
1 cup low-fat milk
dietary supplements

Morning Snack

Tiger's Milk Nutrition Bar™ or Sports Meal Bar

Lunch

4 to 6 ounces lean broiled meat
1/2 cup carrots
1/2 cup whole-grain pasta
1 medium hard roll
1 teaspoon low-fat spread
1 apple
12 ounces of sport drink

Afternoon Snack

protein drink, such as UltraWhey Pro, Extreme Whey, or LeanPro

Dinner

1 serving baked fish (4 to 6 ounces)
1 medium baked potato
2 tablespoons sour cream, low-fat
1/2 cup fresh green peas
2 medium whole-wheat rolls
2 teaspoons low-fat spread
8 ounces vanilla yogurt, low-fat, with 1/2 cup fresh fruit
dietary supplements

Evening Snack

1 ounce turkey jerky or 2 egg whites or low-calorie protein shake

Just as foods can't do it all, neither can supplements. Supplements are intended to do just what the name implies—supplement your diet. Proper nutrition is *the* most important thing.

Our supplement guidelines are intended for daily use by healthy adults. As you review the chart, notice that the standard Recommended Daily Intake (RDI) is provided for reference. But remember that the RDI is only the minimum needed for survival, and is not intended to promote optimum health. Therefore some of our recommendations are much higher than the RDI. We provide a range of dosages to accommodate a variety of body types and activity levels. Most people should take doses somewhere in the middle of the range.

2,600-Calorie-Per-Day Menu

Breakfast

1 medium grapefruit
2 slices whole-wheat toast
2 teaspoons low-fat spread
1 tablespoon jelly
1 cup low-fat milk
dietary supplements

Morning Snack

Tiger's Milk Nutrition Bar™ or
Sports Meal Bar

Lunch

6 fluid ounces canned vegetable juice
chef salad
    2 ounces turkey
    1 ounce ham
    1½ ounces Swiss cheese
    1½ cups mixed greens
    1½ tablespoons dressing
2 medium corn muffins
2 servings fresh fruit

Afternoon Snack

protein drink, such as UltraWhey Pro,
Extreme Whey, or LeanPro

Dinner

4 to 6 ounces steak, broiled, lean only
1 cup yellow corn, fresh or frozen
½ cup stewed tomatoes, canned, no salt
2 medium whole-grain rolls
1 teaspoon low-fat spread
½ cup lime sherbet
dietary supplements

Evening Snack

1 ounce turkey jerky or 2 egg whites or low-
calorie protein shake

Use the blank columns provided to keep track of your total daily supplement intake and to ensure that you are not overdoing something that may have adverse effects over the long term. Recordkeeping will become important when you increase your daily intake of certain nutrients for special reasons, which we'll discuss in chapter 11. Take the time to read the detailed information in chapter 11 on each ingredient to insure its proper use.

Try to take your supplements at the same time every day. If you skip a dosage or a day or two, you can simply resume your program the next day. You don't have

3,400-CALORIE-PER-DAY MENU

Breakfast

$1/2$ medium cantaloupe
2 medium bran muffins (200 to 240 calories)
2 teaspoons low-fat spread
2 teaspoons jelly
3 to 4 eggs (egg whites)
1 cup whole milk
dietary supplements

Morning Snack

Tiger's Milk Nutrition Bar™ or
Sports Meal Bar

Lunch

6 to 8 ounces chicken breasts
1 cup carrot
1 cup whole-grain rice
1 medium hard roll
1 teaspoon low-fat spread
1 apple
12 fluid ounces sport drink

Afternoon Snack

1 serving protein drink such as Muscle
   Builder, LeanPro, Dynamic Weight
   Gainer, or Complete RX

Dinner

6 to 8 ounces baked fish
2 medium baked potatoes
6 tablespoons low-fat sour cream
1 cup broccoli
4 medium whole-wheat rolls
2 teaspoons low-fat spread
8 ounces vanilla yogurt, low-fat, with $1/2$ cup
   fresh fruit
dietary supplements

Pre-Training Meal

4 slices whole-grain bread
1 serving energy drink

Evening Snack

1 serving Protein Drink such as Muscle
Builder, LeanPro, Dynamic Weight Gainer,
or Complete RX

3,400-CALORIE-PER-DAY MENU

Breakfast

1 medium grapefruit
4 slices whole-wheat toast
2 teaspoons low-fat spread
1 tablespoon jelly
1 cup low-fat milk
4 to 6 ounces lean meat, baked
dietary supplements

Morning Snack

Tiger's Milk Nutrition Bar™ or
Sports Meal Bar

Lunch

6 fluid ounces vegetable juice
luncheon salad
    4 ounces roast beef
    2 ounces turkey
    1 1/2 ounces American cheese
    1 1/2 cups lettuce
    2 tablespoons dressing
2 medium corn muffins
2 servings fruit

Afternoon Snack

1 serving protein drink such as Muscle
    Builder, LeanPro, Dynamic Weight Gainer,
    or Complete RX

Dinner

6 to 8 ounces lean steak, broiled/baked
1 cup yellow corn
1 cup stewed tomatoes, canned, no salt
2 medium whole-grain roll
1 teaspoon low-fat spread
1 cup sherbet
dietary supplement

Pre-Training Meal

4 servings whole-grain bread
1 serving energy drink

Evening Snack

1 serving protein drink such as Muscle
    Builder, LeanPro, Dynamic Weight Gainer,
    or Complete RX

to be concerned about catching up. Your goal should be consistency when taking supplements, as well as eating right to begin with. Finally, don't be frustrated if you can't find one dietary supplement that contains all the recommended nutrients in the suggested daily intake ranges. You will probably have to select two or more products to meet your optimum supplement goals. For example, you might take one or two multivitamins almost every day, while individual ones will be added periodically depending on emotional, physical, and seasonal factors. This may mean

DYNATRITION DIETARY SUPPLEMENT GUIDELINES

For your daily essential nutrient supplement program. These supplement ingredient ranges are for both men and women.

IU= International Units, mg = milligrams, mcg = micrograms.

Nutrient	Reference Daily Intake For Adults	Effective Daily Supplement Dosage Range	Comments on Select Nutrients. *(Refer to Chapter 11 for comprehensive information on other nutrients.)*	Your Personal Daily Supplement Intake Notes Section
The Vitamins:				
Vitamin A (from acetate and palmitate)	5,000 IU	1,000 IU to 10,000 IU	Because vitamin A from acetate and palmitate has the potential to build up in your body and cause side effects, most people should stay in this range. Women who are planning to become pregnant should keep under 2,500 IU per day. If you want to increase your vitamin A intake, take supplements with pro-vitamin A, beta-carotene.	
Beta-carotene	None established	2,500 IU to 30,000 IU		
Vitamin D	400 IU	200 IU to 800 IU	Take higher levels of vitamin D (600 IU to 800 IU) as you get older, or if you do not spend much time exposed to the sun. (Exposure to sunlight stimulates natural vitamin D production in your body.)	

Nutrient	Reference Daily Intake For Adults	Effective Daily Supplement Dosage Range	Comments	Your Personal Daily Supplement Intake Notes Section
The Vitamins:				
Vitamin E	30 IU	100 IU to 1,000 IU	The most recent research indicates that a daily intake of vitamin E between 200 IU and 800 IU is best.	
Vitamin K	80 mcg	20 mcg to 180 mcg	Vitamin K seems to play a role in bone health and aids in blood clotting.	
Vitamin C	60 mg	250 mg to 2,000 mg	The most recent research confirms that consistent intake of 1,000 mg per day has been shown to improve immunity and reduce risk of infectious diseases.	
Vitamin B_1	1.5 mg	1.5 mg to 60 mg		
Vitamin B_2	1.7 mg	1.7 mg to 60 mg		
Vitamin B_3 (niacin)	20 mg	10 mg to 100 mg		
Vitamin B_6	2 mg	2 mg to 100 mg		
Folate	400 mcg	200 mg to 1,000		
Vitamin B_{12}	6 mcg	6 mcg to 200 mcg		
Biotin	300 mcg	20 mcg to 300 mcg		
Pantothenic acid	10 mg	2 mg to 60 mg		

Nutrient	Reference Daily Intake For Adults	Effective Daily Supplement Dosage Range	Comments	Your Personal Daily Supplement Intake Notes Section
The Minerals:				
Calcium	1,000 mg	500 mg to 1,500 mg	Take a supplement containing 1,000 to 1,200 mg of calcium each day for bone health.	
Phosphorus	1,000 mg	20 mg to 800 mg	Most supplements don't contain phosphorous because it is readily available in the diet.	
Magnesium	400 mg	100 mg to 600 mg		
Iron	18 mg	4 mg to 25 mg		
Zinc	15 mg	5 mg to 35 mg		
Iodine	150 mcg	30 mcg to 300 mcg		
Selenium	70 mcg	20 mcg to 300 mcg		
Copper	2 mg	0.5 mg to 4 mg		
Manganese	2 mg	0.5 mg to 30 mg		
Chromium	120 mcg	60 mcg to 300 mcg		
Molybdenum	75 mcg	25 mcg to 150 mcg		
Sodium	3,400 mg	None or less than 200 mg	Sodium is not usually contained in supplements because most people get plenty from their diet.	
Chloride	3,400 mg	None or less than 200 mg	Chloride is not usually contained in supplements because it is readily found in foods.	

Nutrient	Reference Daily Intake For Adults	Effective Daily Supplement Dosage Range	Comments	Your Personal Daily Supplement Intake Notes Section
Potassium	3,500 mg	20 mg to 400 mg	Potassium is usually obtained from foods but occurs in some supplement formulas, tablets, and powdered drinks.	
Boron		0.5 mg to 6 mg		
Choline		20 mg to 400 mg		
Inositol		20 mg to 400 mg		
Bioflavonoids		20 mg to 600 mg	Bioflavonoids are usually present in multinutrient supplement formulas from different sources, such as rutin, quercitin, pycnogenol, activin, curcumin, green tea extract, and grape seed extract.	
The New Antioxidants, compounds and botanicals:			Antioxidants are vital for antiaging and protect cells from elevated exercise-induced free-radical damage. They also protect the cardiovascular system and other body systems.	
Alpha-lipoic acid		5 mg to 30 mg	Alpha-lipoic acid is an antiaging antioxidant now being added to some multinutrient supplements and to super antioxidant formulas; it can also be taken as a separate product.	

Nutrient	Reference Daily Intake For Adults	Effective Daily Supplement Dosage Range	Comments	Your Personal Daily Supplement Intake Notes Section
Co-enzyme Q_{10}		15 mg to 30 mg		
Grape seed extract		10 mg to 100 mg		
Green tea extract		20 mg to 300 mg		
Milk Thistle		20 mg to 80 mg		
Turmeric		20 mg to 80 mg		
Ginkgo leaf extract		15 mg to 60 mg		
N-acetylcysteine		20 mg to 60 mg		
Lutein		5 mg to 40 mg		
The Fatty Acids:				
EPA		50 mg to 250 mg		
DHA		50 mg to 250 mg		
Alpha-linolenic acid		500 mg to 2,000 mg		
Linoleic acid		200 mg to 1,000 mg		
Gamma-linolenic acid		40 mg to 300 mg		
Glucosamine		500 mg to 1,500 mg		
Chondroitin sulfate		500 mg to 1,500 mg		

Nutrient	Reference Daily Intake For Adults	Effective Daily Supplement Dosage Range	Comments	Your Personal Daily Supplement Intake Notes Section
The Probiotics: Lactobacillus and bifidobacterium		2 to 10 billion cells		

every day for some people, or four to six days a week for others. Whatever you personal strategy is, remember that consistency is a vital factor.

Refer to the specific entries in chapter 11 for details on these nutrients and special concerns. Guidelines for other nutrients not included in this table, like amino acids, botanicals, and metabolites, are covered in their respective sections in chapter 11. Special Dynatrition sports supplement recommendations for competitive athletes are presented in chapter 8.

MACRONUTRIENT SUPPLEMENTS

Depending on your nutritional requirements and athletic goals, you may find it useful to take dietary supplement products that contain macronutrients such as fiber or protein. Protein supplements are very popular and there are a number of good ones on the market. Soy protein powdered beverages, whey, casein, and egg-white-containing protein supplements are considered very high-quality protein sources. Remember that they do add calories to your diet, so keep track of them just as you would other foods.

When mixed with water, most protein supplements will contain between 80 to 240 calories per serving. They are convenient and can be taken with meals or between meals as a nutritious snack. If you like to take protein powder with you to eat

The Healing Power of Antioxidants

Longevity researchers continue to confirm the health-promoting power of antioxidants. A recent study found that people who lived to be 100 years old had higher blood levels of antioxidants, such as vitamins E and C. Antioxidants reduce damage from naturally occurring and artificially occurring chemicals found in the body. They also neutralize "free radicals," compounds in the body that are unstable and need to react with other substances in the body. Unstable free radicals damage healthy molecules, cell membranes, the circulatory system, and nerves. In our modern environment, which is often contaminated by chemicals and pollutants, we probably need higher levels of antioxidants than food alone can deliver from an average diet. Research shows that supplementing with a variety of antioxidants, like vitamins E and C, may have anti-aging effects and prevent diseases such as cancer.

The Dietary Supplement Guidelines chart in this chapter includes some familiar antioxidants, like vitamins C and E, beta-carotene, and selenium, but we also list some compounds that are now receiving attention from researchers, such as botanical substances like bioflavonoids and polyphenols, lipoic acid, botanical extracts like green tea leaf, bilberry fruit, ginkgo, and grape seed, and a group of antioxidant-containing herbs. New understanding of how herbal compounds function as antioxidants in the body has evolved during the past 20 years. Bioflavonoids show tremendous antioxidant power. When you take into consideration that plants sit in strong sunlight all day absorbing UV light that forms free radicals, it's no surprise that they are loaded with antioxidant compounds.

Furthermore researchers are discovering that different plant compounds have different antioxidant powers. For example, there are actually seven primary kinds of free radicals: hydrogen peroxide, hydroxyl radical, organic or fatty acid hydroperoxide, oxidized protein, polyunsaturated fatty acid radical, singlet oxygen, and superoxide anion radical. It makes sense, then, that a variety of vitamin and herbal antioxidants are needed to combat these different types of free radicals.

Additionally, antioxidants appear to exhibit free radical scavenging activity that is specific to different parts of the body. Vitamin E's antioxidant activity is beneficial to the circulatory system and skin. As for herbs, turmeric benefits the liver, bilberry, the eyes, soy isoflavones, breast tissue, and lycopene, the prostate. Research continues, so keep on the lookout for additional beneficial antioxidants.

on the road or at work, you don't need to pay extra money for single-serving pouches. Instead, purchase a large-sized container of your supplement when it is on sale, and make your own single servings by measuringing a serving into a plastic bag. This will save you a small fortune in the long run.

Carbohydrate supplements give you an energy boost during or after exercise, and they usually contain other nutrients, such as electrolytes and B vitamins. Like protein powders, they contain calories and can cause weight gain like anything else if eaten to excess.

Finally, you might try adding essential fatty acids as a supplement if you don't feel you are getting enough from your diet. You must reduce your fat intake from other food sources, since there is no extra benefit to taking essential fatty acids if you are overeating other types of fats in your diet. Essential fatty acid–containing oils, such as flaxseed oil and evening primrose oil, are high in calories—about 120 calories per tablespoon. As a rule of thumb, you should be keeping your total daily fat intake under 30 percent and in most cases between 20 and 25 percent of total daily calories.

As you age, and depending upon your health status and family history, you may need to take other types of supplements aimed at enhancing your cardiovascular system, your immune system, your energy, your memory, your digestive system, and your skeletal system, for example.

Another very popular class of supplements are those aimed at protecting and revitalizing joint function, like glucosamine. Glucosamine is the single most important substance in the synthesis of connective tissue. More than 30 years of research has gone into understanding glucosamine, and scientists have long known that simply ingesting purified glucosamine from connective tissue allows the body to bypass the step of converting glucose to glucosamine. Glucosamine as a supplement clearly aids in connective tissue synthesis. All athletes need such a substance, as the repair and growth of connective tissue is neverending.

This is just the start of your quest to improve performance through nutrition. Even conservative scientists are finally catching on to what many progressive health experts and athletes have been practicing for ages—the use of special diets and supplements to enhance athletic performance. As research continues, you can expect health-care practitioners everywhere to become more knowledgeable about the complex subject of sports nutrition. The important thing to remember is to stick to the nutrition practices currently supported by scientific research and to avoid looking for a "magic bullet" to cover all your specific nutritional needs. Your dedication to a good sports nutrition program is the only way you will succeed and achieve maximum performance. With knowledge and practice, you can have the best of both worlds: good health and optimum performance.

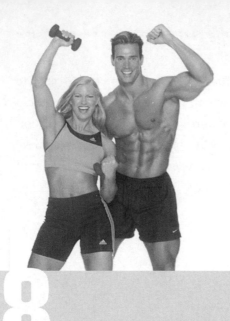

8

Sports-Specific Dynatrition Plans

When you engage in athletic training, competition, and exercise for fitness, the demands of your physical activity will create special nutrition needs. In other words, your athletic conditioning determines what food and supplements will work best for your specific physical conditioning program. For example, a marathon runner needs to eat different amounts of protein, carbohydrates, and fat than a powerlifter does. However, all athletes need to follow the rules of healthy eating, as well as modify their dietary intake to enable them to achieve maximum performance. This chapter is dedicated to addressing the essential issues regarding sports nutrition, and adjusting your nutrition to meet those demands.

EATING TO MATCH YOUR ATHLETIC PERFORMANCE-FITNESS GOALS

When you train for a particular sport, you are conditioning your muscles to produce strength and contractions, which generate motion specific to your sport objectives. For example, a marathon runner needs to display a lower intensity muscular output that can be sustained for long time periods. Compare this to the explosive strength needed for a sprinter to run 100 meters as fast as humanly possible. The sprinter's muscles are much larger and his muscle output is high in intensity over a very short period of time. This explosive strength generates tremendous power. His physical conditioning results in specific performance abilities and shapes the size and bioenergetic conditioning of his muscles. It determines what type of muscle fibers he develops as well as his metabolic anatomy and physiology. Like the sprinter, you have to know what your body needs before you can figure out what to eat.

DYNATRITION EATING PLANS FOR ATHLETES AND PERFORMANCE FITNESS

We're going to put together some of the things you've learned from pervious chapters about nutrition and training to help you meet your energy, growth, recovery, and performance demands. These categories serve as a starting point, but each individual will have slightly different needs. Our Dynatrition model guarantees a high success rate and should spare you years of unscientific trial and error.

Step 1: Determine your body composition. Keep track of any changes in your body weight. Retest yourself periodically to determine if changes come from loss of fat or muscle growth.

Step 2: Determine your daily caloric expenditure range. Your daily energy needs will vary with your daily activities. Determining your approximate energy needs will give you a good starting point. You can then fine-tune your caloric consumption based on how your body responds to your nutrition plans. If your goal is to build muscle and trim the fat, pay close attention to changes in your body weight and body composition. If your goal is to maximize performance and not make any changes in your body composition or body weight, then follow a diet for weight maintenance.

Step 3: Pick your sport/activity category from the examples provided in the table that follows: Anaerobic—Immediate Energy System; Anaerobic Glycolytic; Anaerobic Glycolytic—Oxidative Glycolytic; and Oxidative.

Step 4: Assess your daily protein needs and select the foods and supplements to achieve them.

Step 5: Assess your daily carbohydrate needs and select the foods and supplements to achieve them. Include any carbohydrate beverages you may drink before, during, and after exercise.

Step 6: Regulate your fat consumption and choose foods and cooking methods to keep intake low. Achieving a level of 30 percent of total daily calories will be an ongoing struggle. Try your best, and don't admonish yourself if you slip up now and then. Just make sure you stick to your performance-fitness eating plan during your competition season.

Step 7: Maintain proper fluid and supplement intake to meet your daily needs, as determined by the amount of your physical activity, environmental factors, and your specific training and health needs.

PERFORMANCE NUTRITION PLAN	SPORT TYPE
15% Fat **30% Protein** **55% Carbohydrates**	**Anaerobic–Immediate** **Energy Sports**
Baseball Bodybuilding Boxing Football Gymnastics Martial Arts Powerlifting Running, Sprinting Skiing, All Downhill Events Swimming, Sprint Events Track & Field, Power/Sprint Events Weight Lifting Wrestling	Sports that demand explosive strength and power (immediately available ATP and CP); anaerobic energy is used. Large muscles comprised of mostly fast-twitch muscle fibers. High protein is required to maintain positive nitrogen balance and repair fragile fast-twitch muscle fibers. Low-fat, high-carbohydrate intake is suggested, because these athletes utilize energy mostly from muscle glycogen to replenish ATP and CP stores.

PERFORMANCE NUTRITION PLAN	SPORT TYPE *(continued)*
20% Fat **25% Protein** **55% Carbohydrates**	**Anaerobic Glycolytic** **Sports**
Basketball Bowling Cycling—Sprint & Middle Distance Dancing, Power Equestrian, Power Field Hockey, Power Players Fitness, Power Exercisers Golf Hockey, Ice Motor Sports Racket Sports Rock Climbing Running, Mid-distance Skiing, Mid-distance Soccer, Power Positions Swimming, Mid-distance Tennis Track & Field, Mid-distance Events Volleyball	Sports that require explosive strength and power on a highly repetitive basis. Muscle glycogen is a primary source of energy. High protein is required to maintain positive nitrogen balance and repair fast-twitch muscle fibers.
20% Fat **20% Protein** **60% Carbohydrates**	**Anaerobic Glycolytic–** **Oxidative Glycolytic Sports**
Cycling, Long-distance Dancing, Stamina	Sports where the aerobic pathway is the predominant energy source, but glycolysis is also

PERFORMANCE NUTRITION PLAN	SPORT TYPE *(continued)*
20% Fat **20% Protein** **60% Carbohydrates**	**Anaerobic Glycolytic—** **Oxidative Glycolytic Sports (continued)**
Equestrian, Mid-distance Field Hockey, Mid-distance Players Fitness, Stamina Exercisers Soccer, Mid-distance Positions Swimming, Long-distance	relied upon. Fatty acids and muscle glycogen therefore become important energy sources. Moderate protein intake is required to maintain positive nitrogen balance and repair muscle fibers. This is a good daily intake macronutrient composition for cross-training sports, or multienergetic sports, as well as for general health and fitness.
25% Fat **15% Protein** **60% Carbohydrates**	**Oxidative Sports**
Fitness, Endurance Exercisers Running, Long-distance Skiing, Long-distance Track & Field, Long-distance Events Triathlon	Sports where oxidative endurance is required for long-distance events. Slow-twitch muscle fibers predominate. High carbohydrates are required to maintain glycogen stores. As endurance athletes utilize a high amount of fatty acids for energy, moderate dietary fat intake is recommended. Protein intake is lowest for this group, but is about twice as high as for nonathletes.

TAILOR-MADE SPORTS-NUTRITIONAL PLANS FOR PEAK PERFORMANCE

We have found that most prescribed diet plans found in books and articles do not work because they are difficult to follow over the long term. Many include recipes and special foods that are not practical for busy individuals. Let's face it, if you don't enjoy the food on a plan, you're not going to follow it for very long. It seems that unless you are confined to an institution, where someone else is preparing all your meals every day, it's hard to follow most prescribed diets. Finally, when confronted with real life situations (eating out, eating over at friends' houses, or traveling) it's close to impossible to follow a month-long eating plan that someone else created without knowing your individual preferences.

With these pitfalls of plans in mind, we have deleloped some simple daily meal examples and food category lists to assist in selecting foods to meet your sport-specific fat, protein, and carbohydrate goals. The daily diet examples show you how to spread out your caloric intake on training days, and gives examples of foods you can eat to meet your sport-specific daily nutrient requirements. Additionally, there are two caloric examples for each of the four different menus: 2,500 calories per day and 3,500 calories per day. The examples are dynamic and you can easily add or subtract foods to match your needs. If your sport has enormous daily caloric demands (like 5,000 to 7,000 calories per day) you can simply double the portions in the other examples.

To be successful, you will have to do some planning to make sure that your refrigerator and pantry are well stocked with the foods you need. Meeting your daily nutrition goals may also mean packing a brown bag meal to take with you while out of the house.

We've purposely included common foods to get you started and ones that are considered wholesome, for the most part. To make the plans work best, add your favorite foods to the list and figure out how much to allow yourself. Most grocery foods have the nutrition information on their labels, but ideally you should visit your local health-food store and include more of these foods in your performance diet.

Another thing to remember when constructing your personal nutrition plans is not to become overly concerned if you find that you cannot exactly get the foods to meet your target caloric and macronutrient goals. You have to be a little flexible. Even when scientists calculate the energy and macronutrient content of foods, they make a lot of assumptions and an acceptable range of error is to be expected.

Finally, if you are following a 15-30-55 diet, this does not mean that each meal consists of 15 percent fat, 30 percent protein, and 55 percent carbohydrates; rather this refers to the total daily intake goal. Most athletes can follow a 20 percent to 30 percent fat, 15 percent to 20 percent protein, and 55 percent to 60 percent carbohydrate diet during the off-season. Because long-distance athletes tend to train all year round, you can stick to the 25 percent fat, 15 percent protein, and 60 percent carbohydrate diet all year, except as otherwise directed by your coach or health practitioner.

The tables that follow each plan provide some guidelines that can be useful when planning your daily dietary supplement intake. They are intended for information purposes only, for healthy adult athletes. Always check with your health-care practitioner before taking supplements or following a new nutrition plan, especially if you are pregnant or breastfeeding, chronically ill, elderly, under 18 years old, or taking any medications. These guidelines may not be suitable for everybody, and are intended for short-term use during the athletic season. Use supplements only as directed by the manufacturer.

15% FAT, 30% PROTEIN, 55% CARBOHYDRATE DYNATRITION PLAN FOR ANAEROBIC/IMMEDIATE ENERGY SPORTS

The 15 percent fat, 30 percent protein, 55 percent carbohydrate daily nutrition plan is recommended for massive, power athletes, driven by the very short-term, immediate energy system. Athletes such as football players, powerlifters, sprinters, and bodybuilders will do best following this nutrition plan during the season. When training or competing, these athletes rely primarily on the immediate, and to a lesser extent the glycolytic, energy systems. They have massive muscles, with highly developed fast-twitch muscle fibers. Because of this, these athletes require a high amount of protein to maintain positive nitrogen balance and to repair their fragile fast-twitch muscle fibers. Since muscle glycogen is the primary energy source used for replenishing the ATP and CP stores, a diet that is low in fat and rich in carbohydrates is indicated. Low in fat, because not much fat is used up during training and competition. Rich in carbohydrates, because the muscle's supply of glycogen needs to be restored every day, or performance and recovery will be impaired. The proper profile of micronutrients and ergogenic nutrients from supplements needs to be just right for optimum performance of the explosive-power athlete.

DAILY DIETARY SUPPLEMENT GUIDELINES

Nutrient	Range of Intake	Personal Notes
Vitamin A	8,000–16,000 IU	
Vitamin A (as beta-carotene)	20,000–30,000 IU	
Vitamin B$_1$ (thiamin)	30–120 mg	
Vitamin B$_2$ (riboflavin)	30–120 mg	
Vitamin B$_3$ (niacin)	40–80 mg	
Vitamin B$_5$ (pantothenic acid)	20–100 mg	
Vitamin B$_6$ (pyridoxine)	20–80 mg	
Vitamin B$_{12}$ (cobalamin)	12–120 mcg	
Biotin	125–175 mcg	
Folate	400–800 mcg	
Vitamin C	800–2,000 mg	
Vitamin D	400–800 IU	
Vitamin E	200–600 IU	
Vitamin K	60–160 mcg	
Boron	2–8 mg	
Calcium	800–1,500 mg	
Chromium	200–500 mcg	
Copper	1–4 mg	
Iodine	100–200 mcg	
Iron	15–50 mg	
Magnesium	250–650 mg	
Manganese	12–35 mg	
Molybdenum	100–200 mcg	
Phosphorus	150–800 mg	
Potassium	50–1,000 mg	
Selenium	100–200 mcg	
Zinc	15–50 mg	
L-arginine	1,000–4,000 mg	
L-glutamine	1,000–5,000 mg	
L-ornithine	1,000–4,000 mg	
Alpha-linolenic acid	1,000–2,000 mg	
Docosahexaenoic acid (DHA)	250–750 mg	
Eiocosapentaenoic acid (EPA)	250–750 mg	
Gamma-linolenic acid (GLA)	400–800 mg	
Linoleic acid	3,000–6,000 mg	

DAILY DIETARY SUPPLEMENT GUIDELINES

Nutrient	Range of Intake	Personal Notes
Beta-hydroxy beta-methylbutyrate	1,500–3,000 mg	
Bioflavonoids	200–800 mg	
Choline	100–600 mg	
Creatine monohydrate	5,000–10,000 mg	
Ferulic acid	100–200 mg	
Inositol	100–600 mg	
L-carnitine	750–2,000 mg	

2,500 CALORIES PER DAY	3,500 CALORIES PER DAY
15% fat, 375 cals, 42 grams 30% protein, 750 cals, 188 grams 55% carbohydrates, 1,375 cals, 344 grams	15% fat, 525 cals, 58 grams 30% protein, 1,050 cals, 263 grams 55% carbohydrates, 1,925 cals, 481 grams
Training Days	**Training Days**
Breakfast	Breakfast
Meal goal: 500 cals, 40g P, 62.5g C, 10g F Take vitamin, mineral, ergogenic supplements	Meal goal: 573 cals, 51g P, 64g C, 13g F Take vitamin, mineral, ergogenic supplements
2 cups egg alternative (as Fleishmann's Egg Beaters) vegetable omelet, 200 cals, 28g P, 20g C, 0g F	2 1/2 cups egg alternative (as Fleishmann's Egg Beaters) vegetable omelet, 250 cals, 35g P, 25g C, 0g F
1 slice lean Canadian bacon, 86 cals, 12g P, 0g C, 4g F	1 slice lean Canadian Bacon, 86 cals, 12g P, 0g C, 4g F
4 oz boiled potato, pulp, 117 cals, 2g P, 28g C, 0g F	4 oz boiled potato, pulp, 117 cals, 2g P, 28g C, 0g F
1/2 tbsp butter or olive oil margarine, 50 cals, 0g P, 0g C, 6g F	2/3 tbsp butter or olive oil margarine, 81 cals, 0g P, 0g C, 9g F
6 oz grapefruit juice, 60 cals, 0g P, 15g C, 0g F	12 oz grapefruit juice, 120 cals, 0g P, 15g C, 0g F

2,500 CALORIES PER DAY	3,500 CALORIES PER DAY
Morning Snack Protein nutrition bar, low calorie, about 225 cals, 30g P, 15g C, 5g F. Tiger's Milk, Fi-Bar or Sports Meal	**Morning Snack** Protein nutrition bar, medium calorie, about 470 cals, 40g P, 64g C, 6g F. Tiger's Milk, Fi-Bar or Sports Meal
Lunch Meal goal: 500 cals, 40g P, 62.5g C, 10g F Take vitamin, mineral, ergogenic supplements 1 orange, medium, 62 cals, 1g P, 13g C, 0g F 2 slices bread, whole-grain, 170 cals, 8g P, 34g C, 3g F 4 oz chicken breast, no skin, 124 cals, 26g P, 0g C, 2g F 1 tbsp salad dressing (Seven Seas), oil & vinegar, 45 cals, 0g P, 1g C, 4g F 2 oz iceberg lettuce, trimmed, 8 cals, 0.5g P, 1.5g C, 0g F 4 oz broccoli spears (Birds Eye), 30 cals, 4g P, 6g C, 0g F 2 oz carrot, raw, 24 cals, 1g P, 6g C, 0g F	**Lunch** Meal goal: 573 cals, 51g P, 64g C, 13g F Take vitamin, mineral, ergogenic supplements 1 orange, medium, 62 cals, 1g P, 13g C, 0g F 2 slices bread, whole-grain, 170 cals, 8g P, 34g C, 3g F 6 oz chicken breast, no skin, 186 cals, 39g P, 0g C, 2.5g F 1½ tbsp salad dressing (Seven Seas), oil & vinegar, 67 cals, 0g P, 1.5g C, 6g F 2 oz iceburg lettuce, trimmed, 8 cals, 0.5g P, 1.5g C, 0g F 4 oz broccoli spears (Birds Eye), 30 cals, 4g P, 6g C, 0g F 2 oz carrot, raw, 24 cals, 1g P, 6g C, 0g F
Pre-Training Snack 2½ hours before training Protein drink, low calorie, 225 cals, 30g P, 15g C, 5g F	**Pre-Training Snack** 2½ hours before training Protein drink, medium calorie, 470 cals, 40g P, 55g C, 10g F
Then BCAAs (branched-chain amino acids) supplement 30 minutes before workout, with water Carbohydrate sports drink during workout, high calorie, 16 oz, 400 cals, 0g P, 100g C, 0g F	**Then** BCAAs (branched-chain amino acids) supplement 30 minutes before workout, with water Carbohydrate sports drink during workout, high calorie, 20 oz, 500 cals, 0g P, 125g C, 0g F

2,500 CALORIES PER DAY	3,500 CALORIES PER DAY
Dinner	**Dinner**
Meal goal: 650 cals, 48g P, 87.5g C, 12g F _Take vitamin, mineral, ergogenic supplements_	Meal goal: 914 cals, 81g P, 100g C, 20g F _Take vitamin, mineral, ergogenic supplements_

1 pork chop (Master Choice), 220 cals, 22g P,
    0g C, 4g F
8 oz baked beans, barbecue (B&M), 260 cals,
    15g P, 48g C, 6g F
6 oz spinach, 36 cals, 5g P, 6g C, 0.6g F
1 tomato, 26 cals, 1g P, 5.7g C, 0.4g F
8 oz skim milk, 86 cals, 8.4g P, 11.9g C, 0.4g F
4 oz fruit cocktail, canned, in light syrup,
    65 cals, 0.5g P, 16.9g C, 0.1g F
	2½ pork chops (Master Choice), 550 cals,
	    53g P, 0g C, 10g F
	8 oz baked beans, barbecue (B&M), 260 cals,
	    15g P, 48g C, 6g F
	6 oz spinach, 36 cals, 5g P, 6g C, 0.6g F
	1 tomato, 26 cals, 1g P, 5.7g C, 0.4g F
	8 oz skim milk, 86 cals, 8.4g P, 11.9g C, 0.4g F
	4 oz fruit cocktail, canned, in light syrup,
	    65 cals, 0.5g P, 16.9g C, 0.1g F

Optional Evening Snack—nutrition bar or
    protein shake
	Optional Evening Snack—nutrition bar or
	    protein shake

20% FAT, 25% PROTEIN, 55% CARBOHYDRATE DYNATRITION PLAN FOR ANAEROBIC-GLYCOLYTIC SPORTS

The 20 percent fat, 25 percent protein, 55 percent carbohydrate daily nutrition plan is recommended for individuals who participate in sports and fitness activities that require explosive strength and power on a sustained or highly repetitive basis. When training for or during competition, these individuals rely primarily on the glycolytic energy systems. Muscle glycogen is their primary source of energy. These individuals need to consume large amounts of protein to maintain a positive nitrogen balance and to repair their fragile fast-twitch muscle fibers.

DAILY DIETARY SUPPLEMENT GUIDELINES

Nutrient	Range of Intake	Personal Notes
Vitamin A	8,000–16,000 IU	
Vitamin A (as beta-carotene)	20,000–30,000 IU	
Vitamin B$_1$ (thiamin)	30–120 mg	
Vitamin B$_2$ (riboflavin)	30–120 mg	
Vitamin B$_3$ (niacin)	40–80 mg	
Vitamin B$_5$ (pantothenic acid)	20–100 mg	
Vitamin B$_6$ (pyridoxine)	20–80 mg	
Vitamin B$_{12}$ (cobalamin)	12–120 mcg	
Biotin	125–175 mcg	
Folate	400–800 mcg	
Vitamin C	800–2,000 mg	
Vitamin D	400–800 IU	
Vitamin E	200–600 IU	
Vitamin K	60–160 mcg	
Boron	2–8 mg	
Calcium	800–1,500 mg	
Chromium	200–500 mcg	
Copper	1–4 mg	
Iodine	100–200 mcg	
Iron	15–50 mg	
Magnesium	250–650 mg	
Manganese	12–35 mg	
Molybdenum	100–200 mcg	
Phosphorus	150–800 mg	
Potassium	50–1,000 mg	
Selenium	100–200 mcg	
Zinc	15–50 mg	
L-glutamine	1,000–5,000 mg	
Alpha-linolenic acid	500–1,000 mg	
Docosahexaenoic acid (DHA)	250–750 mg	
Eiocosapentaenoic acid (EPA)	250–750 mg	
Gamma-linolenic acid (GLA)	100–400 mg	
Linoleic acid	2,000–4,000 mg	
Bioflavonoids	200–800 mg	
Choline	100–600 mg	

DAILY DIETARY SUPPLEMENT GUIDELINES		
Nutrient	**Range of Intake**	**Personal Notes**
Creatine monohydrate	4,000–8,000 mg	
Ferulic acid	50–100 mg	
Inositol	100–600 mg	
L-carnitine	750–1,500 mg	
Octacosanol	3,000–6,000 mg	

2,500 CALORIES PER DAY	3,500 CALORIES PER DAY
20% fat, 500 cals, 56 grams **25% protein, 625 cals, 156 grams** **55% carbohydrates, 1,375 cals, 344 grams**	**20% fat, 700 cals, 78 grams** **25% protein, 875 cals, 219 grams** **55% carbohydrates, 1,925 cals, 481 grams**
Training Days	Training Days

Breakfast
 	
Meal goal: 465 cals, 27g P, 60g C, 13g F
Take vitamin, mineral, ergogenic
   supplements
 	
1 cup egg alternative (as Fleishmann's Egg
   Beaters) vegetable omelet, 100 cals, 14g P,
   10g C, 0g F
1 slice lean Canadian bacon, 86 cals, 12g P,
   0g C, 4g F
4 oz boiled potato, pulp, 117 cals, 2g P,
   28g C, 0g F
2/3 tbsp butter or olive oil margarine, 81 cals,
   0g P, 0g C, 9g F
9 oz grapefruit juice, 90 cals, 0g P, 22.5g C, 0g F
	Breakfast
	
	Meal goal: 579 cals, 38.5g P, 61g C, 18.5g F
	Take vitamin, mineral, ergogenic
	   supplements
	
	1 1/2 cups egg alternative (as Fleishmann's Egg
	   Beaters) vegetable omelet, 150 cals, 21g P,
	   15g C, 0gF
	1 slice lean Canadian bacon, 86 cals, 12g P,
	   0g C, 4g F
	4 oz boiled potato, pulp, 117 cals, 2g P,
	   28g C, 0g F
	1 tbsp butter or olive oil margarine, 100 cals,
	   0g P, 0g C, 9g F.
	6 oz grapefruit juice, 60 cals, 0g P, 15g C, 0g F
	4 oz milk, 2%, 60 cals, 4g P, 5.5g C, 2g F

2,500 Calories Per Day	3,500 Calories Per Day
Morning Snack	**Morning Snack**
Protein nutrition bar, low calorie, approximately 225 cals, 30g P, 15G C, 5g F; Tiger's Milk, Fi-Bar, or Sports Meal	Protein nutrition bar, medium calorie, approximately 470 cals, 40g P, 64g C, 6g F; Tiger's Milk, Fi-Bar, or Sports Meal
Lunch	**Lunch**
Meal goal: 465 cals, 27g P, 60g C, 13g F Take vitamin, mineral, ergogenic supplements 1 orange, medium, 62 cals, 1g P, 13g C, 0g F 2 slices bread, whole-grain, 170 cals, 8g P, 34g C, 3g F 2 oz chicken breast, no skin, 62 cals, 13g P, 0g C, 1g F 2 tbsps salad dressing (Seven Seas), oil & vinegar, 90 cals, 0g P, 1g C, 8g F 2 oz iceberg lettuce, trimmed, 8 cals, 0.5g P, 1.5g C, 0g F 4 oz broccoli spears (Birds Eye), 30 cals, 4g P, 6g C, 0g F 2 oz carrot, raw, 24 cals, 1g P, 6g C, 0g F 1 tomato, 4.75 oz, 26 cals, 1g P, 5.7g C, 0.4g F	Meal goal: 579 cals, 38.5g P, 61g C, 18.5g F Take vitamin, mineral, ergogenic supplements 1 orange, medium, 62 cals, 1g P, 13g C, 0g F 1 roll, hoagie, 210 cals, 8g P, 34g C, 5g F 4 oz chicken breast, no skin, 124 cals, 26g P, 0g C, 2g F 3 tbsps salad dressing (Seven Seas), oil & vinegar, 135 cals, 0g P, 3g C, 12g F 2 oz iceburg lettuce, trimmed, 8 cals, 0.5g P, 1.5g C, 0g F 4 oz broccoli spears (Birds Eye), 30 cals, 4g P, 6g C, 0g F 2 oz carrot, raw, 24 cals, 1g P, 6g C, 0g F
Pre-Training Snack	**Pre-Training Snack**
2½ hours before training Protein drink, low calorie, approximately 225 cals, 30g P, 15g C, 5g F	2½ hours before training Protein drink, medium calorie, approximately 470 cals, 40g P, 55g C, 10g F
Then	**Then**
BCAAs supplement 30 minutes before workout, with water Carbohydrate sports drink during workout, high calorie, 16 oz, approximately 400 cals, 0g P, 100g C, 0g F	BCAAs supplement 30 minutes before workout, with water Carbohydrate sports drink during workout, high calorie, 20 oz, approximately 500 cals, 0g P, 125g C, 0g F

2,500 Calories Per Day	3,500 Calories Per Day
Dinner	Dinner
Meal goal: 724 cals, 42g P, 94g C, 20g F Take vitamin, mineral, ergogenic supplements	Meal goal: 901 cals, 62g P, 98g C, 29g F Take vitamin, mineral, ergogenic supplements
3 oz beef, bottom round, prime, untrimmed, 192 cals, 17.1g P, 0g C, 13.2g F 2 oz pasta, 210 cals, 9g P, 41g C, 1g F 4 oz pasta sauce (Ragu), Mushroom Thick and and Hearty, 100 cals, 2g P, 15g C, 3g F 12 oz spinach, 72 cals, 9.6g P, 12g C, 1.2g F 8 oz milk, skim, 86 cals, 8.4g P, 11.9g C, 0.4g F 4 oz fruit cocktail, canned, in light syrup, 65 cals, 0.5g P, 16.9g C, 0.1g F	5 oz beef, bottom round, prime, untrimmed, 225 cals, 31g P, 0g C, 10.5g F 2 oz pasta, 210 cals, 9g P, 41g C, 1g F 1/2 tbsp olive oil, 60 cals, 0g P, 0g C, 7g F 4 oz pasta sauce (Ragu), Mushroom Thick and and Hearty, 100 cals, 2g P, 15g C, 3g F 12 oz spinach, 72 cals, 9.6g P, 12g C, 1.2g F 8 oz milk, whole, 150 cals, 8g P, 11g C, 8g F 4 oz fruit cocktail, canned, in light syrup, 65 cals, 0.5g P, 16.9g C, 0.1g F
Optional Evening Snack—nutrition bar or protein shake	Optional Evening Snack—nutrition bar or protein shake

20% FAT, 20% PROTEIN, 60% CARBOHYDRATE DYNATRITION PLAN FOR ANAEROBIC-GLYCOLYTIC/OXIDATIVE-GLYCOLYTIC ATHLETES

The 20 percent fat, 20 percent protein, 60 percent carbohydrate daily nutrition plan is recommended for individuals who participate in sports or fitness activities that require explosive strength and power on a sustained or highly repetitive basis. While these individuals rely to some extent on the glycolytic energy systems, they depend primarily on the oxidative energy systems. Fatty acids as well as muscle glycogen are their primary fuel sources during activity. Therefore, these athletes need to consume just moderate amounts of protein to maintain positive nitrogen balance and to repair their fragile fast-twitch muscle fibers.

DAILY DIETARY SUPPLEMENT GUIDELINES

Nutrient	Range of Intake	Personal Notes
Vitamin A	8,000–16,000 IU	
Vitamin A (as beta-carotene)	30,000–60,000 IU	
Vitamin B$_1$ (thiamin)	100–250 mg	
Vitamin B$_2$ (riboflavin)	100–200 mg	
Vitamin B$_3$ (niacin)	10–20 mg	
Vitamin B$_5$ (pantothenic acid)	100–200 mg	
Vitamin B$_6$ (pyridoxine)	20–80 mg	
Vitamin B$_{12}$ (cobalamin)	12–120 mcg	
Biotin	125–200 mcg	
Folate	400–800 mcg	
Vitamin C	1,000–2,000 mg	
Vitamin D	400–800 IU	
Vitamin E	400–1,000 IU	
Vitamin K	60–160 mcg	
Boron	2–8 mg	
Calcium	800–1,500 mg	
Chromium	200–500 mcg	
Copper	1–4 mg	
Iodine	100–200 mcg	
Iron	15–50 mg	
Magnesium	250–650 mg	
Manganese	12–35 mg	
Molybdenum	100–200 mcg	
Phosphorus	150–800 mg	
Potassium	50–1,000 mg	
Selenium	100–200 mcg	
Zinc	15–50 mg	
L-glutamine acid	1,000–1,500 mg	
L-glutamine	1,000–5,000 mg	
Alpha-linolenic acid	500–1,000 mg	
Docosahexaenoic acid (DHA)	400–1,000 mg	
Eiocosapentaenoic acid (EPA)	400–1,000 mg	
Gamma-linolenic acid (GLA)	200–500 mg	
Linoleic acid	500–1,000 mg	
Bioflavonoids	500–1,000 mg	
Choline	500–1,000 mg	

DAILY DIETARY SUPPLEMENT GUIDELINES		
Nutrient	**Range of Intake**	**Personal Notes**
Coenzyme Q_{10}	60–120 mg	
Inositol	500–1,000 mg	
L-carnitine	1,000–3,000 mg	
Octacosanol	1,000–2,000 mg	

2,500 CALORIES PER DAY	3,500 CALORIES PER DAY
20% fat, 500 cals, 56 grams **20% protein, 500 cals, 125 grams** **60% carbohydrates, 1,500 cals, 375 grams**	**20% fat, 700 cals, 78 grams** **20% protein, 700 cals, 175 grams** **60% carbohydrates, 2,100 cals, 525 grams**
Training Days	**Training Days**

Breakfast
 	
 Meal goal: 474.5 cals, 23.5g P, 67g C, 12.5g F
 Take vitamin, mineral, ergogenic
    supplements
 	
 3 pancakes, buttermilk, Hungry Jack, prepared,
    200 cals, 6g P, 28g C, 7g F
 3 oz ham, fresh, trimmed, 117 cals, 18g P,
    0g C, 4.5g F
 8 oz vegetable juice (V8), 35 cals, 1g P,
    8g C, 0g F
 2 tbsp pancake syrup (Hungry Jack), lite,
    87.5 cals, 0g P, 24g C, 0g F
	Breakfast
	
	 Meal goal: 489 cals, 36g P, 52.5g C, 15g F
	 Take vitamin, mineral, ergogenic
	    supplements
	
	 3 pancakes, buttermilk, Hungry Jack, prepared,
	    200 cals, 6 P, 28g C, 7g F
	 4 oz ham, fresh, trimmed, 156 cals, 24g P,
	    0g C, 6g F
	 8 oz skim milk, 86 cals, 8g P, 11.9g C,
	    0.4g F
	 3 1/2 tbsp pancake syrup (Hungry Jack), lite,
	    50 cals, 0g P, 14g C, 0g F

Morning Snack
 	
 1 Nutrition Bar approximately 270 cals, 12g P,
    45g C, 5g F; Tiger's Milk, Fi-Bar, or Sports
    Meal
	Morning Snack
	
	 1 Nutrition Bar approximately 440 cals, 16g P,
	    68g C, 12g F; Tiger's Milk, Fi-Bar, or Sports
	    Meal

2,500 Calories Per Day	3,500 Calories Per Day
Lunch	Lunch

Meal goal: 474.5 cals, 23.5g P, 67g C, 12.5g F
Take vitamin, mineral, ergogenic
    supplements
	Meal goal: 489 Cals, 36g P, 52.5g C, 15g F
	Take vitamin, mineral, ergogenic
	    supplements

½ oz American cheese, 55 cals, 3g P, 0.5g C,
    4.5g F
1 sandwich roll, 123 cals, 4.5g P, 21.6g C, 3.3g F
3 slices turkey (Tyson), 60 cals, 12g P, 0.9g C,
    1.2g F
2 oz iceberg lettuce, trimmed, 8 cals, 0.6g P,
    1.2g C, 0.2g F
3 tsp mustard, 48 cals, 3g P, 3g C, 3g F
2 oz apricot, dried (Del Monte), 140 cals, 2g P,
    35g C, 0g F
	½ oz American cheese, 55 cals, 3g P, 0.5g C,
	    4.5g F
	1 sandwich roll, 123 cals, 4.5g P, 21.6g C, 3.3g F
	6 slices turkey (Tyson), 120 cals, 24g P, 1.8g C,
	    2.4g F
	2 oz iceburg lettuce, trimmed, 8 cals, 0.6g P,
	    1.2g C, 0.2g F
	3 tsp mustard, 48 cals, 3g P, 3g C, 3g F
	1 banana, w/o skin, 105 cals, 1.2g P, 26.7g C,
	    0.6g F

Pre-Training Snack	Pre-Training Snack

2½ hours before training
Protein drink, low calorie, approximately
    225 cals, 30g P, 15g C, 5g F
	2½ hours before training
	Protein drink, high calorie, approximately
	    548 cals, 30g P, 80g C, 12g F

Then	Then

BCAAs supplement 30 minutes before
    workout, with water
Carbohydrate sports drink during workout,
    high calorie, 16 oz, approximately 300 cals,
    0g P, 100g C, 0g F
	BCAAs supplement 30 minutes before
	    workout, with water
	Carbohydrate sports drink during workout,
	    high calorie, 20 oz, approximately 400 cals,
	    0g P, 125g C, 0g F

Dinner	Dinner
Meal goal: 748 cals, 36g P, 106g C, 20g F Take vitamin, mineral, ergogenic supplements	Meal goal: 932 cals, 57g P, 122g C, 24g F Take vitamin, mineral, ergogenic supplements

4 oz tuna, bluefin, 164 cals, 26.4g P, 0g C,
    5.6g F
1 tomato, 4.75 oz, 26 cals, 1g P, 5.7g C, 0.4g F
8 oz iceberg lettuce, trimmed, 32 cals, 2.4g P,
    4.8g C, 0.8g F
	6 oz tuna, bluefin, 246 cals, 39.6g P, 0g C,
	    8.4g F
	1 tomato, 4.75 oz, 26 cals, 1g P, 5.7g C, 0.4g F
	8 oz iceberg lettuce, trimmed, 32 cals, 2.4g P,
	    4.8g C, 0.8g F

2,500 Calories Per Day	3,500 Calories Per Day
Dinner (continued)	Dinner (continued)
2 oz onion, trimmed, 22 cals, 0.6g P, 4.8g C, 0.2g F 3 oz brown rice, 309 cals, 6.9g P, 66g C, 3g F 6 oz cauliflower, 42 cals, 2.4g P, 8.4g C, 0.6g F 2 tbsp salad dressing (Seven Seas), oil and vinegar, 90 cals, 0g P, 2g C, 8g F 3 oz grape juice, 60 cals, 0g P, 15g C, 0g F	2 oz onion, trimmed, 22 cals, 0.6g P, 4.8g C, 0.2g F 1 oz garbanzo bean, 103 cals, 5.5g P, 17.2g C, 1.7g F 3 oz brown rice, 309 cals, 6.9g P, 66g C, 3g F 6 oz cauliflower, 42 cals, 2.4g P, 8.4g C, 0.6g F 2 tbsp salad dressing (Seven Seas), oil and vinegar, 90 cals, 0g P, 2g C, 8g F 3 oz grape juice, 60 cals, 0g P, 15g C, 0g F
Optional Evening Snack—nutrition bar or protein shake	Optional Evening Snack—nutrition bar or protein shake

25% FAT, 15% PROTEIN, 60% CARBOHYDRATE DYNATRITION NUTRITION PLAN FOR OXIDATIVE SPORTS

The 25 percent fat, 15 percent protein, 60 percent carbohydrate daily nutrition plan is recommended for individuals who participate in aerobic sports or fitness activities. When training or during competition, these individuals rely primarily on oxidative energy systems. Their muscles are composed of highly developed slow-twitch muscle fibers. Because of this, these individuals need to consume large amounts of carbohydrates to maintain their glycogen stores, due to the long duration of training and events. However, fatty acids are their primary source of energy, so they should consume a moderate amount of healthy fats and oils. The amount of protein for this group of individuals is the lowest of the four plans, but is still about two times more than non-athletes require.

DAILY DIETARY SUPPLEMENT GUIDELINES

Nutrient	Range of Intake	Personal Notes
Vitamin A	8,000–16,000 IU	
Vitamin A (as beta-carotene)	35,000–60,000 IU	
Vitamin B$_1$ (thiamin)	100–250 mg	
Vitamin B$_2$ (riboflavin)	100–200 mg	
Vitamin B$_3$ (niacin)	10–20 mg	
Vitamin B$_5$ (pantothenic acid)	100–200 mg	
Vitamin B$_6$ (pyridoxine)	20–80 mg	
Vitamin B$_{12}$ (cobalamin)	12–120 mcg	
Biotin	125–200 mcg	
Folate	400–800 mcg	
Vitamin C	1,000–2,000 mg	
Vitamin D	400–800 IU	
Vitamin E	400–1,000 IU	
Vitamin K	60–160 mcg	
Boron	2–8 mg	
Calcium	800–1,500 mg	
Chromium	200–500 mcg	
Copper	1–4 mg	
Iodine	100–200 mcg	
Iron	15–50 mg	
Magnesium	250–650 mg	
Manganese	12–35 mg	
Molybdenum	100–200 mcg	
Phosphorus	150–800 mg	
Potassium	50–1,000 mg	
Selenium	100–200 mcg	
Zinc	15–50 mg	
L-glutamine acid	1,000–1,500 mg	
L-glutamine	1,000–2,000 mg	
Alpha-linolenic acid	500–1,000 mg	
Docosahexaenoic acid (DHA)	400–1,000 mg	
Eiocosapentaenoic acid (EPA)	400–1,000 mg	
Gamma-linolenic acid (GLA)	200–500 mg	
Linoleic acid	500–1,000 mg	
Bioflavonoids	500–1,000 mg	
Choline	500–1,000 mg	

DAILY DIETARY SUPPLEMENT GUIDELINES		
Nutrient	**Range of Intake**	**Personal Notes**
Coenzyme Q_{10}	60–120 mg	
Inositol	500–1,000 mg	
L-carnitine	1,000–3,000 mg	
Octacosanol	1,000–2,000 mg	

2,500 CALORIES PER DAY	3,500 CALORIES PER DAY
25% fat, 625 cals, 69 grams **15% protein, 375 cals, 94 grams** **60% carbohydrates, 1,500 cals, 375 grams**	**25% fat, 875 cals, 97 grams** **15% protein, 525 cals, 131 grams** **60% carbohydrates, 2,100 cals, 525 grams**
Training Days	**Training Days**
Breakfast	Breakfast
Meal goal: 464 cals, 20g P, 58.5g C, 16.5g F Take vitamin, mineral, ergogenic supplements	Meal goal: 590.5 cals, 24g P, 77.5g C, 20.5g F Take vitamin, mineral, ergogenic supplements
3 pancakes, buttermilk, Hungry Jack, prepared, 200 cals, 6 P, 28g C, 7g F 2 oz ham, fresh, trimmed, 78 cals, 12g P, 0g C, 3g F 12 oz vegetable juice (V8), 70 cals, 2g P, 16g C, 0g F 2 tbsp pancake syrup (Hungry Jack), lite, 50 cals, 0g P, 14g C, 0g F 1/2 tbsp butter, 50 cals, 0g P, 0g C, 5.5g F	3 pancakes, buttermilk, Hungry Jack, prepared, 200 cals, 6 P, 28g C, 7g F 3 oz ham, fresh, trimmed, 117 cals, 18g P, 0g C, 4.5g F 12 oz vegetable juice (V8), 70 cals, 2g P, 16g C, 0g F 4 tbsp pancake syrup (Hungry Jack), lite, 100 cals, 0g P, 25g C, 0g F 2/3 tbsp butter, 81 cals, 0g P, 0g C, 9g F
Morning Snack	Morning Snack
1 Nutrition Bar approximately 230 cals, 10g P, 45g C, 2.5g F; Tiger's Milk, Fi-Bar, or Sports Meal	1 Nutrition Bar approximately 440 cals, 16g P, 68g C, 12g F; Tiger's Milk, Fi-Bar, or Sports Meal

2,500 CALORIES PER DAY	3,500 CALORIES PER DAY
Lunch	**Lunch**
Meal goal: 464 cals, 20g P, 58.5g C, 16.5g F	Meal goal: 590.5 Cals, 24g P, 77.5g C, 20.5g F
Take vitamin, mineral, ergogenic supplements	Take vitamin, mineral, ergogenic supplements
1 oz American cheese, 110 cals, 6g P, 1g C, 9g F	1 oz American cheese, 110 cals, 6g P, 1g C, 9g F
1 sandwich roll, 123 cals, 4.5g P, 21.6g C, 3.3g F	1 sandwich roll, 123 cals, 4.5g P, 21.6g C, 3.3g F
2 slices turkey (Tyson), 40 cals, 8g P, 0.6g C, 0.8g F	3 slices turkey (Tyson), 60 cals, 10g P, 0.6g C, 1.2g F
2 oz iceberg lettuce, trimmed, 8 cals, 0.6g P, 1.2g C, 0.2g F	2 oz iceburg lettuce, trimmed, 8 cals, 0.6g P, 1.2g C, 0.2g F
2 tbsp mustard, 32 cals, 2g P, 2g C, 2g F	2 tbsp mustard, 32 cals, 2g P, 2g C, 2g F
2 oz apricot, dried (Del Monte), 140 cals, 2g P, 35g C, 0g F	2 oz apricot, dried (Del Monte), 140 cals, 2g P, 35g C, 0g F
	1/3 tbsp safflower oil, 40 cals, 0g P, 0g C, 4.5g F
	6 oz grapefruit juice, 60 cals, 0g P, 15g C, 0g F
Pre-Training Snack	**Pre-Training Snack**
2 1/2 hours before training	2 1/2 hours before training
1 Nutrition bar approximately 270 cals, 12g P, 45g C, 6g F; Tiger's Milk, Fi-Bar, or Sports Meal	Protein drink, high calorie, approximately 548 cals, 30g P, 80g C, 12g F
Then	**Then**
BCAAs supplement 30 minutes before workout, with water	BCAAs supplement 30 minutes before workout, with water
Carbohydrate sports drink during workout, high calorie, 16 oz, 300 cals, 0g P, 100g C, 0g F	Carbohydrate sports drink during workout, high calorie, 20 oz, 400 cals, 0g P, 125g C, 0g F
Dinner	**Dinner**
Meal goal: 743 cals, 32g P, 93g C, 27g F	Meal goal: 924 cals, 37g P, 122g C, 32g F
Take vitamin, mineral, ergogenic supplements	Take vitamin, mineral, ergogenic supplements
3 oz tuna, bluefin, 123 cals, 19.8g P, 0g C, 4.2g F	3 oz tuna, bluefin, 123 cals, 19.8g P, 0g C, 4.2g F

2,500 CALORIES PER DAY	3,500 CALORIES PER DAY
Dinner *(continued)*	Dinner *(continued)*
1 tomato, 4.75 oz, 26 cals, 1g P, 5.7g C, 0.4g F	1 tomato, 4.75 oz, 26 cals, 1g P, 5.7g C, 0.4g F
4 oz iceberg lettuce, trimmed, 16 cals, 1.2g P, 2.4g C, 0.4g F	4 oz iceberg lettuce, trimmed, 16 cals, 1.2g P, 2.4g C, 0.4g F
2 oz onion, trimmed, 22 cals, 0.6g P, 4.8g C, 0.2g F	2 oz onion, trimmed, 22 cals, 0.6g P, 4.8g C, 0.2g F
3 oz brown rice, 309 cals, 6.9g P, 66g C, 3g F	4 oz brown rice, 412 cals, 9.2g P, 88g C, 4g F
6 oz cauliflower, 42 cals, 2.4g P, 8.4g C, 0.6g F	6 oz cauliflower, 42 cals, 2.4g P, 8.4g C, 0.6g F
4 tsp salad dressing (Seven Seas), oil and vinegar, 180 cals, 0g P, 4g C, 16g F	5 tsp salad dressing (Seven Seas), oil & vinegar, 225 cals, 0g P, 5g C, 20g F
Optional Evening Snack—nutrition bar or protein shake	Optional Evening Snack—nutrition bar or protein shake

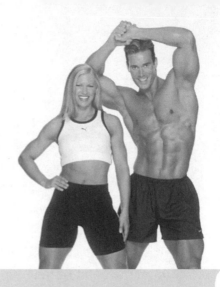

Fat Loss and Body Weight Maintenance

9

ou may be surprised to find that the topic of fat loss and body weight maintenance comes so late in *The Edge*. After all, deep down inside we all want to be trim. But so often the quest to be thin outweighs common sense and most people go on severely reduced-calorie diets, characterized by unbalanced nutrition that has a negative impact on overall health. We purposely focus first on building a strong healthy body, using good nutrition habits and effective weight-lifting technique. Now that you have a foundation, you can use the information in this chapter if weight loss really is a concern.

You will be pleased to know that in our experience, just following the exercise and nutrition guidelines presented in the previous chapters will start to trim down the unwanted body fat and shape your physique. But this chapter will provide additional guidelines if losing excess body fat is your primary goal. In your battle of the bulge, the most important ammunition is establishing and maintaining proper eating habits, appetite control, and regular exercise. While it is true that exercise and certain supplements can help with appetite control and improve and maintain a vigorous metabolism, a proper eating plan must be the foundation.

People are usually overweight because they eat the wrong foods and eat too many of them. Poor daily and weekly eating patterns are also major contributors to being overweight. Many people binge eat, or they skip meals during the day only to overeat at night. Others do okay during the week but live it up with the all-you-can-eat weekend buffet. Overeating at any meal conditions your body to store the excess calories as fat. That is why it is crucial to exercise your willpower at every meal and during snack time. Adopt the grazing mentality and eat a smaller number of calories at each meal, which you will use up for energy rather than store as body fat. As you age, you'll need to work harder because your body burns fewer calories and your metabolic rate slows. But by incorporating the nutrition, supplements, and exercise programs in this book into your life, you can rev up your metabolism and turn your body into a fat-burning machine, instead of a fat-storing machine.

WHY FAD DIETS DON'T WORK

With thousands of foods to choose from, you can easily see how fad diets take hold of people with different food combinations and dieting angles. But upon close examination, many of these trendy diets are deficient in important essential nutrients. Most of them do not provide adequate nutrition and are not meant for individuals who are on a fitness or athletic training program because they are often too low in protein or carbohydrates, and some of them are even too high in fat. They can also leave the dieter in a poor state of health, with a damaged metabolism from a deficit intake of one or more essential nutrients.

Typically the weight lost on fad diets consists of water weight and muscle mass, not just fat. This is where a major problem exists; loss of muscle mass reduces your body's ability to burn calories. So after the dieter has lost weight, his or her body now has a lower capacity to burn calories. As most dieters soon return to their old eating habits, they tend to gain more weight as body fat, and can end up having a higher percentage of body fat, even if they do not return to their previous weight. After dieters take their bodies through a few cycles of fad diets, many of them have a hard time losing weight the second, third, or fourth time around.

CALORIE ECONOMICS

One of the key aspects of body-fat reduction is effective calorie reduction. If you reduce your caloric intake too much, then you will also start to lose muscle mass and water weight. This is exactly what you don't want. A simple way to start is to reduce your caloric intake by about 20 percent of the amount of food you eat to maintain body weight. This will result in a steady rate of fat loss of one to a few pounds a week. A faster rate of fat loss is possible but usually results in a significant loss of muscle mass. This is counterproductive. It will leave dieters with a reduced lean body mass and reduce their ability to burn calories.

In the most recent surveys of people who have successfully lost weight and kept it off for more than five years, women eat less than 1,400 calories on average, and men less than 1,700 calories. If you exercise regularly, your daily caloric rate will need to be higher than this. If you need to fuel performance but still want to reduce calories, you need to increase your dietary fiber intake and keep those high-fat, high-calorie foods out of your house so you won't be tempted to eat them all up in a binge. Stock up on high-volume, low-calorie foods, such as vegetables, where a pound only contains about 160 calories and plenty of fiber.

PUT PROTEIN FIRST

Never cut calories from the protein portion of the food you eat. Lean protein should be the heart of every meal, thus ensuring you get enough to maintain muscle. If you are already following a healthy nutrition plan, then you have already taken care of reducing your possible overconsumption of total fat and saturated fats. You know what's coming next—watch those carbohydrates! Begin with a 20-percent re-duction in carbs to see how your body responds. If you need to reduce further, slowly work your way to a maximum 30-percent reduction. Double-check to make sure that you are not overconsuming fats and oils. One tablespoon of oil adds about 120 calories to your diet.

EATING, DAY AND NIGHT

We all burn calories better during the day, as our metabolic rate slows down at night. It makes sense, then, to control your food intake at dinner and try to elimi-nate the after-dinner snack. This also means cutting back on the amount of com-plex carbohydrates (from pasta, bread, and rice) that you eat in the evening. Many people who are overweight develop a condition that the medical community refers to as insulin resistance. Insulin is the hormone in your body that is needed to stim-ulate the passage of nutrients from the blood stream into your cells. When you are insulin resistant, your body does not do this job efficiently, and many of the nutrients you eat, especially the ones from carbohydrates, end up back to the liver, where they are converted to fat. If you find that your rate of weight loss is slow, instead of reducing the calories even further, try cutting back on your daily servings of carbohydrate foods for a week or two. Substitute a vegetable serving in place of a grain/bread/cereal/rice serving, especially in the evenings. This, along with a regular exercise program, can improve your insulin resistance condition in a few weeks, assuming you are otherwise healthy and do not have any serious medical conditions, like diabetes.

Remember that eating out does not mean pigging out; the calories are not free. Too many people with weight problems simply blow it when they eat out. They stick to their eating plan, lose weight, then chose to reward themselves with a fat-laden, calorie-rich feast. This makes no sense at all. If you have a problem with weight maintenance, you need to stick to your eating plan all the time. Yes you can eat out in fancy restaurants. But you can't eat all the rolls, salad with cream dressing, appetizers, entree, and dessert, and expect to stay trim. Create a new strategy when eating out.

A little advance meal planning can really add to your weight-loss success. If you plan your eating, then you increase your chances of sticking to your plan and not throwing meals together in a last-minute frenzy to satisfy your hunger. You

---

BEWARE OF PERFORMANCE TRADE-OFFS

Any time you go on a body-fat reducing plan, chances are that your physical performance will suffer. Most often, from total calorie reduction and carbohydrate reduction, you will reduce the carbohydrate stored in your body in the form of muscle glycogen. When you do this, your ability to do physical work is reduced. If you are athletic, we suggest trying only a 10-percent reduction in calories from carbohydrates. At this level, you may still be able to sustain your capacity to do physical work. However, if you are a competitive athlete who needs to maintain maximum physical performance, then reduction of body fat is best performed during the off-season or early pre-season. In the case of bodybuilding, getting lean for a contest is part of the sport, so this is an exception to the rule.

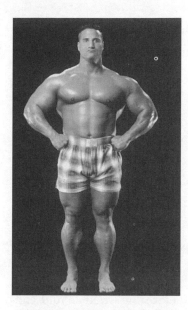
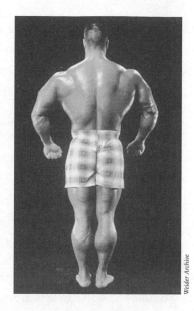

Before photos of bodybuilding champion Mike Matarazzo

Weider Archive

These before and after photos of professional bodybuilding champion Mike Matarazzo illustrate how using training and nutrition can be used to develop a massive physique and significantly reduce body-fat composition. In the before photos, Mike's body fat is ideal by most standards. However, to prepare for a bodybuilding competition, an important part of his contest training includes reducing body-fat mass to much lower levels to reveal fine details of his muscle development. Of course athletes and fitness enthusiasts do not need to reduce their body fat to the same low levels that competitive bodybuilders do. Keep in mind that bodybuilders are fantastic athletes, but physical performance is not a primary factor for their competitions, and achieving and maintaining such low body-fat levels places demands on the energy systems that would significantly reduce athletic performance in other sports. However, just as we turned to our bodybuilding experience to discover muscle-building insights, working with bodybuilders during their contest preparation phase has revealed important information about reducing body-fat levels with nutrition and dietary supplements while maintaining muscle mass. We then incorporate these findings into the weight-loss plans to lose body fat as fast as possible while building and maintaining muscle mass.

After photos of bodybuilding champion Mike Matarazzo

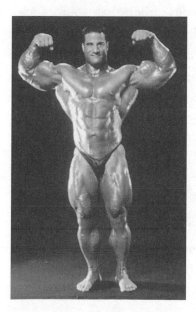
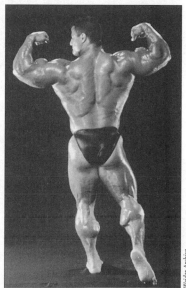

Weider Archive

should eat three small meals and two or three snacks each day. Write out your menus for the day and week ahead. Have a healthy snack in your car for the times when you are on the run, such as a sports nutrition bar. This is a much better alternative than pulling into a fast-food restaurant where you will end up eating over 1,000 fat-laden calories. Be prepared, plan ahead.

Here are some simple steps for creating a personalized body-fat reduction plan.

1. **Take inventory of your food consumption.** Using the Food Log in Appendix B, start to write down everything you drink and eat every day. This is not a test, so don't worry about including foods that you might not want to admit you eat. The purpose is to examine your eating patterns.

2. **Evaluate and modify your eating patterns.** Make sure that your calorie intake is what it should be. Make an attempt to determine whether your consumption of protein, carbohydrates, and fats is within the proper ranges. Make a shift from eating fast foods and junk foods to eating more healthy whole foods. Put whole-grain foods, lean protein sources, vegetables, low- and non-fat dairy, and fruit on the top of your food list. If you are in the habit of skipping meals, make an effort to spread your food intake out over five to seven smaller meals and snacks per day. If you find that you are eating a lot of sweets, try eating some low-calorie vegetables first to fill up on, then only a few bites of your favorite sweet.

3. **Eat more fibrous carbohydrate sources,** such as beans, whole-grain rice and pasta, boiled potatoes, oatmeal, and the like. Reduce your consumption of processed grains, such as white-flour-based food, and white rice. Increasing fiber and complex carbohydrates will result in improved appetite control, better maintenance of blood-sugar levels, sustained energy levels, and reduced cravings for sweets.

4. **Increase your aerobic exercise.** While you should maintain your weight-training schedule, increasing the amount of aerobic exercise will help your body build more fat-burning enzymes and increase its fat-burning rate.

5. **Cycle your fat loss with periods of weight maintenance.** As you lose body fat, your body sends chemical messages to its control center that body weight is being lost. The body may respond by slowing your metabolism down in an

effort to put the brakes on weight loss. Exercise will help prevent this, as will maintaining an adequate intake of protein, carbohydrates, and fats. However, just as people plateau when building muscle mass, they often reach a plateau when losing weight. If this happens to you, then return to a weight-maintenance diet (where calorie intake is balanced with daily caloric expenditure) for a week before returning to the reduced-calorie diet. This process will keep your metabolism active.

6. **Use nutritional supplement fat-loss aids.** Numerous scientific studies have been conducted on losing body fat. Many of these weight-loss studies have found that certain dietary supplements can be used to help control your appetite and increase your rate of losing body fat. But keep in mind that what we have found works best is to follow the Dynatrition plan, use your regular nutritional supplements, engage in regular exercise, and follow the fat-loss tips mentioned above. If you still find that you are having trouble losing body fat, then start to include some of the weight-loss supplements into your program.

   The best supplements to start with are high-quality protein meal-replacement drinks and nutrition-bar meal replacements. These drinks are packed with protein and other essential nutrients, and are low in fat. There is a wide range of these protein meal-replacement drinks to suit your nutritional needs and budget. Some are high in carbohydrates, while others are lower in carbohydrates. During your weight-loss program, we recommend that you try using protein meal replacements that are lower in carbohydrates and total calories. Some types are also especially designed to include other fat-burning nutrients, discussed below. Start using a protein meal-replacement to substitute a meal that you may be skipping, or a meal when you tend to overeat, or as a nutritious snack. You can also use meal-replacement nutrition bars in a similar manner. However, make sure you read the labels and check that the sugar and saturated fat content is not too high. They should be high in protein and low in calories—120 to 320 calories per bar. If a brand you like is high in protein and low in carbohydrates and fats, but high in calories because it is a large bar, then just eat a third or half of it at a time.

   There are many supplements that help improve your body's metabolic rate. Even some simple vitamins and minerals will help. Chromium is a trace mineral which has been shown to assist insulin in moving nutrients into your cells instead of being stored as excess body fat. Insulin is the hormone that signals cells to let in nutrients that are circulating around the bloodstream after a meal. Getting adequate chromium will allow insulin to function at full capacity. This means getting more nutrients into your cells, where they can be used for energy and growth, instead of being circulated back to the liver and converted to fat.

Natural appetite suppressants are leading the category of weight-loss supplements. A relative newcomer, 5-HTP, which is used primarily to ease anxiety, also helps with appetite control. An amino acid called L-phenylalanine is also reported to help reduce cravings and appetite. Next on the list is Garcinia camobgia, also called Brindall berry. This botanical can help control appetite and may also block the formation of fat from carbohydrates in the liver.

Then there is the group of supplements sold under the heading of lipotropics and fat metabolizers. These diet supplements contain ingredients that help stimulate the body to use more fat for energy. Recent clinical studies revealed that along with diet and exercise, taking L-carnitine supplements resulted in losing more fat than was lost from diet and exercise alone. L-carnitine has also been shown to help the rate of fat loss in some people. When fatty acids enter the cell, carnitine carries them into a special cellular structure where fats are used to make energy. In this way, supplemental amounts of carnitine help stimulate your fat-burning metabolism, and you lose fat at a faster rate. Other fat-fighting nutrients to look for include choline, inositol, and L-methionine.

Supplement companies also offer botanical diuretics to help reduce excess water weight. Traditionally, diuretics are used in the treatment of menstrual distress, edema, and hypertension. Dieters have also turned to diuretics to help reduce edema and the bloated feelings common to being overweight. As a result of this, you can find on the shelves weight-loss aid supplements containing botanical diuretics, such as uva ursi, buchu, cornsilk, juniper berry, and hydrangea. We don't advocate the use of these types of supplements unless under a doctor's supervision. While it is satisfying to see quick results on the scale, remember that much of the weight lost is from water and will return as fast as you lost it.

Fiber and fat-absorbing supplements are a better weight-loss aid category. Eating more fibrous foods, such as non-starchy vegetables, and taking fiber supplements, like psyllium, guar gum, and citrus pectin, will help improve your digestion and appetite control. Studies have shown that a special "marine fiber" concentrate called chitosan can help absorb and lock on to ingested fats, thereby keeping some of them from entering your body. Nutritionists have concluded that as you increase your fiber intake, you decrease the amount of calories absorbed into the body. This is true for all kinds of diets. So, increase fiber intake.

The last major weight-loss aid supplement category has been the subject of controversy in the media and by the FDA for several years. This category includes the so-called "thermogenic aids." Just as exercise will boost your calorie-burning rate, so can some of the foods and botanical supplements you eat. Thermogenic supplements stimulate your body to burn up more fatty acids, increasing your metabolic rate. Many people also experience improved appetite control. They include guarana, ginseng, mustard seed, cinnamon, and cayenne. These are considered the safe thermogenic aids. Then there is the champion of thermogenic aids, ephedra, which is widely sold and used by millions. Use of ephedra supplements has attracted much controversy. But in spite of this, it is one of the best-selling weight-loss supplements. In fact, during the writing of this book, a major scientific study was released on the weight-loss benefits of ephedrine-caffeine combination products. A joint research project conducted by Columbia University and Harvard University found effectiveness for fat loss, with slight side effects. Use caution, however, because there are special concerns and potential harmful side effects for some people when using supplements containing ephedra—especially for people with any disease condition or who are on medication, inactive people, obese people, and young adults and children.

When losing weight, remember these important guidelines:

- Do so under a doctor's supervision.

- Do not overeat.

- Do not skip meals.

- Spread your calories over five to seven meals and snacks.

- Follow a nutritionally balanced, low-fat diet.

- Exercise regularly.

- Take your nutrition supplements.

- Maintain a healthy rate of weight loss—one to three pounds per week.

- Eliminate foods you are allergic to.

- Have fun. Eating less is not more work, but it can be less expensive!

SUMMARY OF WEIGHT-LOSS NUTRITION AND DIETARY SUPPLEMENT PRODUCTS

These diet aids will help you stick to a reduced-calorie diet, or increase the amount of fat lost while on a calorie-restricted diet. Always consult your doctor prior to starting a weight-loss program, and to help you monitor your progress.

Supplement	Daily Dosages	Comments
Multivitamin/mineral supplements, essential fatty acids	See chapters 11 and 12	
High-protein meal replacements and nutrition bars	At least 15 grams of protein per serving	Choose brands that are low-fat, low-carbohydrate, and 120 to 220 calories per serving.
L-carnitine 5-HTP Garcinia	1g to 3g 50 mg to 100 mg 500 mg to 750 mg, three times a day with meals.	Helps to burn more fat Helps control appetite Helps control appetite and slows the conversion of carbohydrates to fats in the liver
Extra chromium Fiber supplements L-tyrosine	400 mcg to 600 mcg 5g to 20g 500 mg to 1,500 mg	Take with meals Helps with appetite control

Summary of Weight-Loss Nutrition and Dietary Supplement Products

Supplement	Daily Dosages	Comments
L-phenylalanine	500 mg to 1,500 mg	Helps with appetite control
Chitosan	Use as directed with meals	Helps absorb fat in the digestive system
CLA (Conjugated Linoleic Acid) Caffeine-containing thermogenic aids	1g to 2g Use as directed by manufacturer	Reported to reduce fat accumulation Helps increase your metabolic rate (increases the calories you burn)
Ephedrine-containing thermogenic aids	Use as directed by manufacturer	Helps increase your metabolic rate (increases the calories you burn). Check with your doctor first. Side effects are possible.
7-KETO	50 mg to 200 mg	A new compound shown to aid in weight loss by stimulating thermogenesis without stimulant side effects

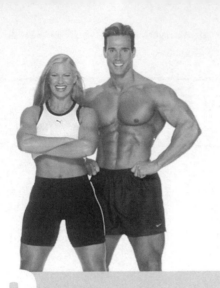

10

Technique and Skill: Mastering Performance Fitness

Now that you know enough about proper nutrition and weight-training methods for peak performance to fill your own book, let's not forget the third side of the Weider Triangle—technique or skill. Good technique is acquired by perfecting the things that affect your health and performance and applying them to all areas of your training. Luckily, skill training has progressed significantly over the last several decades. It is easy to see this when you compare old news-reel footage of sporting events filmed in the early 1900s with the athletes of today. There have been no genetic changes in the human body during this period, so the factors causing these significant improvements clearly stem from nutrition, weight training, and mastering technique.

This is a short chapter to help you become a master of your game and achieve your performance goals. After a lifetime committed to the bodybuilding lifestyle, we know the key to turning a dream into a reality is perseverance and belief in your goals. Perseverance and confidence will win the day.

SELECTING THE SPORT AND FITNESS
ACTIVITY THAT IS RIGHT FOR YOU

Aside from being optimistic, you must also be open-minded and realistic, especially when it comes to competitive sports. Genetics play an important part in deciding just what sport can best benefit a particular aspiring athlete. Body size is an obvious variable you have some control over. Champion weight lifters and football players used to be big and fat. Now to be a champion in these sports you still have to be big, but big and muscular. Overly fat bodies have little chance at today's standards of peak performance. But given the basic size, with correct coaching in modern nutrition, weight training, and advanced skill training, the overly fat body can be transformed into a sleek, functional physique.

Scientific discoveries have also led us to understand how genetic variables much less obvious than size can affect your potential for peak performance in a particular sport. Muscle-fiber types is one example. People who are born with a preponderance of slow-twitch muscle fibers will be able to do better in long-distance sports. People with more fast-twitch muscle fibers tend to be better suited for power sports. Agility is another trait that comes in many ranges. So, working with your coach, you need to decide if the sport you have picked is best for you.

DEVELOPING TO YOUR POTENTIAL

While it is true that size and your physiology may be bound by certain genetic limitations, there is more to winning than just genetics. Between two individuals of equal size and strength, the one with better skills, motivation, focus, and competitive awareness will prevail. Motivation and a positive attitude are extremely important. After you set your goals and develop strategies to attain them, then being positive and staying motivated will be the forces that complete your drive for success. Another key characteristic to develop is patience. You may want to lose in 10 days the weight it took 10 years to gain. Be realistic and patient. You may want to build a body like Mr. Olympia's, but want to do it over the summer. Be realistic and patient. The problem with most people is that they give up on their goals if it starts taking too much time to achieve them. Well, let us be very direct on this point: When you give up on your goals you give up on yourself. Champions don't give up.

MASTERING TECHNIQUE

Building the strength, speed, stamina, and endurance of your muscles to match your sport-specific needs will always help you apply greater functional force, whether to an object, an opponent, or the ground. This is a major reason for improving strength using weight training. Therefore, sport-specific weight training is a skill you must master in order to develop the muscles that will work best for execution of your athletic performance. Once you have used weight training to develop functional muscles, training to make them work together to enhance your sport is vital. In order to train your muscles to be activated or inhibited in the proper sequence, which involves accurately judging such factors as position, direction, timing, rate, speed, and effect of force application, it takes practice. Neuromuscular training is a key to developing your motion skills.

For many sports this means performing movements over and over again until they become instinctive, like a reflex. This is where a good coach comes in. But with all this said, you must begin to think long term, and plan out each year for maximum improvements. During the past three decades a sophisticated athletic-training planning method was developed to help accomplish this. It is called periodization, and as you will discover below, it helps to focus your skill-building efforts during different seasons of the year, culminating in attaining the best sports technique possible in that year during your competition season.

If your goal is to become the best athlete you can be, you must skill train all year long. With periodization, the year is divided into phases or seasons called *macrocycles,* with specific training goals set for each period of training. Four macrocycles are usually used, with each one lasting one to four months. Often, the macrocycles are further divided into *mesocycles,* which are several weeks long, and *microcycles,* which are several days long. Your specific sport, your skills, and your goals will determine how your year should be divided.

In general, a periodized training program includes the following:

Macrocycle I. Developmental phase, four months long.

The training focus of this macrocycle should be on developing skills, defining physical-performance parameters, adjusting body composition, and improving weaknesses as well as strengths. The training intensity should be moderate, and this is a good time to increase your muscle mass and reduce your body fat.

Macrocycle II. Preparation phase, three months long.

This macrocycle immediately preceeds the competitive season. The training focus should be on making final adjustments to body composition (preferably early in the macrocycle) and honing skills. The training intensity should go from moderate to high over the course of the macrocycle. Perform repetitions in a rhythmic fashion, and avoid going to negative failure. The emphasis is building speed of muscle movement and strength. Make any final adjustments to your body weight early in this macrocycle to avoid the need for weight-loss dieting during the competitive phase, which will reduce your athletic performance.

Macrocycle III. Competition phase, four months long.

This is the macrocycle during which all the attention to training and good nutrition pays off. The training focus should be on improving skills and physical performance factors that were found to be lacking after the first few competitions. The training intensity should remain very high throughout the macrocycle. Only perform weight training as directed or approved by your coach and trainer.

Macrocycle IV. Recovery phase, one month long.

The goal of this macrocycle is to maintain fitness and flexibility. The training focus should be on healing injuries using professionally supervised therapeutic and nutrition programs. The training intensity should be low. During this macrocycle, plans for the following year's Macrocycle I should be made with input from the coach, trainer, and team physician.

If your season runs longer or shorter than the typical four months used in this example, adjust your schedule by modifying macrocycles I and IV. Do not change Macrocycle II, which should always be three months long for the best results.

A year-round training program will help you make steady progress toward your ultimate performance goals. The top athletes in the world train year-round to be their best. If being the best is your goal, find a good coach to help you construct a periodized training program appropriate for your sport, skills, and goals.

COACHING SUPPORT

A good coach should also be a good mentor—someone who will invest time in answering your questions and work with you to develop an annual plan to improve your sports performance. To hone your skills, find the best coach that you can. This may mean traveling to sports camps, but when you have the right coaching, it will make all the difference in your athletic career. In the off-season, join a local sports club to maintain your physical conditioning. Read every book you can on your sport, as well as biographies of champion athletes and coaches. If you approach your athletic career with realistic expectations and follow a methodical approach, you will soon be on the road to achieving sports excellence.

HEALTH-PROFESSIONAL SUPPORT

Health-professional support is very important for peak athletic performance. Follow-up visits to a doctor, chiropractic adjustments, and prescription medications are sometimes indicated for athletes in heavy training who have come down with a medical problem. Only qualified sports-medicine specialists should prescribe such support. Do not hesitate to seek a second opinion if you are not satisfied with a diagnosis or course of treatment prescribed by one doctor. If you have a serious injury, seek the advice of a sports doctor who specializes in your particular injury. Sports medicine is a highly diversified and complex field.

Preventive medicine is also important. More and more research supports the practice of visiting your doctor on a regular basis to keep track of your state of health. In addition, you should also regularly visit a chiropractor and masseuse as part of your preventive program. Keep good records of everything you do. Whirlpools, electrical muscle stimulation, massage, ultrasound, intense light, and a host of other therapeutic modalities can have a very positive effect on your training efforts, both directly (the degree of your force output) and indirectly (how quickly you recover from your workout). In other words, pamper yourself. Use these therapeutic modalities to your advantage. When you are hurt, tend to your injury immediately. Utilize all the medical and therapeutic help that you can. There is nothing macho about letting your injuries go unattended. It is much smarter to deal with an injury when it occurs than to suffer with the consequences when it heals incorrectly. Better yet, make your preferred therapeutic modalities a part of your preventive program. Taking time during training for injury prevention may seem bothersome, but it will pay off in the long term.

KEEPING A JOURNAL

Keeping a daily nutrition and training log book is vital to your success. While this is mandatory for athletes, it is also beneficial for nonathletes following the WTM. To assist you in this endeavor, pages 345 through 348 contain log-book templates for you to photocopy and use daily. Create a training and nutrition loose-leaf notebook, where you can also collect articles on training and nutrition for your reference. Don't just write in your book without glancing back through the pages and charting your improvements. Evaluation of how your body composition and performance respond to your nutrition and training programs is vital to continued success.

PSYCHOLOGICAL TECHNIQUES

Self-hypnosis, mental imagery, meditation, visualization, and a number of other "mind strategies" can help you improve your strength and performance in competition and training. They can help you develop a mental edge and a winning mind-set.

Until recently, the powers of the human mind were generally overlooked by our society. Other cultures also place limitations on individuals and restrict their mental potential. The human mind has the capacity to store trillions of bits of information, more than the most powerful computers. In fact, according to one progressive educational authority, the human brain has a greater storage capacity than the U.S. National Archives. Sadly, however, most people utilize only a small percentage of their mind's capacity.

When you start to understand what you can do with your mind, you can begin to open your mind to new thoughts and information and expand its utilization. Your mind is more than just a storehouse for knowledge. Your mind also regulates your emotions, your ego, your physical abilities, and your overall vim and vigor. Some medical research suggests that the mind even has the ability to heal the body.

For athletes, the mind is a powerful piece of sports equipment. Knowing how to maximize and control your internal forces can offer you a big advantage in sports and life. Most athletes practice some kind of mental technique, even if it is just "psyching themselves up" before a competition. Among the more popular techniques practiced by athletes are meditation and visualization.

MEDITATION

Meditation has been practiced since the beginning of recorded history. However, while the Asian societies and primitive cultures of the world have held onto the practice of meditation as a way of life and health, Western society parted ways with meditation many years ago. Luckily, Westerners are now once again beginning to realize the importance of meditation. In its most fundamental sense, meditation is a technique in which you elevate your state of mind above the conscious to the un-conscious. In other words, you clear your mind of all conscious thoughts and enter an altered state of consciousness, a state of relaxation and mental imagery.

Many practitioners look at the anatomical divisions of the brain and ascribe the power to meditate to the right hemisphere. In the contemporary model of the brain, the mind's logical functions (such as speaking, writing, calculating, and worrying) take place in the left hemisphere, while the more creative, visually ori-entated operations take place in the right hemisphere. Although this simple model of the human brain is constantly being updated and revised, of practical interest to us here is that even modern science recognizes the function and power of the cre-ative right hemisphere. To put it in more practical terms, most people tend to func-tion from the left hemisphere, always preoccupied with jealousy, insecurity, anger, and other negative thoughts that adversely affect their overall state of health and well-being. By meditating, you can open up and develop your powerful creative mind and use techniques such as visualization to help improve your athletic per-formance and health.

If you are interested in trying meditation, seek the guidance of a trained pro-fessional. In addition, read through the following guidelines:

- Plan to meditate at a time of day when you can relax and when you are not under the influence of a mood-altering substance such as alcohol, a medication, or a recent meal.

- Find a quiet place away from distractions. Turn off the phone and create a comfortable, relaxing environment.

- Turn down the lights and sit in a comfortable position. If you wish, meditate in the dark while lying down.

- To meditate, first clear your thoughts. If you have trouble, try repeating the same word to yourself or focusing, with your eyes closed, on a bright object that you picture in your mind. Even beginners will find themselves slipping in and out of the meditative state. Your goal is the state between consciousness and unconsciousness, the point where the conscious and unconscious meet.

- Work up to meditation sessions lasting thirty to sixty minutes.

Whatever the exact physiological condition is that your body enters into during meditation, one thing is certain—when you are done meditating, you will feel relaxed, refreshed, and renewed. And each time you meditate, the benefits will accrue. You will eventually find your general state of mind to be more controlled and less stressful. Meditation, therefore, is an important stepping stone in the path to total empowerment. When you learn to control your thoughts and emotions, you will be on your way to mastering your sport and defeating your opponents. You will be on your way to success in life.

VISUALIZATION

Visualization is the technique of using mental imagery to picture yourself accomplishing a stated purpose. It is almost like daydreaming, but more intense. You can practice it as part of your meditation, or you can use it to help reach the meditative state.

Before you begin a visualization session, you must state your purpose. For example, your purpose may be to master a certain move or to prepare yourself mentally for a competition. Once you have stated your purpose, you must set your stage—that is, you must establish your setting and point of view before you bring on the "players." Then begin the visualization, running a picture of yourself accomplishing your purpose over and over again in your mind. Visualize everything—all the sights, sounds, smells, and feelings. If you are preparing for a contest, visualize the specific moves you will use to defeat your opponent. Visualize everything you anticipate happening.

Visualization can be a powerful tool. Practice it on a weekly basis, for about 30 to 60 minutes per session. Increase your sessions to once a day during the week before an event.

PUTTING THE PERFORMANCE-FITNESS TRIANGLE ALL TOGETHER

Now you have a thorough understanding of the three sides of the Weider Triangle Method for Peak Performance-Fitness: Dynatrition, Variable Weight Training, and Technique. To cover each exhaustively would take several volumes. However, you can keep advancing your knowledge on the latest discoveries in bodybuilding and sports nutrition by reading one of our monthly magazines that suits your athletic and personal fitness goals the best, or visit our health and fitness websites daily for the most up-to-date information.

You have learned how sound nutrition integrated with training is essential to build strength, muscle, energy and endurance. You have also learned how new advances in nutrient supplementation are helping athletes and fitness exercisers take maximum advantage of their skill training and weight training by extending training times, decreasing muscle fatigue, and increasing energy levels by providing the optimum micronutrient environment for the growth of muscle and strength. Finally, you have seen how the Weider Triangle Method integrates the three components so that the right skill combines with the right bodybuilding and the right nutrition to produce champions. Now all that's missing is you.

For updated information on fitness and nutrition topics you can refer to the following websites:

www.fitnessonline
www.ifbb.com
www.supplementfacts.com
www.dynatrition.com

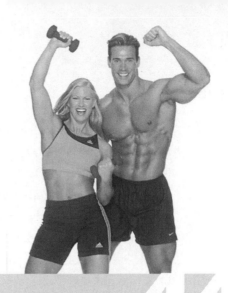

Nutritional
Supplement Review

S electing and using sports supplements can be a real chore these days, with so many products on the market. Chapters 6 and 7 provided some basic guidelines on the primary essential supplement nutrients to use: vitamins, minerals, fatty acids, and amino acids, for example. In addition to these, you will encounter a variety of other supplement ingredients, including metabolites—substances made by the body like creatine and carnitine—and a growing selection of botanical ingredients.

The following information will provide a short overview of the ingredients most often used in sports and fitness supplements. Dosage and use guidelines are provided for most of the ingredients. For essential vitamins and minerals, daily performance-fitness intake guidelines are provided. These represent common ranges of intake from food and supplements for most active and healthy male and female adults. Keep in mind that ideal dosages and ingredient usage will always depend on your individual condition of health and the advice of your health-care practitioner.

ALANINE

Alanine is found in high concentrations in most muscle tissue and is grouped with the nonessential amino acids because it can be manufactured by the body. Alanine is involved in an important biochemical process during exercise called the "glucose-alanine cycle." In the muscle, when glycogen stores are broken down to glucose and then to a three-carbon molecule called pyruvate, some of this pyruvate is used directly for energy by the muscles. However, pyruvate is converted to alanine, which is transported through the bloodstream and to the liver, where it is made back into glucose. This glucose is then transported back to the muscle and used for energy. The glucose-alanine cycle serves to conserve some of the energy in the form of carbohydrates through this recycling process. Sports physiologists believe that this helps maintain glucose levels during prolonged exercise. In this way, alanine may be useful in the same way as branched-chain amino acids—to help diminish muscle tissue breakdown during exercise and to spare the liver's glycogen.

ALKALINIZERS, BLOOD BUFFERS

Most of the research on blood buffers has centered on sodium bicarbonate (baking soda). Studies performed on sprinters, 800-meter racers, and world-class rowers have all shown improved performance among individuals who carry out repeated maximum workloads for durations ranging from seconds to several minutes. Large amounts of sodium bicarbonate are needed, however—about 0.1 g for every pound of lean body mass. For a person with 150 pounds of lean body mass, the amount would be approximately $150 \times 0.1 \text{ g} = 15 \text{ g}$. Most sodium bicabonate products recommend a maximum daily dosage of 4 g per day, as higher amounts may cause side effects such as diarrhea, nausea, cramps, or flatulence. Sodium bicarbonate can be taken on an empty stomach one hour before strenuous activity. If you find that you suffer gastrointestinal side effects, start two hours before your activity and take a quarter of the dosage with water every 15 minutes. Sodium bicarbonate loading will also load you up with a few grams of sodium, so use caution if you have blood-pressure problems or hypertension. To avoid injury to the gastrointestinal system, make sure the powder is completely dissolved, and do not take sodium bicarbonate when you are overly full. Do not take sodium bicarbonate for more than a few days at a time. Because sodium bicarbonate is considered an antacid, it may interact with other drugs. Consult your doctor immediately if gastrointestinal pain and discomfort persist.

ANDROSTENEDIONE

Androstenedione has gained attention and is widely used by strength-training athletes. Androstenedione is a male hormone, androgen. It is naturally produced by the body, and its function is to promote the characteristics that define masculinity: muscular build, deep voice, sex drive, and body hair. Androstenedione can be converted to either testosterone or estrone (an estrogen). This makes androstenedione a direct precursor of testosterone production. Testosterone can then go on to promote anabolic and androgenic functions, or it can be converted to another hormone called dihydrotestosterone. Too much dihydrotestosterone in the body is associated with causing male pattern baldness, abnormal prostate growth, and increase in body hair. It is important to realize that indiscriminate use of a hormone (pro-hormone) supplement may not be without undesireable side effects, in both men and women. Increased levels of testosterone sometimes results in the formation of another estrogen, estradiol, which has been shown to cause gynecomastia, activation and development of breast tissue in males. As far as the research is concerned, there are not compelling studies yet on the effect androstenedione supplementation has on body mass, strength, or performance. The study that is cited in many advertisements for androstenedione supplements was conducted on women, where a increase in testosterone levels was observed. One study does report an increase in testosterone levels in one male subject. Androstenedione can be converted to testosterone, but more research is needed to determine how much is the best dosage, what the side effects are, whether the increased testosterone occurs in healthy, active subjects, and whether the increased testosterone results in any body composition or performance effects. Products on the market typically contain daily dosages of 20 mg to 100 mg of androstenedione. Individuals using hormone supplements like androstenedione and DHEA should do so under the supervision of a physician, and get regular examinations and blood tests to monitor the effects. Some other compounds related to androsenedione that you may find used in supplements include: 19-Norandrostenediol, 19-Norandrostenedione, and 4-androstenediol.

ARGININE

Arginine is another nonessential amino acid that influences several metabolic factors important to athletes. Arginine is most well known for stimulating human growth hormone (somatotropin) release. Several studies have measured the ability of arginine, both alone and with other amino acids, to increase growth hormone levels in people taking supplemental arginine. Potential benefits of increased growth hormone levels include a reduction in body fat, improved healing and recovery, and increased muscle mass. Research has also been conducted on different forms of arginine, such as L-arginine-pyroglutamate combined with lysine hydrochloride. One study used 1,200 mg of each and reported significant elevation of growth hormone levels over either compound taken alone. This particular study has been criticized by other scientists unable to replicate its findings, however, so the safety of these concoctions has not yet been clearly determined. Nor have the exact benefits for athletes.

A second important function of arginine is its role as a precursor in creatine production. Creatine combines with phosphate and is an important energy source during high-intensity sports, like weight lifting and sprinting. Ingestion of 4 g per day of arginine and glycine was shown to cause a small increase in body creatine stores. This may help improve performance for power athletes. A third function of arginine that may benefit athletes is its role in ammonia detoxification. Arginine is an intermediate in the urea cycle. It converts ammonia to the waste product urea, which can then be excreted from the body. Ammonia is toxic, and levels increase with exercise. Scientists speculate that the potential ammonia-lowering effects of arginine may be beneficial to athletes. While more studies are needed to determine the exact effectiveness, safety level, and appropriate dosage of arginine, athletes may benefit from arginine supplementation due to its ability to reduce ammonia levels, increase growth hormone, and increase creatine. Arginine supplementation may be of special interest to athletes undergoing strenuous sports and training. Furthermore, arginine has been found to increase wound healing and immune system function.

BETA-ECDYSTERONE

Ecdysterone is of plant origin and is being touted as a phytochemical that may potentially enhance muscle-building. While the details of how beta-ecdysterone functions need to be worked out, initial research indicates that it can help improve nitrogen retention when consumed with protein.

BETA-HYDROXY BETA-METHYLBUTYRATE (BHMB)

BHMB (also just HMB) is one of the newer metabolite supplements to gain immediate popularity and use in weight-lifting and bodybuilding circles. It is being touted as an aid to muscle gain when used in association with a weight-lifting program. BHMB seems to be a breakdown product of the amino acid leucine and may play an important role in protein metabolism. Studies have reported that when BHMB is taken in supplemental amounts, it boosts nitrogen retention, thereby helping the body to retain more amino acids, which are necessary for muscle growth and repair. BHMB therefore may be useful for individuals training to increase or maintain muscle mass. According to studies, amounts ranging from 1,500 mg to 4,000 mg yield positive results.

BIOFLAVONOIDS

This is a group of naturally occurring plant compounds that improve vitamin C absorption. Bioflavonoids are part of a larger group of plant compounds called flavonoids. Flavonoids that influence the human body in some way are called bioflavonoids. There are thousands of them, and researchers are confirming the many benefits bioflavonoids have to offer in improving health and performance. They have been proven to strengthen capillary walls and thereby prevent capillary damage. Bioflavonoids may also have an anti-inflammatory effect and show anti-cataract activity. Bioflavonoids exhibit antioxidant activity and help maintain vitamin C potency. The major bioflavonoids found in supplements are rutin, hesperidin, citrus, quercetin, flavones, and flavonols. Quercetin has been studied for its ability to reduce inflammation as well as reducing LDL oxidation. Hesperidin also helps lower LDL and triglycerides and raise HDL (the good lipoproteins). Hesperidin also has anti-inflammatory and analgesic effects. Some new types of bioflavonoid ingredients appearing on the shelves in the late 1990s include epigallocatechin gallate in green tea, which prevents the oxidation of LDL cholesterol; soy flavonoids genistein and daidzein, which are powerful antioxidants and cancer inhibitors (lowering risks for breast and prostate cancer); anthocyanidins found in many plants; curcuminoids in turmeric, which exert anti-infammatory and antimicrobial effects; ginkgoflavon-glycosides, which improve blood flow to the brain; and silymarin, which acts as an antioxidant and helps protect the liver while boosting the immune response.

In general terms, bioflavonoids are the brightly colored chemical constituents found in most fresh fruit, vegetables, and herbs; for example, citrus fruits, grapes, plums, apricots, cherries, blackberries, rose hips, leaves, broccoli, greens, soy products, and grains. Ergogenic effects of bioflavonoids have not yet been tested, but the benefits listed above clearly make this group of plant compounds a must in your daily nutrition plan. Bioflavonoids have been noted to improve recovery and provide nutritional support for athletes recovering from injury. Daily recommended supplement amounts range from 200 mg to 2 g, depending on the product. Refer to manufacturer's instructions on dosages. Higher amounts are usually indicated when under the stress of intensive training or healing an injury.

BIOTIN

Biotin is a water-soluble vitamin of the B vitamin family. It is a sulfur-containing vitamin that is involved in energy metabolism, urea formation, protein synthesis, glucose formation, and fatty acid synthesis. Biotin is manufactured by intestinal bacteria. At this time, there are no reports on any ergogenic effects of biotin. Biotin plays an important role in energy production and fat metabolism. It functions in the biosynthesis of fatty acids, the replenishment of the tricarboxylic acid cycle, gluconeogenesis, and amino acid metabolism, and it acts as a coenzyme for a number of carboxylase enzymes. The performance-fitness intake guideline for men and women who are healthy and actively training is 125 mcg to 300 mcg per day. The 1989 adult estimated safe and adequate daily dietary intakes of biotin is 30 to 100 mcg. The RDI for biotin is 300 mcg. Use of biotin in amounts up to 10 mg (10,000 mcg) per day has been reported with no side effects observed.

BORON

Boron is an ultra-trace mineral, one which occurs in the body in small amounts. It has been established as an essential mineral in humans. Boron appears to have several functions, including influencing calcium, phosphorus, and magnesium metabolism; parathormone action; functionality of membranes; and bone formation. Recent attention by athletes has been directed toward boron as a result of its alleged role in increased testosterone production. In 1987, a study was published reporting increased testosterone levels in postmenopausal women. Translating this effect to younger adult males and females is speculative at best. One study in 1992 was conducted with bodybuilders taking 2.5 mg of boron per day for seven weeks. The subjects did not report any increases in testosterone levels, nor significant increases in lean body mass or strength over the placebo group. While further research is needed to determine boron's exact benefits for athletes, megadosing is not recommended or supported by the research.

Boron intake is required daily for health and performance, but like the other minerals, side effects can occur if too much boron is taken. The estimated safe intake range for boron in healthy adults is daily amounts up to 40 mg. Side effects of overconsumption have been observed with amounts ranging from 5 to 10 g and include nausea, vomiting, diarrhea, dermatitis, lethargy, nervous system irritability, renal failure, and shock. There are many supplements now being marketed containing high amounts of boron, some above 1 g, which should be avoided until further research determines if these high amounts of intake are indeed safe and effective. Boron trichelate is a preferred boron supplement form. The performance-fitness intake for men and women who are healthy and actively training is 6 to 12 mg per day from food and supplements.

BOSWELLIA (BOSWELLIA SERRATA)

Boswellia is an herb used in the traditional Ayurvedic medicine of India. Boswellic acid, one of the active phyto-nutrients found in Boswellia, exhibits anti-arthritic and anti-inflammatory properties. Boswellia is primarily used as a medicinal herb for its anti-inflammatory actions. Used in clinical studies, Boswellia extract has been shown to be effective in the treatment and management of osteoarthritis, rheumatoid arthritis, gout, low-back pain, myositis, fibrositis, and injury, and for the treatment of chronic inflammatory conditions. High-quality supplements contain standardized Boswellia serrata extract (40 to 65 percent Boswellic acids). Medical studies have shown that effective dosages of Boswellia are between 100 and 400 milligrams of standardized Boswellia per day. In clinical studies for treatment of arthritis and other severe conditions, 200 milligrams, taken 3 times per day for 4 weeks, produced improvements in the majority of subjects tested. Its use in the treatment and management of inflammatory diseases should be done under doctor supervision. In clinical studies, Boswellia has been shown to be safe and effective when used properly.

BRANCHED-CHAIN AMINO ACIDS (BCAAS)

BCAAs—isoleucine, leucine, and valine—are all essential amino acids that make up about 35 percent of the amino acids in muscle tissue and can also be used for energy. Studies confirm that under conditions of stress, injury, or exercise, a disproportionately high amount of the BCAAs are required to maintain nitrogen balance. Studies also indicate that leucine is used at up to two or more times the rate of isoleucine or valine. Many formulas on the market will typically have about twice as much leucine as the other BCAAs.

BCAAs have a history of use in hospital situations where patients are in stressed states (burn victims, surgery, trauma, starvation). Intravenous feeding of BCAAs is used to stimulate protein synthesis and nitrogen balance. During the 1980s, sports-nutrition companies picked up on this clinical practice, and research on animals and athletes revealed that the BCAAs are used for energy. The researchers hypothesized that taking supplements of BCAAs would then compensate for the BCAAs used for energy, promote muscle growth, and restore nitrogen balance. Additionally, leucine exerts other growth-related metabolic effects, such as growth hormone release and insulin release. Although athletes widely use BCAAs, there are no good studies that have been performed testing them with athletes.

Dosages of BCAAs vary depending upon the products available. Some products contain just the BCAAs, others have a few more ingredients, and still others contain a full spectrum of 18 amino acids with extra amounts of the BCAAs plus cofactors. Athletes, especially bodybuilders, report muscle growth and strength benefits when taking effective BCAA formulations. However, BCAAs are not just for power athletes. On the contrary, endurance athletes can also benefit from

BCAA supplementation. Research has determined that as much as 90 percent of the total daily leucine intake can be used for energy purposes in endurance athletes. This means that several times the normal amount of protein needs to be eaten to maintain nitrogen balance. But an alternative method can be to fortify the base diet of food proteins with a BCAA supplement. New research has also demonstrated a beneficial effect on endurance when BCAAs are ingested before and during exercise in a beverage form.

How much of the BCAAs are needed? The exact answer to this question has not been determined as of yet, but the following guidelines are based on available research and experience. You can either take a combination formula of just the BCAAs and a few cofactors, take a full-spectrum amino acid along with the BCAAs, or take a full-spectrum amino acid supplement with extra BCAAs. Formulations with the BCAAs, vitamin B_6, and glutamic acid are best. Supplemental amounts of the BCAAs should range from 1.5 g to 6 g for leucine and 800 g to 3 g for isoleucine and valine. Cofactors should be present, like vitamin B6 (pyridoxine) and glutamic acid. Split the dosage over two servings per day. Take them 30 to 60 minutes before exercise, directly after exercise on training days, and along with meals to fortify base proteins on non-training days. BCAAs may compete for absorption with other amino acids like tyrosine, phenylalanine, and methionine. If you are taking supplemental amounts of these amino acids, do so in the evening and mornings, at least three hours after BCAA supplement intake.

BROMELAIN (ANANAS COMOSUS)

Bromelain is a proteolytic enzyme contained in plant extracts derived from pineapple fruit. Proteolytic enzymes digest or break apart proteins. In fact, bromelain and other proteolytic enzymes are used in food tenderizers to soften meat. In the body, bromelain decreases fibrin by enhancing fibrinolytic action (which breaks fibrin down). While fibrin plays a vital role in the body as a clotting agent, after an injury occurs, too much fibrin in the damaged tissues can block blood flow, resulting in poor oxygen supply, build-up of metabolic waste products, and increased swelling and inflammation. Bromelain can function to minimize fibrin buildup in injured tissues and increase recovery time from injury. Bromelain can also aid in the digestion of proteins when taken with meals. Concerning injury recovery, bromelain has been shown in clinical studies to shorten recovery time from injury;

reduce swelling, inflammation, and pain; and accelerate tissue repair. As a digestive aid, for regular use, bromelain is included in dietary supplements in amounts ranging from 5 to 30 milligrams per dosage; along with other digestive enzymes. For nutritional support as part of a total treatment for injuries, the dosage found to be effective in clinical studies is 500 milligrams of standardized bromelain, 3 times per day, taken 30 minutes before meals. Use under doctor supervision to insure proper treatment of injuries. Use a high-quality Bromelain-containing supplement that has a guaranteed potency—for example, 2,400 gelatin-digesting units—or other equivalent enzyme activity. Use of bromelain is not recommended for individuals with known gastrointestinal disorders. Bromelain can cause reversible side effects such as gas, nausea, diarrhea, and allergic skin reaction. Use of bromelain for treating injury should be conducted under doctor supervision. Only use bromelain as directed, and for short periods of time in high dosages, up to a few weeks at a time.

CAFFEINE

Caffeine is a naturally occurring compound that belongs to a group of substances called methylxanthines. It is found in coffee, tea, chocolate, cola, and botanical supplement products, such as guarana, yerba mate, and green tea. Although caffeine is naturally occurring, it is also sold as a nonprescription drug, as an alertness aid and stimulant. Caffeine has several main effects. It increases alertness by stimulating the nervous system; it acts as a diuretic; it stimulates cardiac muscle tissue; it increases lipolysis; and it stimulates thermogenic activity. Almost the entire world relies on a daily caffeinated beverage to get the day started. However, for the athlete, caffeine offers much more than a good morning drink. Studies clearly show that intakes of caffeine can have beneficial effects on performance. Caffeine causes the body to use fatty acids rather than glycogen for energy, which in turn has a glycogen-sparing effect. Caffeine as a nervous system stimulant provides a mental boost to help the athlete through rigorous training sessions. Research shows that caffeine can even increase the rate of fat loss. The downside of caffeine is that it can cause dependency and alter your physiology. For this reason, it is banned by some sports groups and by the Olympics at certain blood levels. Caffeine works by stimulating the nervous system to increase production of excitatory neurotransmitters. If an individual takes too much caffeine, or takes it for prolonged periods of time, the precursor nutrients that produce these excitatory neu-rotransmitters become depleted, and cause a mentally burned-out feeling. Caffeine's diuretic effects are most detrimental to endurance athletes. Caffeine should be used sparingly by athletes, and only periodically to provide a mental boost to en-hance workouts. Also, some studies indicate that heavy caffeine intake over long periods of time may deplete the body of calcium; therefore, adequate calcium in-take is mandatory for caffeine users, and heavy caffeine use should be avoided for this and other reasons. Check first on the legality of caffeine in your sport before taking it before competition as an ergogenic aid. Researchers recommend 200 to 400 mg (about three to five cups of coffee) one hour before competition, but make certain that you are well hydrated to offset the diuretic effects of caffeine. Also, note that studies indicate that caffeine may reduce absorption and utilization of creatine.

CALCIUM

The role calcium plays in bone formation is well known, but calcium has other very important functions as well. Calcium plays essential roles in nerve conduction, transmission of nerve impulses, normal heartbeat, muscle contraction, membrane permeability, and blood clotting. Calcium also functions as an enzyme cofactor. Recently, calcium has been connected to controlling blood pressure in some indi-viduals. While calcium is a primary nutrient in bone formation and maintenance, other nutrients are also important in bone formation and the proper utilization of calcium. They include vitamin D, copper, zinc, manganese, and boron. Mineral-ization of bone requires a positive calcium balance; that is, more calcium must be absorbed than excreted. This is important to maintain during growth years and also during adulthood. Until recently, most medical authorities believed that once an individual attained the ripe old age of 30, it was not possible to build more bone tissue. But recent research has finally proven what many sports fitness scientists already knew: Exercise and proper dietary intake of calcium will result in increased bone mass in adults. The benefits are obvious for everyone who wants to maintain a healthy body. High-intensity exercise, such as weight lifting, appears to stimulate increase in bone mass more than aerobic exercise. From an athlete's standpoint, adequate calcium must be maintained all year long, from childhood through adult-hood. This means eating a diet high in calcium and taking a comprehensive supplement with the other nutrients, good sources of calcium, and the calcium cofactors. Dietary surveys have determined that both athletes and nonathletes exhibit inadequate calcium intake. This results in poor bone formation or onset of a bone disease, such as osteoporosis. Poor calcium intake also results in muscle cramping and reduced energy levels. Rickets and stunted growth are also potential disorders related to a calcium-deficient diet.

Besides being low in most diets, the calcium in many diets is in a form that is poorly absorbed. That's right. Like other minerals, different forms of calcium will be absorbed by the body better than others. In fact, the 1989 RDA book estimated that young adults absorb only 20 to 40 percent of their ingested calcium. This is another reason to take a good calcium supplement every day. Excess calcium taken during short or long periods of time normally does not cause major side effects in adults, aside from constipation and an increased risk of urinary-stone formation. A high calcium intake can interfere with the absorption of iron, zinc, magnesium, and other minerals. Very high calcium intake for long periods of time can lead to renal function problems. Studies support the adequate daily intake of calcium for maintenance of overall health and performance; the research does not report benefits of mega-dosing calcium for increased performance. The performance-fitness intake guidelines for men and women who are healthy and actively training is: 1,200 mg to 2,600 mg per day from food and supplements. The estimated safe range of intake is 1,200 mg to 4,000 mg or more, depending on the individual.

L-CARNITINE / ACETYL-L-CARNITINE

Carnitine is made by the body and its primary role is the transportation of fatty acids into mitochondria. Research has demonstrated certain athletic performance improvements with carnitine supplementation. Athletic benefits include increased endurance, improved oxygen uptake, reduced lactate levels during exercise, and improved anaerobic strength output. Studies support the use of carnitine supplementation for intensively training, competitive athletes. Benefits are not reported for low-intensity activities. Carnitine may also be useful in increasing the rate of fat loss, but more studies need to be undertaken to clearly establish this. L-carnitine supplementation of 1 to 3 g per day is reported to yield performance enhancing results, taken several weeks before competition, or carnitine loading of 2 to 5 g per day, one week before events. Both endurance and strength athletes can benefit from L-carnitine supplementation.

CHITOSAN

Chitosan is a fibrous substance of animal origin. It is derived from a compound called chitin, found in the exoskeletons of shellfish, such as crabs, lobsters, and shrimp. Chitosan absorbs fats in the digestive system, thereby reducing the calories from fats which may have entered into the bloodstream. Some studies show that taking chitosan with meals reduces the absorption of cholesterol and fats from the digestive system into the body. Chitosan helps maintain healthy cholesterol levels. It binds to fats, and can function as a nutritional weight-loss aid for people who are overweight due to consumption of a diet high in fats or low in dietary fiber. Studies have shown that taking 500 to 1,500 mg three times a day with main meals can be effective as a diet aid or cholesterol-lowering agent. Due to the fact that chitosan may absorb nutrients, taking a multivitamin/mineral supplement is mandatory to ensure adequate nutrient bioavailability. Chitosan is considered nontoxic but should not be overused, as nutrient deficiencies may develop. It is for use by adults only. Although most chitosan is highly purified, it comes from sources like shrimp shells; therefore, persons who are allergic to shrimp, lobster, crabs, and the like should use it cautiously and consult a doctor before using or if a reaction occurs. Not for use by children or pregnant or lactating women unless under a doctor's supervision.

CHOLINE

Choline is involved in fatty acid metabolism. The term "lipotropic" was used to describe the effects of choline and other substances that prevent deposition of fat in the liver. Choline is a component of the phospholipid phosphatidylcholine (lecithin) and is a part of all cell membranes and lipoproteins. Choline is also used by the body to make the neurotransmitter acetylcholine, which is critical for optimum nervous system functioning. Exercise can deplete the supply of choline and this may theoretically reduce acetylcholine amounts in the nervous system. More research on the exact performance effects is needed. Choline deficiency can have major consequences on the liver, memory, nerve functioning, and normal growth. Excess intakes of choline, 2 or more grams per day, can result in diarrhea, depression, and dizziness. The normal diet contains about 400 to 900 mg of choline per day. Performance-fitness intake of choline is 600 mg to 1,200 mg daily.

CHONDROITIN SULFATE (CS)

Chondroitin sulfate is a biological polymer that is an important component of connective tissues. It gives cartilage and ligaments their flexibility and attracts water to these tissues, maintaining proper hydration. CS is also an important component of the circulatory system. During the aging process, connective tissues become increasingly worn, causing joint mobility problems and degenerative diseases. CS supplementation has been shown to improve the condition of connective tissues, improve tissue repair and healing of wounds, treat osteoarthritis by restoring joint function and reducing pain, and cause improvements in circulatory system wellness by increasing the structure of the inner lining of blood vessels. CS is derived from cartilage from different animal sources. Purity and quality vary considerably. Select products that contain purified CS or hydrolyzed chondroitin sulfate. For nutritional support of joint and cardiovascular system health, use 400 to 600 mg per day. Concerning therapeutic use of CS, several clinical studies have reported that taking 600 to 1,200 mg per day caused improvements in joint function in cases of osteoarthritis and rheumatoid arthritis, and promoted faster healing of injuries. Minor side effects observed with long-term use include allergic reactions and gastrointestinal upset. Take with meals to reduce gastrointestinal upset.

CHROMIUM

Chromium's major role is helping insulin work in your body. Chromium also plays a role in the metabolism of nucleic acids (DNA and RNA) and helps to maintain their structure and gene expression. Chromium aids in fatty acid and cholesterol formation in the liver, and some studies have shown a lowering of cholesterol with chromium supplementation. Furthermore, chromium-deficient diets are linked to higher incidence of diabetes and heart disease. It is chromium's role as an insulin potentiator that has brought it so much recent media attention. Early researchers found that chromium exhibited a lowering of blood glucose levels. Because of this characteristic, chromium is referred to as a glucose tolerance factor. The glucose tolerance test is a test used to determine how well a person can remove high levels of glucose from the blood stream. The subject being tested is fed high amounts of glucose, and the blood levels are tested over several hours. The test is used for determining diabetes and hypoglycemia. It is also used to measure the efficacy of nutrients and drugs that possess blood-glucose-removal properties, like chromium. Due to chromium's role as a potentiator of insulin function, glucose and amino acids that circulate in the blood stream after ingestion have a higher rate of uptake by the cells. This does not necessarily mean that the levels of insulin are increased. And it does not mean that chromium has a direct effect on muscle building (like testosterone) or fat loss (like growth hormone). It just means that increasing dietary chromium levels will improve the functioning of insulin, which should result in a higher rate of cellular uptake of glucose and amino acids into the cells. For the athlete, adequate chromium intake is essential. Several studies have shown that individuals taking supplemental amounts of chromium in association with training and a good diet have been able to increase the rate of muscle gains and increase the rate of fat loss. Studies support the adequate daily intake of chromium for maintenance of overall health and performance. The research doesn't report benefits of mega-dosing chromium supplements for increased performance. The performance-fitness intake guideline for men and women who are healthy and actively training is: 200 mcg to 600 mcg per day from food and supplements. The estimated safe range of intake is up to 1,000 mcg (1 mg) per day.

COENZYME Q_{10} (Ubiquinone)

CoQ_{10} has a history of use in clinical application for people suffering from cardiovascular disorders. Its safety and effectiveness are well established, and studies on athletes report ergogenic effects, such as improved physical performance in endurance events. CoQ_{10} is a coenzyme found in every cell's mitochondria. It participates in the manufacturing of ATP, appearing along the energy-producing pathway and the electron-transport system. This is an oxidative pathway. Q_{10} has been thought of as a limiting factor in this energy-producing pathway. Q_{10} has also recently been identified as an exhibitor of powerful antioxidant activity, and a stabilizer of cellular membranes. As an endurance-enhancing supplement, Q_{10} will mostly benefit long-distance athletes. Ergogenic dosages range from 60 mg to 300 mg. All athletes will benefit from the antioxidant effects of Q_{10}; daily dosages for this purpose range from 10 to 60 mg per day.

CONJUGATED LINOLEIC ACID (CLA)

The fatty acid CLA occurs naturally in a number of foods, primarily beef and dairy products. The word "conjugated" in its name refers to the variation in chemical structure that sets it apart from the essential fatty acid linoleic acid. A slight change in the double bonds that hold its atoms together transforms it from linoleic acid to CLA. This small molecular reconfiguration has profound effects on its function; in particular, CLA has been shown in some studies to increase the body's ability to burn fat while maintaining lean body mass. Research has also shown that CLA acts as a powerful antioxidant, benefits the immune system, and possesses anticarcinogenic properties. CLA may have value for people who need to burn fat while preserving muscle mass, particularly athletes. Based upon the research to date, the recommended daily dose of CLA ranges from 2 to 5 gm per day.

COPPER

Copper is an essential mineral with several important functions. Copper is present in many enzymes, and it is part of the antioxidant SOD; it is important in the formation of collagen; and it is involved in energy production, melanin pigment synthesis, myelin formation, immune function, glucose metabolism, and cholesterol metabolism. Some attention was directed toward copper by athletic researchers as a result of copper's role in energy production. Copper is part of cytochrome oxidase, an enzyme that is found in the electron-transport system. Because dietary surveys indicate that many athletes, especially endurance athletes, have inadequate copper intake, the addition of supplemental amounts of copper have been researched. The role copper plays as a component of antioxidant SOD is again vital for the protection of the body at the cellular level, for improved performance, and for shorter recovery times after exercise. The performance-fitness daily intake for men and women who are healthy and actively training is 3 mg to 6 mg per day. Estimated safe range of intake: up to 10 mg per day.

CORDYCEPS (CORDYCEPS SINENSIS)

In 1993, the women of China's national track-and-field team broke the record for the 10,000-meter run by 40 seconds. They also improved on the previous world records for the 1,500- and 3,000-meter events and went on to set further record times at the Asian Games in Japan in 1994. Since then, many articles have been written about a tonic mushroom that was attributed with having a large impact upon their performance. The mushroom, known as the caterpillar fungus, or cordyceps, has been widely used by millions of Chinese for thousands of years. Cordyceps grows not on trees but on the living bodies of certain moth larvae. The mushroom organism, in the form of fine threads, penetrates the larva, eventually killing and mummifying it. The mushroom is cultivated because it is in great demand as a supertonic that builds physical stamina, mental energy, and sexual power. Chinese doctors say that it is simultaneously invigorating and calming, as well as life-prolonging. Chinese people usually buy it in its whole dried form, consisting of the mummified larva and attached fruiting body of the mushroom, which they add to a soup or stew. In addition, extract of cordyceps is included in many compound tonic formulas. Cordyceps is considered safe and gentle, indicated for both men and women. One way cordyceps is thought to exert beneficial effects is to increase testosterone production. Consult specific products for proper dosage and use.

COROSOLIC ACID (GLUCOSOL)

Clinical studies have revealed that an extract of the leaves of *Lagestroemia speciosa,* which contains corosolic acid, can significantly lower blood-sugar levels in people with high blood-sugar levels. The primary active ingredient in the dietary supplement Glucosol is corosolic acid. Glucosol is considered to be an insulin-like herb or phytoinsulin, but it differs in two important ways from the pancreatic hormone. First, Glucosol can be given by mouth in order to lower blood-sugar levels. Second, oral doses of Glucosol have not resulted in any observable side effects in study participants. Research indicates that Glucosol, especially when given in the form of a soft gelatin capsule, can lower blood sugar to normal levels, produce weight loss (even after a person stops taking the extract), reduce the classic symptoms of diabetes, act as a strong antioxidant, and promote normal blood pressure in some people. Aside from being a potential weight-loss aid and having possible benefits for diabetic athletes, the applications for healthy athletes are not clear at this time, as the blood-sugar-lowering effect may cause hypoglycemia and impair athletic performance. People with diabetes should consult their doctor about using Glucosol to help maintain desirable blood-sugar levels.

CREATINE MONOHYDRATE

Creatine monohydrate has been used nutritionally to increase the amount of creatine and high-energy creatine phosphate in muscle tissue. Creatine is present in food and is manufactured in the body. It occurs in animal products, such as meat and fish. One pound of raw steak contains about 2 g of creatine. But, it should be noted that cooking will convert the creatine into an inactive form, which is quickly excreted from the kidneys. In the body, creatine is made from the amino acids glycine, arginine, and methionine. Normal daily dietary creatine requirements are estimated at 2 g per day in nonathletic individuals.

As you recall, ATP and CP are stored in muscle cells and function as a pool of immediate energy. The bigger the amounts in the muscles, the more the muscle can lift and perform short-term maximum-strength performance. CP is used to quickly replenish ATP in fast-twitch glycolytic muscle fibers. This process takes only a fraction of a second. The more CP the muscles have on hand, the more ATP can be replenished during bursts of all-out effort. Creatine loading can therefore result in improving training intensity and recovery in anaerobic sports by increasing the muscles' resting reserve of creatine phosphate.

Of the dozens of studies conducted on creatine supplementation during the 1990s, improvements in strength performance were observed mostly in sports that exhibited all-out effort for under 30 seconds. For example, creatine supplementation of 1,000 mg improved perfomance in weight lifting, powerlifting, football, short-duration track and field events (sprinting, jumping, throwing, etc.), vertical jump performance, 300-meter sprint, and short rowing events. Increases in VO_2 max have been observed in a limited number of studies on untrained and moderately active individuals. However, no performance improvements have been measured in endurance events.

Studies have also been conducted to see how creatine supplementation affects body mass. Not all studies on body mass have shown significant changes following creatine supplementation. Several studies *have* shown creatine to significantly increase body mass. Scientists speculate, however, that much of the increase in lean body mass is due to water retention rather than increased contractile protein, at least in the short-term studies lasting one to six weeks. Another factor that can be responsible for an increase in lean body mass is that when a large amount of creatine is ingested, the amino acids needed to make creatine are now available for other functions. This means that glycine, arginine, and methionine are available in surplus amounts for other anabolic functions. Dosages ranging from 1 to 40 g per day have been reported; higher dosages were only tested for short periods of time, one to two weeks. For long-term building up of creatine levels, use 8 mg per pound of lean body mass (about 1 to 2 g per day). For short-term creatine loading, taking 80 to 160 mg per pound of lean body mass (10 to 24 g per day) for several days will increase creatine levels in the body.

The conventional loading method used in studies and recommended by manufacturers is intake of 20 to 25 g of creatine for seven to 14 days, followed by a lower maintenance dose of 5 to 10 g per day during competition season and training. Studies by A. L. Green in 1996 demonstrated that combining creatine with a simple carbohydrate, such as glucose, will increase creatine transport into the muscle. The solution that was tested consisted of 5 g of creatine and 90 g of glucose, consumed four times per day. When tested against creatine alone, the creatine-carbohydrate supplement increased total muscle creatine and creatine phosphate levels significantly more.

The scientific studies conducted over short periods of time, up to eight weeks, have not reported any severe side effects. One hypothetical health concern is with the breakdown product of creatine metabolism, creatinine. Because creatinine is quickly excreted by the kidneys, this extra demand may cause problems with individuals with impaired kidney function. This extra excretion also increases the demand for proper water intake to maintain optimum levels of hydration. There have also been anecdotal reports of individuals complaining about mega-dose creatine ingestion causing muscle cramps and strains. This can be attributed to the increase of muscle water content, which causes intracelluar swelling. The extra cellular water content can also upset electrolyte balance.

CURCUMIN (also known as Turmeric, Curcuma longa)

Curcumin has a long history of use in Ayurvedic medicine and as a spice. Recently, scientists have determined that phytonutrients in curcumin have various beneficial health effects, such as antioxidant function, anti-inflammatory action, anti-platelet aggregation activity, and as a natural antiseptic. Curcumin is considered to be very safe; recent research indicates that it is a natural alternative to expensive and potentially harmful COX-2 inhibitor prescription drugs. Curcumin has also been tested in clinical studies and found to be an effective anti-inflammatory agent, useful in injury recovery and supportive therapy for rheumatoid arthritis. In Europe, curcumin is used to treat peptic disorders. For best results, choose supplements containing standardized curcumin root extract (85 to 98 percent curcuminoids). As a dietary supplement for daily use, 50 to 200 mg, two to three times a day, of standardized curcumin root extract is beneficial. For short-term nutritional therapeutic use as an anti-inflammatory agent, higher dosages in the range of 250 to 500 mg, three times per day, have been shown to be safe and effective. Curcumin use is contraindicated in cases of obstructed bile ducts and gallstones; in these cases as well as with any medical condition, doctor supervision is required. If you are suffering from inflammatory conditions, make sure to let your doctor know that you are using curcumin, to ensure adequate medical supervision. Keep in mind that curcumin's anti-inflammatory action will take several days to become apparent. There is some indication that regular intake of curcumin, as a supplement or spice, can help reduce the risk of certain degenerative conditions and protect against cancers.

DEHYDROEPIANDROSTERONE (DHEA)

DHEA entered the dietary supplement market in the mid 1990s as a longevity substance, then to promote increases in testosterone levels, which in turn may benefit strength sports. However, DHEA is not for everyone; most health authorities do not recommend it for individuals under the age of 40. The DHEA levels declines with age, and younger people do not seem to benefit from supplemental DHEA because their bodies are already making enough. Note, too, that DHEA is banned by many sports governing organizations. DHEA is a hormone produced mainly by the adrenal glands. In men, it is also produced in the testes as an intermediate in testosterone production, and in women, it is also produced in the ovaries as an intermediate in estrogen production. DHEA seems to exert weak androgen (a steroid hormone that promotes masculine characteristics) activity, and it has also been reported to induce growth of body hair in men and women. However, in a study of men between the ages of 20 and 25, supplemental DHEA did not increase testosterone levels, but it did help cause a decrease in body fat and increase lean body mass. Conversely, in another study, an increase in androgen levels was reported in postmenopausal women given DHEA supplements, as was an increase in body-hair growth during the study period. Another study, this one using both men and women, did not report any significant changes in lean body mass or body fat, but did report an overall improvement in the feeling of well-being. Going by the results of the studies just mentioned, medically unsupervised DHEA use by young male athletes is not warranted, though use by female athletes and by male athletes over age 40 may experience some beneficial physical and physiological effects. Other reported benefits of DHEA include immune-system enhancement, anticancer activity, antidepressant action, enhancement of mental functioning, and longevity in laboratory animals. The amounts used in studies have varied, but benefits have been reported in the 25 mg to 100 mg dosage range. A word of caution: Do not take DHEA supplements if you are a man who may have prostate cancer or a woman who may have breast cancer, a reproductive cancer, or a reproductive disorder.

ECHINACEA (Echinacea purpurea, E. angustifolia)

Echinacea is a well-established botanical that stimulates the immune system. The main active ingredients found listed on labels of standardized echinacea extracts are phenolics, echinacosides, or sesquiterpene esters, standardized to about 4 percent. Taking 200 to 400 mg two to three times per day is an effective dosage for stimulating the immune system. Stimulation of the immune system is useful for the treatment of colds and flus. Some recent research performed on athletes in the early part of the athletic season show that athletes taking echinacea experienced fewer upper respiratory infections when compared to athletes not taking echinacea. Echinacea is taken in repeating cycles of 14 to 21 days at a time, with several days off so as to not overstimulate the immune system all of the time.

EPHEDRA (Ma Huang, Ephedra sinica, and other Ephedra species)

The plant ephedra is now a common ingredient in dietary supplements. Ephedra contains naturally occurring substances called ephedrine alkaloids, which include primarily ephedrine. Ephedra has been traditionally used in China for thousands of years for the treatment of bronchial asthma, diseases of the respiratory tract, and related ailments. Ephedrine is also a nervous-system stimulant. The use of the combination of the drugs ephedrine and caffeine as weight-loss agents actually started in Europe by accident, when doctors observed that patients taking a drug preparation for bronchial asthma containing ephedrine and caffeine lost weight. Scientists subsequently conducted studies using ephedrine and caffeine together and apart to determine their effects on losing body fat. While both substances increase the rate of fat loss, along with a reduced-calorie diet, ephedrine was observed to increase fat loss at a faster rate. The research using these drugs prompted development of dietary supplements naturally containing these substances, such as ephedra for natural ephedrine, and guarana for natural caffeine. Ephedrine appears to work by increasing total calorie burning rate, increasing the rate of fat burning, and controlling appetite. Also note that the plants contain other natural substances that are believed to exert additional effects.

In addition to using products containing ephedra for weight loss, studies show that ephedrine, like caffeine, can improve athletic performance for some athletes. Details about these effects are unimportant, as most athletic organizations ban the use of both ephedrine and caffeine during sporting events. So if you are using a botanical supplement product with ephedra, guarana, or other botanicals reported to be weight-loss aids or stimulants, make sure that it (and any other drugs you may be using) does not contain substances banned by your athletic organization.

It is estimated that millions of Americans take supplements containing ephedra to achieve their weight-loss goals and boost energy levels. Adding to two decades of existing studies, researchers at Columbia and Harvard universities recently completed a six-month study using an ephedra-containing product to determine its safety and effectiveness as a weight-loss aid on healthy male and female overweight subjects. These researchers reported that, under the conditions of their study, the ephedra supplement, which also contained natural caffeine, resulted in improved reduction of body fat, and was safe and effective during the study period. The herbal supplement supplied 90 mg of ephedrine per day, and 192 mg of caffeine per day, taken in divided dosages, three times per day. Mild side effects observed included a temporary increase in blood pressure, persistent increase in heart rate, dry mouth, heartburn, and insomnia in some of the research subjects. To further evaluate the ephedra safety issue, in December 2000 a group of medical experts determined, after a review of numerous research studies and case studies, that ephedra-containing products are safe at a total daily dosage of up to 90 mg of ephedrine alkaloids, taken in a few smaller individual doses of up to 30 mg each. Findings are based on the conclusions of a comprehensive, science-based risk analysis performed by Cantox Health Sciences International, a world-renowned, independent scientific consulting firm. Cantox assessed all available scientific information—focusing on nineteen clinical trials. Other key data included adverse event reports (AERs) collected by the Food and Drug Administration (FDA). The committee reported that three conditions for safe ephedra-supplement use are dosage limits, effective labeling, and post-market monitoring. A total daily intake of 90 mg of ephedrine, taken in divided doses of up to 30 mg, caused no observed adverse effects, which is called the No Observed Adverse Effect Level (NOAEL). The report also identified a 150 mg total daily dosage as the lowest level at which moderate adverse effects were first observed—the Lowest Observed Adverse Effect Level (LOAEL). State lawmakers in Ohio also determined ephedra's safe use limits. They passed regulations that allow for a single dosage containing less than 25 mg of ephedrine alkaloids, and less than 100 mg of ephedrine alkaloids in a twenty-four-hour period, for not more than twelve weeks for a healthy adult. Experts advise that people using ephedra products pay close attention to the directions on the labels of the products they are using to ensure maximum safety and effectiveness. Improper use of ephedra products may be harmful to your health. Consult the product labels for proper use instructions and caution statements. It is best to consult your doctor if you have any questions about using ephedra-containing products, are on medication, have a medical condition, or have a family history of medical problems.

ESSENTIAL FATTY ACIDS

The three fatty acids that make up a triglyceride molecule will vary in composition. Composition depends upon whether their origin is from plants or animals. Of the many fatty acids, only two are of essential dietary concern and one is conditionally essential in the diet. Linoleic acid is a primary essential fatty acid that the body cannot manufacture. It therefore has to be obtained from the diet for normal growth and health. However, recent research indicates that diets too high in linoleic acid may cause the metabolism to be sluggish and promote a tendency toward developing a condition that favors storage of body fat. A major researcher in this area of fatty acid balance and obesity, Artemis P. Simopoulos, M.D., believes that our food supply may be too high in linoleic acid (an omega-6 fatty acid) and too low in alpha-linolenic acid (an omega-3 fatty acid). She contends that humans evolved on a diet that was much higher in protein, lower in carbohydrates, but higher in fruits and vegetables and much lower in saturated fat than today's conventional diets. Furthermore, the consumption of refined carbohydrate products, such as sugar, fructose, high-fructose corn syrup, and trans-fatty acids from hydrogenated vegetable oils and margarines, adds to the metabolic disruption. The issues of proportions of dietary fat, carbohydrate, and protein are more involved for athletic performance, and guidelines are presented in chapters 6 through 8, in the Dynatrition program.

Recently a modified form of linoleic acid, called conjugated linoleic acid (CLA), has emerged on the shelves of health-food stores. The marketers promote CLA as having fat-metabolizing effects that result in burning more fat, thereby increasing lean body mass and decreasing body fat. CLA products are typically taken in dosages that range from 1 to 3 g. Another fatty acid, arachidonic acid, is made in the body from linoleic acid. Arachidonic acid only becomes essential when linoleic acid deficiency exists. However, because arachidonic acid has to be made from linoleic acid and arachidonic acid is a polyunsaturated fatty acid, the presence in the diet will have a linoleic sparing effect. This may be beneficial to the athlete because arachidonic acid is also an important structural fatty acid that is present in cell membranes.

Alpha-linolenic acid is the other essential fatty acid (an omega-3 fatty acid). It is similar to linoleic acid in structure. Alpha-linolenic acid has several functions, is important in growth, and is the precursor of two other important fatty acids (EPA and DHA) discussed in chapter 6. The body would rather use the essential fatty acids, like protein/amino acids, for growth and functional needs instead of fuel needs. A diet that is high in essential fatty acids and low in nonessential fatty acids will therefore increase metabolism and discourage increased body-fat formation, assuming that you are not overeating. Remember, excess carbohydrates and amino acids can be converted to body-fat stores. Flaxseed oil, fish, and poultry are good foods to eat to increase your intake of alpha-linolenic acid. The functions of the essential fatty acids are important to existence and performance. Some of the specific functions of the essential fatty acids include their presence in phospholipids, which are important for maintaining the structure and function of cellular and subcellular membranes; their function as precursors for eicosanoids, which are important in regulating a wide diversity of physiological processes; and their involvement in the transfer of oxygen from the lungs through the alveolar membrane, the formation of a structural part of all cells, the reduction of the time required for the recovery of fatigued muscles after exercise by facilitating the clearance of lactic acid buildup, the maintenance of proper brain and nervous system function, the formation of healthy skin and hair, wound healing, and growth enhancement.

ELECTROLYTES (Sodium, Chloride, and Potassium)

Sodium, chloride, and potassium are collectively referred to as the electrolytes. While the other minerals may have electrolyte activity, these three are generally considered the main electrolytes in the body. Magnesium is sometimes grouped with these three electrolytes by some authorities, but it is treated separately here due to its unique functions and supplement requirements. The main function of these electrolytes is maintenance of the balance of fluids in the body between cells and the bloodstream, including the uptake of some nutrients in intestines, muscle contraction, and nerve impulse transmission, among others. Deficiency of the electrolytes can occur under conditions of severe dehydration, during prolonged periods of exercise without proper hydration or electrolyte replenishment, and in conditions of kidney disease. Side effects of electrolyte deficiency include dizziness, fainting, and reduced performance. Excessive intake of sodium and chloride (because they occur together in food) causes hypertension, fluid balance problems, and edema. High potassium intake, 18 g or more, will lead to acute hyperkalemia, which can cause cardiac arrest and prove fatal.

These three electrolytes occur in all foods. Sodium and chloride are supplied by food mostly as sodium chloride, though sodium bicarbonate and monosodium glutamate also contribute to dietary sodium intake. Table salt (sodium chloride) and processed foods are by far the largest contributors. Potassium is present in all foods but is particularly high in fruits and vegetables. In fact, while the typical daily intake of potassium is 2,500 mg to 3,400 mg, some individuals on high fruit and vegetable diets maintain a potassium intake as high as 8 to 11 g per day. Most individuals want to maintain moderate sodium and chloride intake and maintain higher potassium intake. Athletes especially have higher demands of these minerals due to excessive sweating and increased physical activity. But do not think you have to load up on table salt. The higher food intake of athletes usually compensates for higher electrolyte demands.

Many sports drinks on the market contain water, carbohydrates, and electrolytes. Use of these drinks is recommended for active athletes. Drink them during and after exercise. Long-distance and ultra-long-distance athletes need to make sure they are first maintaining adequate water and carbohydrate intake and then maintaining appropriate levels of electrolytes. Drinks with low levels of electrolytes are best during exercise, because high electrolyte concentrations will delay gastric emptying and impair hydration and carbohydrate supply during physical activity.

Supplement intake of sodium and chloride are not usually required. There is typically more than enough in most diets. Athletes wishing to add more sodium or chloride to their diets can do so with the addition of table salt to their foods. However, excess intake of sodium chloride is usually the condition with most diets. Potassium, on the other hand, can range quite considerably in the diet. Individuals concerned with possible low potassium intakes should look for multivitamin/ mineral supplements which contain some potassium as potassium chloride.

The performance-fitness intake guideline for men and women who are healthy and actively training is: sodium, 1,500 mg to 4,500 mg; chloride, 1,500 mg to 4,500 mg; potassium, 2,500 mg to 4,000 mg (all per day from food and supplements).

FOLATE

Folate and folacin are general terms used to describe compounds that have nutritional properties similar to those of folic acid. Folate is another water soluble B vitamin. Folate compounds function metabolically as coenzymes that transport carbon molecules from one compound to another in amino acid metabolism and nucleic acid synthesis. In this way, folate is very important as a cofactor in DNA (deoxynucleic acid) and RNA (ribonucleic acid) formation, protein synthesis, and cell division. Folate also stimulates the formation of red blood cells and vitamin B_{12}. In particular, folate affects tissues that grow rapidly, such as the skin, the lining of the gastrointestinal tract, bone marrow where blood cells are formed, and regenerating muscle tissue. Studies have also indicated that increasing the intake of folate during pregnancy reduces the incidence of premature births and birth defects. Tests of athletic performance using high dosages of folate have not revealed immediate performance-enhancing effects. Mega-dosing folate is not recommended, nor is it readily possible, as supplements containing over 800 mcg of folate per dosage need a prescription. Obviously, those individuals wanting higher dosages of folate can simply take multiple dosages of supplements consisting of 800 mcg or lower per dosage. All athletes will benefit from higher-than-average folate intake, and bodybuilding athletes may find faster recovery and growth rates with even higher amounts of folate. Deficiency of folate can result in anemia, birth defects, sore tongue, digestive problems, growth problems, fatigue, poor memory, and megoblastic anemia. Excessive folate intake may stimulate convulsions in persons with epilepsy, kidney damage, and lower zinc levels. The performance-fitness intake guideline for men and women who are healthy and actively training is: 400 to 1,200 mg per day from food and supplements. The RDI for folate is 400 mcg. Safe levels have been estimated to be 1,200 mcg per day, or slightly more depending on body weight and physical activity.

GAMMA-LINOLENIC ACID (GLA)

Gamma-linolenic acid is another important fatty acid that can be made in the body from the main essential fatty acid, linoleic acid. GLA is an important precursor for the series 1 prostaglandins, which regulate many cellular activities. The series 1 prostaglandins keep blood platelets from sticking together, control cholesterol formation, reduce inflammation, make insulin work better, improve nerve function, regulate calcium metabolism, and are involved in immune system functioning. While studies on athletes have not confirmed any performance-enhancing effects, ingestion of foods and supplements high in GLA will benefit overall health. However, getting GLA through foods is not that simple. GLA is not found in many foods. In fact, the major sources are evening primrose oil, borage oil, and black currant oil.

These oils are also high in linoleic acid. Dosages of 100 to 400 mg of GLA per day, in association with the essential fatty acids and omega-3 fatty acids, may benefit physical performance and health, especially during your athletic season.

GAMMA ORYZANOL AND FERULIC ACID (FRAC)

Gamma oryzanol is a substance extracted from rice bran oil which has been reported to promote a variety of metabolic effects, including increased endorphin release, antioxidant action, stress reduction, and growth hormone stimulation. Ferulic acid is actually a part of the gamma oryzanol molecule that is also available as a supplement. Improvements include increased strength, fast muscle recovery from training, reduced muscle soreness, reduced sensation of fatigue, and decreased catabolic effects of cortisol. Dosages of 10 mg to 60 mg of ferulic acid per day and/or 300 to 900 mg of gamma oryzanol per day have been reported as having no side effects. While research is sparse, athletes report beneficial results from the supplemental use of gamma oryzanol and ferulic acid. Ferulic acid is reported to be about 30 times more bioavailable then gamma oryzanol. However, the sterol molecule to which the ferulic acid is bound is believed by some scientists to be integral to the efficient transport of the ferulic acid molecule. The substance is usually taken before workouts, and in the morning on nontraining days.

GARCINIA (Garcinia cambogia)

The primary active ingedient in garcinia is called hydroxycitric acid (HCA). HCA is reported to block an enzyme in your liver that converts carbohydrates to fatty acids in your body. This means that more carbohydrates will be available for cellular energy. Most supplements contain garcinia which is standardized to an HCA content between 50 percent and 80 percent. Dosages found to be effective are 500 mg to 1000 mg, three times per day, before meals. Garcinia is primarily used as a weight-loss aid. It is also reported to control appetite, along with suppressing the formation of fat and cholesterol in the liver. No side effects from taking garcinia supplements at common dosage levels are reported.

GARLIC (Allium sativum)

Garlic is best known for its ability to lower the bloodstream's cholesterol level. It also is reported to help keep the arteries flexible. Garlic has also been reported to help protect from some infections, and is particularly useful for digestive system health. The best garlic supplements are standardized to about 1 percent allicin. The effective daily dosage range of garlic is 600 mg to 1,200 mg. No known toxicity, except rare gastrointestinal distress. Garlic is of particular interest for athletes as it helps maintain good circulatory system health, which is vital for athletic performance.

GINKGO (Ginkgo biloba)

Ginkgo is another botanical with reported benefits for improving and maintaining good circulation and also mental function. This would be of special interest to endurance althletes. High-quality ginkgo supplements are standardized to 24 percent flavone glycosides and and 6 percent terpenes. The effective dosage range is 40 mg to 200 mg per day, in divided dosages, but 120 mg per day is the most common. Ginkgo also has powerful antioxidant activity, which will help protect athletes from free radical damage, especially oxygen free radicals. There is no known toxicity, but people on anticoagulant therapy should be cautioned about possible blood-thinning effects.

GINSENGS

There are several types of ginseng that have been in use for thousands of years as an overall promoter of health and energy. The types of ginseng primarily found in supplements are Chinese ginseng (Panax ginseng), American ginseng (Panax quinquefolius), and Siberian ginseng (Eleutherococcus senticosus), which is reported to have effects similar to Chinese or Amercian ginsengs. The "active" components of ginseng are a group of sponin compounds called ginsenosides/ panaxosides, and eleutherosides in Siberian ginseng. Ginseng also contains the trace mineral germanium, which has been shown to exhibit overall health effects and increase the body's supply of oxygen. When using ginseng, look for standardized preparations; 2 percent to 4 percent standardized ginseng products are common. Ginseng combined with royal jelly is a traditional combination for energy. Siberian ginseng has been the favorite of Russian athletes, who use it daily. But Chinese ginseng is also widely used. One study reported improved oxygen utilization, quicker recovery time, increased strength, and better reaction time for Chinese ginseng, but conflicting studies again support the use of Siberian ginseng. Both are recommended. All athletes should use 200 mg to 1 g per day of standardized ginseng or ginseng–royal jelly combination during the season and preseason, and as needed during the off-season. Ginseng is also found in some good quality sports multivitamin/mineral supplements.

GLUCOSAMINE

There are several types of connective tissues. Cartilage, tendons, ligaments, intervertebral discs, pads between joints, and cellular membranes all are comprised of connective tissue. All connective tissues have two common components, chief of which is collagen. One third of your body's total protein volume is comprised of collagen, making it the most common protein in the body. The other component is proteoglycans (PGs). PGs form the framework for collagenous tissue. These huge structural "macromolecules" are comprised mainly of glycosaminoglycans (GAGs)—long chains of modified sugars. The principal sugar in PGs is called hyaluronic acid, 50 percent of which is comprised of glucosamine. The principal amino acids forming collagen are proline, glycine, and lysine. Collagen and PGs must somehow get together during the production of new connective tissue. Of the multitude of biochemical reactions that must take place during the synthesis of connective tissue, there is one critical rate-limiting step that must be reached to guarantee that new connective tissue is being successfully synthesized. That rate-limiting step is the conversion of glucose to glucosamine. Glucosamine, then, is the single most important substance in the synthesis of connective tissue. Over thirty years of research has gone into understanding how glucosamine acts as the precursor of GAG synthesis. Glucosamine is so effective it repairs connective tissue in people with arthritis, and may very well be a way to prevent arthritis from occurring in the first place by maintaining adequate connective tissues in your body. In human clinical trials, glucosamine given orally in doses of 750 to 1500 mg daily was observed to initiate a reversal of degenerative osteoarthritis, and also relieve pain in the knees of athletes. Glucosamine as a supplement clearly aids in connective-tissue synthesis. All athletes need such a substance, as the repair and growth of connective-tissue is neverending.

GLUTAMINE

Glutamine is a nonessential amino acid found in proteins. It is formed from glutamic acid by the addition of ammonia and vitamin B_6. It is a neurotransmitter in the brain and can be converted back to glutamic acid there, where the glutamic acid is essential for brain function. Glutamine is an energy source in the brain and a mediator of glutamic acid and GABA activity. Glutamine is also vital to immunity function. New studies show that cell replication in the immune system requires glutamine. However, most glutamine is made in the muscles, so your muscles have to supply a large amount of glutamine to the immune system. Supplemental use of free-form L-glutamine by athletes is known to have a strong anticatabolic effect that neutralizes the cortisol that accompanies strenuous exercise. Cortisol is highly catabolic. Its anticatabolic action allows anabolism—muscle building—to take place more efficiently. L-glutamine additionally plays an active role in the recovery and healing process. Supplemental glutamine has reportedly been taken in dosages ranging from 500 to over 20,000 mg per day during periods of high stress. Dosages on commercial supplements typically range from 1 g to 10 g, with 2 to 5 g a day being the most common dosage range.

GLUTATHIONE

Glutathione is a tri-peptide commonly thought of as a free-form amino acid. It is a sulfur-bearing tri-peptide consisting of glutamic acid, cysteine, and glycine. The sulfhydryl (thiol) group makes glutathione a very effective antioxidant. Glutathione occurs in plant and animal tissues and is vital to the protection against the effects of oxygen and free radicals. Amounts of glutathione tend to decrease with age, making supplemental amounts particularly important to the adult athlete. Glutathione also acts as a detoxifying agent, aids immune function, helps protect the integrity of red blood cells, and functions as a neurotransmitter.

GLYCEROL

Glycerol is a three-carbon molecule that is the backbone of triglycerides and phospholipids. Triglycerides consist of three fatty acids attached to a glycerol molecule, and phospholipids consist of two fatty acids attached to a glycerol molecule, with a phosphate-containing compound attached to the third carbon atom. When glycerol is removed from these fats by hydrolysis, it is a clear, syrupy liquid. The liquid has been used in a variety of ways over the years, but it is especially popular as an emollient in skin care products and cosmetics and as a sweetening agent in pharmaceuticals. As a supplement, glycerol has been found by researchers to help the body remain better hydrated. Studies have shown that athletes training for prolonged periods (more than one hour) were able to run cooler and longer when they ingested a water-glycerol beverage. Preliminary studies have suggested that glycerol acts like a sponge, absorbing water into the bloodstream and holding it there. However, researchers are still trying to determine appropriate dosages; the current estimates range from 10 to 60 g, taken with the amount of water recommended for the activity, over a period of a few hours. A word of caution: Some side effects, including bloating, nausea, and lightheadedness, have been reported with glycerol use. If you choose to try a glycerol-containing beverage, test it out several times before using it during competition to see how your body reacts to it.

GLYCINE

Glycine is a nonessential amino acid that is synthesized from serine, with folacin acting as a coenzyme. Glycine, a sweet-tasting substance, gets its name from the Greek word meaning "sweet." During rapid growth, glycine demand increases. It is an important precursor for many substances including proteins, DNA, phospholipids, collagen, and creatine. It is also a precursor to the release of energy. Glycine is used by the liver in the elimination of some toxic substances and in the formation of bile salts as well. It is necessary for central nervous system functioning and is an inhibitory neurotransmitter. Too much glycine can displace glucose in the metabolic energy chain and cause fatigue, but just enough can help produce more energy. Some studies have observed a growth hormone–increasing effect of glycine using 7 g per day. Some studies have also shown an increase in strength after glycine ingestion, which may be due in part to its growth hormone–elevating effect. Glycine ingestion has also been shown to increase creatine levels. The long-term effects of supplemental use of glycine are not known. Headaches have been reported to occur with glycine supplementation. Supplemental use of glycine is still in an experimental stage, however 3 to 6 g per day may be beneficial to power athletes, and glycine should be part of a full-spectrum amino acid supplement. Use free-form glycine supplements with caution.

GOTU KOLA (Centella asiatica)

Gotu kola is an ancient botanical which is reported to stimulate connective tissue development and healing, increase skin building, and may improve mental function. These are all functions that can benefit athletes. High-quality gotu kola supplements are standardized to 10 percent to 30 percent asiaticosides. Effective daily dosages range from 50 mg to 150 mg per day. No known toxicity with recommended dosages.

GRAPE SEED EXTRACT (GSE, Vitis vinifera)

The phytonutrients contained in GSE have powerful antioxidant action; inhibit enzymes that break down and damage blood vessels, connective tissues, and skin (that is, inhibit collagenase and elastase); and maintain flexibility of blood vessels. These combined effects promote overall health and circulatory-system function. GSE has also been used as nutritional support for venous/circulatory system diseases. These actions will benefit everyone and are of special interest to long-distance athletes, who depend on a well-functioning circulatory system and who need extra antioxidant protection. Use high-quality supplements containing standarized grape seed extract (50 to 85 percent proanthocyanidins. Daily dosages of standardized GSE commonly used in dietary supplements range from 25 to 150 mg for nutrition purposes. Higher daily dosages are used for nutrition support in circulation disorders, 100 to 200 mg, 3 times per day. Grape seed extract contains phytonutrients, which are similar to those contained in Pycnogenol, which is a pine bark extract used in supplements as a source of OPCs.

GREEN TEA (Camellia sinensis)

Green tea extract is another botanical ingredient that you will find in sports nutrition products. Its main function is as a powerful antioxidant. But recent research has determined that the polyphenols in green tea have a thermogenic effect, which increases the metabolic rate and causes more fats to be used for energy. Green tea also has a mild stimulatory action, due to caffeine content. High-quality green tea products are standardized to 50 to 65 percent catechins/polyphenols. Effective dosage range is 50 mg to 300 mg per day. It has no known toxicity.

GUARANA (Paullinia cupana)

Guarana contains caffeine and other related methylxanthines, such as theobromine and theophylline, which are central nervous system stimulants and have a mild diuretic effect. The methylxanthines also stimulate an increase in your fat-burning rate and reduce appetite in some people. Guarana is used in dietary supplements that are designed for stimulating mental alertness. It is also used in dietary supplement weight-loss aids, as part of a thermogenic herbal blend, to stimulate the metabolism of fats. Use as directed on product labels for best results, as use and dosages vary considerably.

GYMNEMA (Gymnema sylvestre)

Gymnema has been shown to have hypoglycemic activity; that is, it lowers blood-sugar levels by stimulating insulin secretions. It is used in traditional Asian-Indian Ayurvedic medicine in the management of blood-sugar-level disorders; it is reported to be beneficial to individuals with Type I diabetes as supportive therapy (in addition to standard medical treatment). High-quality supplements contain standardized gymnema leaf extract (25 percent gymnemic acids). Gymnema should be used under doctor supervision in the treatment of medical conditions. The Western medical community is slowly but surely widening its nutrition therapies for management of diabetes. If you are diabetic, encourage your doctor to explore some of these alternative-medicine practices. But start slowly, and do not discontinue use of medications until approved by your doctor. Gymnema is sometimes used in weight-loss nutritional aid products for its insulin-boosting effects, with the belief that many people with overweight problems have insulin-secretion or -function problems. If you are using gymnema products, be aware that the hypoglycemic effect causes a rise in insulin, which promotes a more rapid removal of blood sugar and may cause dizziness in some people.

HORSE CHESTNUT (Aesculus hippocastanum)

Horse chestnut seed supplements are known for their vascular system toning effects. These improvements in vascular system structure are thought to be due to horse chestnut seeds' effects on stabilizing cell membranes and normalizing capillary tone. It has been used in clinical studies to treat venous insufficiency, treat edema, and help reduce leg pain. Also, it can be beneficial in the treatment and management of hemorrhoids and varicose veins. These circulatory-system-enhancing effects can be beneficial to both athletes and nonathletes. Choose high-quality supplements with standardized horse chestnut seed extract (13 to 24 percent aescin or triterpene glycosides). Daily dosages of horse chestnut for use as a dietary supplement range from 25 to 150 mg of standardized extracts. In medically supervised clinical studies, 600 mg per day of horse chestnut extract was used safely for 19 weeks and was found to be effective for treating chronic venous insufficiency. The effects of long-term use have not been determined. Do not use if you are on anticoagulant drugs, or use with caution under doctor supervision. The beneficial results from clinical studies and from patient use are impressive. It takes several weeks for the benefits of horse chestnut to be observed.

INOSITOL

Like choline, inositol (correctly myo-inositol) is a lipotropic agent. It is involved in fatty acid metabolism, carbohydrate metabolism, and intracellular calcium mobilization. There is no RDA for inositol, nor have their been reports on the effects of mega-dosing on athletic performance. Deficiency of inositol results in buildup of fat in the liver and may affect nervous system function. Inositol appears to be relatively nontoxic in healthy individuals. The average adult diet contains about 1 g of inositol per day. The supplement intake of inositol ranges from 40 mg to 1,000 mg.

IODINE

The form and function of iodine in the body is the simplest of the minerals. Iodine occurs in two thyroid gland hormones: thyroxin and triiodothyronine. Iodine is therefore required for the proper function of the thyroid gland, which is essential for normal metabolism, energy production, growth, and overall physical performance. Studies support the adequate daily intake of iodine for maintenance of overall health and performance. The research does not currently support mega-dosing iodine for increased performance. The performance-fitness intake guideline for women and men who are healthy and actively training is 200 mcg to 400 mcg per day from food supplements. The RDI value is 150 mcg. The estimated safe range of intake is up to 1,000 mcg per day.

IRON

Iron's well-known function is as a part of hemoglobin, which is a carrier of oxygen in the body. Iron also is a constituent of myoglobin and a number of enzymes. Iron stores mostly occur in the body in bone marrow, the spleen, and the liver. When iron intake is low, these stores are depleted, so that individuals can subsist for a while on a diet low in iron without developing anemia. However, when anemia does occur due to severe depletion, it takes a long time to reverse the condition. For the athlete, this can be extremely detrimental. Dietary surveys have reported many athletes' diets being low in iron. Women athletes, long-distance athletes, and athletes on low-calorie diets are most commonly iron deficient. Studies support the adequate daily intake of iron for maintenance of overall health and performance. The research does not currently report benefits of mega-dosing iron for increased performance. In fact, high dosages of iron (over 200 mg to 300 mg and higher per day) will have detrimental effects. Each year, a few thousand cases of iron poisoning are reported in the United States. Several of these cases result in death. Deaths are usually reported in very small children who eat large quantities of supplements containing iron. The lethal dose for a one- to two-year-old child is about 3 grams, and for adults it ranges from 200 to 250 mg per kg of body weight. Oral dosages of about 200 mg can cause abdominal cramping, constipation or diarrhea, and nausea. It is interesting to note that there are reports of patients under medical supervision who have tolerated up to 300 mg per day of ferrous sulfate three times daily without ill effects. But there are not any practical uses for this amount of iron intake in healthy adults. Excessive iron intake may also cause certain liver disorders. An additional note of caution is directed at some individuals who may have the rare hereditary condition called idiopathic hemochromatosis. When this inherited condition exists, individuals will absorb iron at a higher rate than normal and slowly accumulate high iron content in their bodies. This may lead to problems with liver and other organ functions. Choose multivitamin/mineral supplements with iron as part of the total nutrient profile. Look for supplements that provide iron as iron fumarate (ferrous fumarate) and iron glycinate. The performance-fitness intake guideline for men and women who are healthy and actively training is 25 mg to 60 mg per day from food and supplements. The RDI value is 18 mg. The estimated safe range of intake is up to 80 mg per day, or higher under medical supervision.

ISOLEUCINE

Isoleucine is an essential amino acid that, along with leucine and valine, is one of the branched-chain amino acids. Isoleucine is found in proteins and needed for the formation of hemoglobin. It is involved in the regulation of blood-sugar levels and is metabolized in muscle tissue during exercise for energy. Supplemental intake of isoleucine, along with the other BCAAs, has been shown to help spare muscle tissue, maintain nitrogen balance, and promote muscle growth and healing. See BCAAs for dosage details.

LECITHIN (Phosphatidylcholine)

Lecithin is a type of phospholipid that contains choline attached to the phosphate molecule, plus two fatty acids. It is high in linoleic acid. Lecithin supplies choline, which is essential for liver and brain function. Egg yolk, liver, and soybeans contain high amounts of lecithin. Lecithin is also manufactured by the body. Use of lecithin supplements came into vogue when researchers made the choline-memory link. Choline-deficient diets impair memory function. Lecithin's emulsifying properties are also thought to help keep the blood system clean of fatty deposits. Researchers have documented reduced choline levels among athletes running in the Boston Marathon, and speculate that lower choline levels might adversely affect performance and have detrimental long-term nervous-system effects. Choline is important in creatine synthesis, and is therefore suspected to play a role as a strength-building nutrient. Studies on athletes using dosages of 20 to 30 g of lecithin have produced mixed results, some reporting beneficial effects on muscular power, performance, and endurance.

LEUCINE

Leucine is an essential amino acid found in protein and, like the other BCAAs, it is important in energy production during exercise. For many years, it was assumed that the three BCAAs contributed equally to energy. Recent studies, however, show that both exercising and resting muscle tissues use far more leucine for energy than either of the other two BCAAs. It is estimated that up to 90 percent of the dietary intake of leucine can be used for energy in exercising muscles. This may mean that low levels of leucine will sharply curtail activity unless supplemental amounts are taken to compensate for the leucine lost during exercise. Leucine may also stimulate the release of insulin, which increases protein synthesis and inhibits protein breakdown. Refer to the entry on BCAAs for dosage details.

MAGNESIUM

The majority of magnesium (about 24 g) in the body occurs in the bone, muscles, and soft tissues. Magnesium has many metabolic and structural roles. It constitutes part of bone and teeth, plays a role in muscle and nervous system function, activates enzymes, assists calcium and potassium uptake, assists glycolysis, and aids many biosynthetic processes. Of particular interest to athletes are the several studies which show that supplementing the diet with moderate amounts of magnesium (200 mg to 400 mg) improves several athletic performance factors: physical endurance and strength, for example. Maintenance of bone tissue is also an important function of magnesium that should not be overlooked. In addition, magnesium plays a role in the proper function of smooth muscle tissue. When physical activity is increased, depletion of magnesium is observed, especially among athletes involved in long-distance sports. Studies support the adequate daily intake of magnesium for maintenance of overall health and performance. The research does not currently report benefits of mega-dosing magnesium for increased performance. Large amounts (3 to 5 g) have a laxative effect, and several laxative products contain magnesium compounds for this purpose. Individuals with abnormal renal function can be subject to hypermagnesemia, symptoms of which include depression, nausea, vomiting, and hypotension. Magnesium in supplement form is sometimes present with calcium, in a one to two ratio of magnesium to calcium. Clinical studies have verified that this ratio works best for absorption. The performance-fitness intake guideline for men and women who are healthy and actively training is 400 mg to 800 mg per day from food and supplements. The RDI value is 400 mg.

MANGANESE

Manganese is a trace mineral with several important functions. It is required for energy production, is part of enzymes, aids in bone and connective tissue formation, is part of the antioxidant superoxide dismutase (SOD), aids in collagen synthesis, and facilitates carbohydrate metabolism. The role manganese plays in bone and connective tissue formation and antioxidant activity are of particular importance to athletes. The strength and maintenance of bone and connective tissues is essential for performance. Adequate manganese intake is therefore required. Injury prevention and recovery can be benefited by manganese. Maintaining the body's proper supply of SOD is also an important function linked to manganese. SOD is a powerful antioxidant and helps protect the body from free-radical damage. Studies support the adequate daily intake of manganese for maintenance of overall health and performance. The research does not currently support megadosing of manganese for increased performance. Because of manganese's essential role in bone and cartilage formation, and because of its role as a part of the antioxidant SOD, certain degenerative diseases may be caused from inadequate manganese intake, such as osteoporosis and arthritis. Excessive manganese intake exhibits a relatively low level of toxicity under normal circumstances. Not many cases of nutritional manganese overdosing are currently reported. Preferred supplement sources of manganese are manganese arginate, manganese glycinate, or manganese gluconate. The performance-fitness intake guideline for men and women who are healthy and actively training is 2 to 20 mg per day from food and supplements. The adult RDI value is 2 mg per day. The estimated safe range of intake is up to 50 mg per day.

MEDIUM-CHAIN TRIGLYCERIDES (MCTS)

Medium-chain triglyceride formulas were first made in the 1950s, using coconut oils. MCTs contain saturated fatty acids with a carbon chain length of six to 12 carbon atoms and have attracted recent attention from athletes as MCT supplement liquids have appeared on the market. They occur in milk fat, and especially in coconut and palm kernel oil. MCTs' usefulness was first as a calorie source for individuals having certain pathological conditions that do not allow normal digestion and utilization of long-chain fatty acids. MCT formulations are high in caprylic acid and capric acid, which are saturated fatty acids. MCTs tend to behave differently in the body than long-chain triglycerides. They are more soluble in water, and can be taken up through the intestines right into portal circulation; fatty acids are usually taken up through the lymphatic system. This makes MCTs more easily and quickly digested than LCTs. It has been reported in the medical literature that MCTs are not readily stored in fat deposits and are quickly used for energy in the liver. (However, MCTs can be converted to body fat.) MCTs can also pass freely into the mitochondria of cells, independently of L-carnitine. MCTs are then perhaps a high energy source that is quickly used for energy by the body. They also have a reported thermogenic effect, estimated to be 10 percent to 15 percent higher than their caloric value, but only when the diet's MCTs exceed 30 percent of calories.

These features have recently turned the attention of athletes toward MCTs. Bodybuilders have especially jumped on the MCT bandwagon. The perceived benefit is that MCTs are burned quickly for energy and have a thermogenic effect. This may also benefit bodybuilders' restricted contest preparation diets aimed at losing body fat and sparing muscle tissue. The implications of the use of large amounts of MCT by athletes on restricted diets are not clearly evident. Some bodybuilders report that they are able to get "super ripped," when eating about 400 calories per day of MCT as part of a 2,000-calorie-a-day contest preparation diet. But remember, bodybuilders are not concerned with physical performance for their contests—their contests are judged on physique attributes. Do MCTs have a place in every athlete's diet? More research needs to be gathered to adequately determine the exact benefits that MCTs pose for widespread use by all athletes. While bodybuilders may appear to derive certain benefits for losing body fat while on low calorie/low carbohydrate diets, there can be side effects from eating too much MCT. The most common complaints are gastrointestinal cramps and diarrhea. Prolonged use may also be potentially harmful. MCTs are saturated fatty acids, and consumption of more than 10 percent of daily calories from saturated fatty acids is not recommended because of their link to various cardiovascular diseases and certain cancers. Recent research has determined that individuals ingesting only moderate amounts of MCTs have developed elevated triglyceride and cholesterol blood levels. If you plan to experiment with MCTs, you should use formulations that also contain the essential fatty acids EPA and DHA. MCTs may also have a place in the diets of endurance athletes as part of their pregame meal. It is hypothesized that this quick fuel source may be a better fuel than body stores of fatty acids, and can perhaps spare muscle glycogen. Studies need to be performed on athletes to verify this. A major drawback of MCT metabolism is the conversion of MCTs to ketones in their metabolism. Ketones are acidic and can upset an individual's physiology. Although trained endurance athletes have developed the metabolic pathways to utilize ketones better than untrained individuals, those experimenting with MCTs should do so several weeks in advance of a major event to avoid the possibility of impaired performance due to elevation of ketones in the blood.

MOLYBDENUM

Molybdenum is a trace mineral whose content in the body is extremely low, but it is recognized as an essential nutrient and required by the body for maintenance of good health. Molybdenum is present in enzymes, such as xanthine oxidase, sulfite oxidase, and aldehyde oxidase. These compounds are involved in energy production, nitrogen metabolism, and uric acid formation. Studies support the adequate daily intake of molybdenum for maintenance of overall health and performance. The research does not report benefits of mega-dosing molybdenum for increased performance.

No deficiency of molybdenum in humans has been reported. Because it is required in such small quantities, adequate amounts of molybdenum can be found in most diets. Ingestion of large amounts of molybdenum (15 mg daily for several months) may cause gout, retarded growth, and loss of copper. The performance-fitness intake guidelines for men and women who are healthy and actively training is 100 mcg to 300 mcg per day from food and supplements. The RDI value is 75 mcg. The estimated safe range of intake is up to 600 mcg per day.

MSM (Methylsulfonylmethane)

MSM is a sulfur-containing substance available as a dietary supplement. It occurs naturally in plants and animals. MSM-containing supplements therefore serve as a supply of biological sulfur. Sulfur is part of structural proteins and enzymes. MSM's most noted use as a dietary supplement is in the nutritional treatment of connective-tissue disorders. Studies have shown that MSM stimulates collagen formation. MSM also plays a role in promoting immune system function by supplying the sulfur needed in the formation of IgG, an important immune-system compound. Research also indicates that MSM supplements help build and maintain the linings of the gastrointestinal tract and respiratory tract. MSM supplements promote the growth and maintenance of connective tissucs, resulting in improvements in joints, skin, hair, and other tissues. For best results, consult MSM products for proper use.

NADH

NADH (coenzyme nicotinamide adenine dinucleotide) is present in every living cell and is a vital biochemical required for production of cellular energy. NADH is involved in the production of ATP. Some research has shown that supplemental intake of NADH can improve mental function. NADH increases the production of the neurotransmitter dopamine, which plays a role in short-term memory and muscle function. NADH also enhances the synthesis of norepinephrine, which functions in alertness, concentration, and mental activity. Research on athletes indicates that NADH supplementation enhances work capacity. Oxygen uptake and reaction time was also observed to improve in athletes tested using 5 mg of NADH per day for four weeks. The possible increase of dopamine levels could be used to explain improvements in reaction time, and increases in performance could be due to NADH's role in energy production. More research is needed to determine the exact benefits NADH can offer and the safety of long-term use.

NIACIN

Niacin, vitamin B_3, is a water-soluble vitamin of the B complex family that is used in a general sense for both nicotinic acid and niacinamide (nicotinamide). Niacin is functionally active in the body as two very important coenzymes: NAD (nicotinamide adenine dinucleotide) and NADP (nicotinamide adenine dinucleotide phosphate). NAD and NADP are present in all cells and function in many vital metabolic processes, such as energy production, glycolysis, carbohydrate and protein metabolism, fatty acid synthesis, and reduction of both cholesterol and fatty acids in the blood. Niacin's role as a cholesterol-controlling nutrient brought it major acclaim as a miracle nutrient and resulted in its widespread use in mega-dose quantities. Nicotinic acid seems to perform better than niacinamide for lowering cholesterol and fatty acid blood levels. However, nicotinic acid in amounts over 50 mg causes the blood capillaries to dilate, resulting in what has become known as the niacin flush. This flushing produces red skin, itching, and heating of the skin. This is not observed with the niacinamide form of niacin. Caution: niacin may impair performance. It is interesting to note that although niacin is essential for cellular respiration, energy production research conducted with athletes clearly shows that it reduces performance in some instances. The higher amounts of niacin administered before exercise caused glycogen to deplete at a faster rate and caused earlier onset of fatigue. Niacin apparently blocks the release of fatty acids from adipose tissue, making this source of energy less available during exercise. Thus, niacin megadosing should be avoided by endurance athletes. However, there is some evidence that high dosages of niacinamide given before anaerobic exercise may improve performance due to the fact that these athletes get more energy from stored glycogen and faster glycogen liberation may result in better anaerobic energy. More research is warranted to determine this. Amounts used ranged from 50 mg taken over three days, to 200 mg taken two hours before exercise.

Deficiency symptoms of niacin include depression, confusion, headaches, elevated body fats, fatigue, and development of pellagra. Pellagra is a disease characterized by dermatitis, inflammation of mucous membranes, dementia, and inflamed and discolored skin. Intake of niacin in amounts up to 1,000 mg is considered safe. Higher amounts should only be administered by health professionals. Maintain niacin intake within the PDI guidelines from dietary and supplement sources. Current research does not support mega-dosing; in fact, as noted above, endurance athletes should keep niacin intake below 30 mg per day, especially before events. The performance-fitness intake guideline for intake from food and supplements for men and women who are healthy and actively training is 20 mg to 100 mg. The RDI value for niacin is 20 mg. No toxicity has been reported for niacin. Up to 1,000 mg is considered safe, but should be administered only by health-care practitioners.

OMEGA-3 FATTY ACIDS (EPA AND DHA)

During the 1980s, there was a resurgence of attention focused on two fatty acids belonging to the omega-3 family of fatty acids: eicosapentaenoic acid (EPA) and do-cosahexaenoic acid (DHA). Researchers in the 1950s documented the cholesterol-lowering effects of EPA and DHA. However, it was not until 25 years later, when reports of low rates of cardiovascular diseases were documented among fish-eating Greenland Eskimos, that conclusive proof was found. EPA and DHA can be made in the body from linoleic acid and are found in human tissue as normal components. Even though the body can manufacture EPA and DHA, dietary sources have beneficial effects when part of a diet low in saturated fatty acids. These acids have the tendency to disperse fatty acids and cholesterol in the bloodstream, which seems to be how their presence helps prevent arteries from clogging. They have a blood-thinning effect and discourage excessive blood clotting. They also lower blood triglycerides and raise HDLs (high-density lipoproteins, the good lipoproteins). EPA and DHA exert an anti-inflammatory effect and work by competing with arachidonic acid, which forms pro-inflammatory compounds. Besides all of these known health benefits, recent studies on athletes have documented improvement in athletic performance. Studies using 2 to 4 g per day of EPA and DHA from supplements and fish have reported significant increases in strength and aerobic performance. Improvements include higher repetitions in bench press, an increase in the one-repetition maximum, faster running times, reduction in muscular inflammation, and longer jumping distances. Scientists believe that these improvements in various athletic performance parameters are due to the effects in combination that EPA and DHA have on the body, including growth hormone production, anti-inflammatory action, enhanced aerobic metabolism, lower blood viscosity leading to better oxygen and nutrient delivery to muscles, and improved recovery. EPA and DHA are available in supplement forms, gel capsules, and liquids, and are high in cold-water fish such as cod, salmon, sardines, trout, mackerel, and eel. Aim for a combined intake of 2 to 4 g of EPA and DHA per day from supplements and fish.

ORNITHINE

This nonessential amino acid does not occur in proteins and has gained wide-spread popularity with athletes in recent years due to its role as a growth hormone elevator. Ornithine's primary role in the body is in the urea cycle, which makes it important in the removal of ammonia. Ornithine is formed from arginine in the urea cycle. Like arginine, ornithine has been proven an effective growth hormone releaser. Various amounts of ornithine supplementation have been reported, ranging from 2 to 4 g per day. Studies using ornithine with other amino acids have also been conducted. Recently, a study using 1 g of ornithine and 1 g of arginine per day along with five weeks of weight training showed a decrease in body fat and increase in muscle mass. It is indicated, however, that the effective dosage of ornithine may be as high as 5 g to 15 g per day. The effects of ornithine can be beneficial to bodybuilders, powerlifters, and sprinters. More research needs to be conducted to determine ornithine's exact dosage and benefit. Also refer to the section on ornithine alphaketoglutarate.

ORNITHINE ALPHAKETOGLUTARATE (OKG)

OKG has recently been introduced to bodybuilding and sports circles and is being touted as the hot new performance enhancer. Studies report the use of OKG in Europe for a number of years—as far back as the early seventies—mainly for the treatment of burn victims, trauma, postsurgical healing, and cases of severe malnutrition. OKG consists of two ornithine molecules and one alphaketoglutarate molecule. OKG seems to be a stimulus for a variety of metabolic functions. It acts as an ammonia scavenger; increases the glutamine pool in muscle tissue, thereby reducing muscle breakdown (catabolism); elevates growth hormone levels; increases protein synthesis; increases insulin secretion; plays a role in glutamine and arginine synthesis; and provides an anticatabolic effect. While studies on athletes still need to be conducted, based on clinical use, dosages of 2 to 4 g once or twice a day with meals have been reported to be of potential benefit for bodybuilding and strength athletes. Note that there are much more effective nutrients for recovery and tissue repair like L-glutamine, glucosamine, curcumin, and antioxidant mixtures that have many more studies supporting their use by athletes.

PANTOTHENIC ACID

Pantothenic acid is another B vitamin that does not have an RDA determination. Pantothenic acid plays many important metabolic roles, primarily as a component of coenzyme A. These metabolic reactions are important in the release of energy from carbohydrates and fatty acids. Pantothenic Acid is also involved in steroid and cholesterol synthesis. Studies on athletes have yielded results that indicate pantothenic acid may have performance-enhancing effects when taken by endurance athletes in amounts ranging from 30 mg to 2 g for short periods of time. Short-term mega-dosing of pantothenic acid may be beneficial for endurance athletes for short time periods (seven to 14 days) before athletic competition. Amounts up to 2 grams per day have been reported to increase performance. However, more research is needed to fine-tune the optimum intake for this short-term use. The performance-fitness intake guidelines for men and women who are healthy and actively training is 25 mg to 200 mg per day from food and supplements. The RDI for pantothenic acid is 10 mg per day. The estimated safe range for pantothenic acid is up to 1,000 mg per day.

PHENYLALANINE AND DL-PHENYLALANINE

Phenylalanine is an essential amino acid and a precursor for the nonessential amino acid tyrosine. Ingestion of tyrosine will therefore spare the use of phenylalanine for the formation of tyrosine. Phenylalanine has many functions in the body and is a precursor to several important metabolites. These include the skin pigment melanin and several catecholamine neurotransmitters—like epinephrine and norepinephrine. The catecholamines have many functions in the body and are important in memory and learning ability, locomotion, sex drive, tissue growth and repair, immune system function, and appetite control. Phenylalanine can inhibit appetite by increasing the brain's production of norepinephrine and the hormone CCK (cholecystokinin). CCK is thought to be the hormone responsible for sending out the "I'm full" message. These functions of phenylalanine can be of value to all athletes, especially athletes who need to stimulate mental alertness and those who need to lose weight or maintain low levels of body fat.

Dosages of L-phenylalanine ranging from 100 mg to 500 mg and taken once or twice per day have been reported to have no side effects. Take L-phenylalanine on an empty stomach in the evening and the morning. However, note that dosages over 4 g have been shown to cause headaches in some individuals. Cofactors that appear to be necessary in phenylalanine metabolism include vitamin B_6, vitamin

C, copper, iron, and niacin. The mixture of DL-phenylalanine (DLPA) has been shown useful in combating pain control. This can be beneficial to athletes who suffer from acute or chronic pain from injury. Dosages of DL-phenylalanine of 500 mg to 1.5 g per day have been reported effective for pain control. The theorized mechanism for this pain control effect is that DLPA "protects" endorphins from destruction in the body, thereby allowing the endorphins to distribute their morphinelike pain relief. Endorphins are 1,000 times more powerful than morphine. Remember that more will not be better and if only some pain relief is experienced, contact your doctor to evaluate your condition. Don't begin to megadose phenylalanine, especially without medical supervision.

Some interesting facts concerning phenylalanine should be noted here. The artificial sweetener Aspartame™ is a di-peptide made up of phenylalanine and aspartic acid. You may have seen warnings on soft drinks that contain Aspartame, aimed at phenylketonuria (PKU). This is a disease in which phenylalanine is not properly metabolized, and it can be very damaging. People with phenylketonuria should not take any supplemental phenylalanine. People who drink a lot of beverages containing caffeine or take energy supplements with caffeine-containing herbs, like guarana, may need more phenylalanine. Caffeine tends to cause some of the neurotransmitters that are made with phenylalanine to be depleted in the central nervous system. This is why you may sometimes feel mentally fuzzy after drinking a lot of coffee. Taking phenylalanine supplements can help offset this depletion, or better yet, cut down on caffeine consumption.

PHOSPHATIDYLSERINE (PS)

Recent attention has turned to another phospholipid, phosphatidylserine. In PS, serine is attached to the phosphate molecule. Serine is a nonessential amino acid whose metabolism leads to the synthesis of PS. Serine functions in fat metabolism and is vital to the health of the immune system. Intake of 200 to 300 mg per day of PS has been associated with improved memory, mental acuity, and learning. Intake of higher amounts, up to 800 mg, has been linked to a reduction of cortisol levels in the body. Cortisol is a catabolic hormone, and when its levels are reduced, the anabolic metabolism is improved. This means improved muscle growth and recovery after exercise.

PHOSPHORUS

Like calcium, phosphorus is an important part of bone and plays several other important roles in the body. Phosphorus occurs in bone at approximately a 1 : 2 ratio with calcium. Phosphorus is present in bone, in cellular fluids as phosphate ion, and in lipids, proteins, nucleic acids, ATP, creatine phosphate, etc. Phosphorus is also involved in cell permeability, metabolism of fats and carbohydrates, formation of ATP and high-energy storage, modulation of enzyme activity, and phospholipid transport of fatty acids. The chemical energy of the body is stored in high-energy phosphate compounds, like ATP and CP. Phosphorus also plays a role in collagen synthesis. Most diets normally supply adequate amounts of phosphorus, about 1,500 milligrams per day. Even so, some supplement intake is recommended for athletes, along with a full profile of the other essential vitamins and minerals. Due to the role of phosphorus in cellular energy storage, studies on phosphate loading are traced back to the early 1900s. During World War I, the German troops were fed diets and supplements high in phosphorus to improve physical performance and reduce fatigue. Subsequent research has verified the benefits of short-term phosphate loading, mostly for endurance athletes. The effect on power athletes is less clear, but research indicates that short-term phosphate loading may also improve anaerobic endurance. Studies support the adequate daily intake of phosphorus for maintenance of overall health and performance. The research does report benefits of mega-dosing phosphorus for increased performance, in particular with endurance sports. Studies have used 1 g of sodium phosphate taken four times per day for three days prior to events. Do not phosphate-load longer than three days, as the possible side effects have not been clearly established and blood levels are maintained for several days after loading.

Because phosphorus is readily available in most foods, deficiency is rarely seen in adults. It has been observed in cases of malnutrition and in clinical settings among the ill. Deficiency symptoms over long periods of time include poor bone formation, poor growth, weakness, anorexia, and malaise. Excessive intake of phosphorus has been reported to adversely affect calcium metabolism and stimulate bone loss. Look for multinutrient supplements that contain phosphorus as part of a complete multivitamin/mineral formula. Because phosphorus is plentiful in the diet, supplement with only 100 mg to 300 mg per day, and make sure the supplement also contains calcium. People on low-calorie diets may want to supplement with more phosphorus. The performance-fitness intake guideline for men and women who are healthy and actively training is 800 mg to 1,600 mg per day from food and supplements. The RDI value is 1,000 mg per day. The estimated safe range of intake is up to 4 g per day for short periods.

PROLINE AND HYDROPROLINE

Proline and hydroproline are nonessential amino acids. Proline occurs in high amounts in collagen tissues and can be synthesized from ornithine or glutamine acid. Hydroproline is synthesized from proline in the body and is also abundant in collagen. Proline can be important for maintenance and healing of collagen tissues like skin, tendons, and cartilage. Some studies suggest that taking supplements containing these substances will promote connective-tissue growth.

RIBOFLAVIN

Riboflavin (vitamin B_2) is also involved in energy production and cellular respiration. In the body, riboflavin functions primarily as part of two coenzymes: flavin mononucleotide (FMN) and flavin adenine dinucleotide (FAD). These coenzymes are involved in many oxidation-reduction reactions that produce energy from carbohydrates, fatty acids, and some amino acids. Because of riboflavin's role in energy-producing reactions, it is a vital nutrient for the health of all tissues, in particular the skin, eyes, and nerves. Apart from these essential functions, riboflavin taken in amounts of 10 mg per day was reported to produce a lowering of neuromuscular irritability after electrical stimulation of muscles. This indicates that riboflavin taken in higher amounts may improve muscular excitability and result in better overall performance. The performance-fitness intake guideline for men and women who are healthy and actively training is 30 mg to 300 mg per day from food and supplements. The RDI for riboflavin is 1.7 mg. No toxicity has been observed.

RIBOSE

Researchers have learned that a simple sugar, ribose, can stimulate the body's production of ATP. In fact, ribose is the essential molecule required to make ATP and to maintain high levels of it in the heart and skeletal muscles. Whether you are young or old, healthy or ill, a serious athletic competitor or a weekend athlete, you should understand the role of ATP in your body and its contribution to your health, fitness, and well-being. Many cells actually lose their energy-producing compounds during exercise and do not recover even after three days of rest. This is very important for athletes because studies have shown that repeated high-intensity exercise causes a decrease in resting levels of skeletal muscle ATP. Supplemental ribose, then, can be crucial for recovery.

On average, the human body contains 1.6 mg of ribose in every 100 ml of blood at any given time. Some people do not have any free ribose in their blood, while others have as much as 3.6 mg per 100 ml. There are no foods that provide enough ribose to be helpful. Of course, since all living cells contain ribose, we do take in a small amount whenever we eat. Research has shown that about 3 to 5 g of ribose taken every day should put enough in the bloodstream to ensure that the heart and skeletal-muscle cells have an adequate supply. Serious athletes and people concerned about their circulation may want to take more. In fact, these people may require 10 g or more per day. A good course of action would be to start out with about 5 g of ribose per day. If you feel you need more, increase your dosage by about 2 to 3 g per day. However, do not take more than 15 to 20 g per day. If you are in serious physical training or have concerns about the circulation to your heart or extremities, you may want to take up to 10 g per day to start. If you are not in training but just want to maintain healthy levels of energy in your heart and skeletal muscles, 3 to 5 g per day should be an adequate maintenance dose. If your muscles become sore or cramped after even mild exercise, you may want to modify your supplementation regimen. Try taking 10 g of ribose before beginning any physical exercise and then supplementing with additional doses of 4 g every 30 minutes during and then at the conclusion of the exercise. If this works, you can cut back the amount of ribose you take until you find your proper individual dosage level. Studies have shown that short-term use of ribose is safe.

SAMe (S-adenosylmethione)

SAMe is made in your body from the amino acid methionine. Research indicates that, as some individuals age, their production of SAMe is reduced, which leads to the development of degenerative conditions, mainly arthritis and depression. Clinical studies have shown SAMe supplementation to improve depression as well as rheumatoid arthritis, osteoarthritis, fibromyalgia, and liver function. SAMe promotes connective tissue health and joint function and promotes a positive mood. These benefits are of special interest to athletes who often overtrain, experience mood fluctuations, and exert wear and tear on connective tissues. SAMe's role in the body makes it important in many anabolic biochemical reactions. SAMe works differently from and synergistically with other connective-tissue-building supplements, such as chondroitin sulfate, glucosamine, and MSM. It should not be used in place of these supplements but in addition to. SAMe has been used safely in clinical studies in dosages ranging from 400 mg to 1,600 mg per day, under doctor supervision. In clinical studies, lasting up to two years, SAMe has been shown to be safe and effective, with minor occasional side effects such as gastrointestinal distress. Best used under doctor supervision when a medical condition exists.

SELENIUM

Selenium's role in influencing antioxidant activity in the body is well known. Selenium is a vital component of an antioxidant enzyme called glutathione peroxidase. Glutathione peroxidase protects the body from free radical damage, in particular hydroperoxides. In this role as an antioxidant, selenium helps prevent damage to the body's tissues, cells, and molecules, which can lead to reduced risk of degenerative diseases like coronary heart disease, arthritis, and certain cancers. For athletes, protection against free radicals is important for protection of tissues, shortened recovery times, and protection from the extra added free radical load that exercise causes. The few studies on athletes taking selenium supplements report encouraging findings that indicate a reduction in lipid peroxidation. This translates into less tissue damage. The performance-fitness intake guideline for men and women who are healthy and actively training is 100 mcg to 300 mcg per day from food and supplements. The RDI value is 70 mcg. The estimated safe range of intake is up to 1,000 mcg per day.

TAURINE

This nonessential amino acid is one of the sulfur-bearing amino acids and plays a major role in brain tissue and nervous system function. It is involved in blood pressure regulation and transportation of electrolytes across cellular membranes. It is found in the heart, muscle, central nervous system, and brain. It is also an inhibitory neurotransmitter like GABA. Taurine is also found in the eye and may be important for maintaining good vision and eye function. Taurine is made from cysteine, with vitamin B_6 as a cofactor. Use of supplemental amounts ranging between 500 mg to 5 g per day has been reported, but no research has been done on athletes to determine how supplemental taurine may be part of the athlete's nutrition program.

THIAMIN

Thiamin (as thiamin pyrophosphate or TPP), also called vitamin B_1, is the first of the B vitamins to be discussed. In the body, thiamin joins with phosphate to form thiamin pyrophosphate (TPP) and functions as a coenzyme required in carbohydrate metabolism. Thiamin is water soluble and not readily absorbed by the body. Thiamin is converted into coenzymes that aid in the complete breakdown of carbohydrates, along with other B vitamins. Other functions of thiamin include the production of ribose, which is needed for the synthesis of nucleic acids (RNA and DNA) and appetite stimulation. As athletes eat more carbohydrates, thiamin is in greater need. Additionally, performance improvements have been reported in endurance athletes ingesting higher amounts of thiamin. Maintaining the integrity of nervous system functioning is also of great benefit to any athlete. Some research indicates that endurance athletes may derive acute performance-enhancing effects by ingesting megadoses of thiamin for three to five days prior to competition. Amounts of 300 to 900 mg per day have been reported for this use. However, more research is needed to conclusively verify these effects and determine the exact range of thiamin intake for this purpose. Additional research reports that supplemental thiamine may significantly improve firing accuracy in marksmen. The performance-fitness intake guideline for men and women who are healthy and actively training is 30 mg to 300 mg from food and supplements. The RDI for thiamin is 1.5 mg.

TRIBULUS (Tribulus terrestris)

Tribulus is a botanical with ancient origins as a medicinal herb. Traditionally, tribulus is regarded as an herb that stimulates sexual performance and libido. Clinical studies have confirmed these benefits and have also reported an increase in testosterone levels in men. In both men and women, libido and fertility can be increased by taking tribulus supplements. Due to the reports that tribulus stimulates a rise in testosterone levels, many strength athletes have started using tribulus-containing supplements. Clinical studies are needed to confirm the added muscle-building effects that taking tribulus may offer. Use only quality supplements that contain standardized tribulus root extract (20 to 40 percent furanosterols), and consult the product label for dosage and duration-of-use recommendations.

TYROSINE

Tyrosine is a nonessential amino acid made from the essential amino acid phenylalanine. Tyrosine ingestion can have a sparing effect on phenylalanine, making it available for functions not associated with tyrosine formation. Tyrosine has many functions. It is used to make dopamine and norepinephrine and plays a role in appetite regulation and melanin production. When taken as a supplement, tyrosine has an antidepressant effect and increases sex drive in men. Tyrosine supplementation may be useful for athletes undergoing stress, people who need to lose body fat, or people who want to maintain peak alertness. Dosages ranging from 100 mg to several grams per day have been reported. Tyrosine may, however, trigger migraine headaches when it is broken down into a product called tyramine.

VALINE

Valine is an essential amino acid and a member of the branched-chain amino acids. Like the other BCAAs, isoleucine and leucine, valine is an integral part of muscle tissue and can be used for energy by exercising muscles. Valine is involved in tissue repair, nitrogen balance, and muscle metabolism. See information on BCAAs for more details on dosages.

VANADIUM

Vanadium is another ultra-trace mineral that is now a focus of athletes, especially bodybuilding and strength athletes. This attention is due to its role in glucose metabolism, its role as an insulin cofactor, and even its potential ability to mimic the action of insulin. Marketing companies have taken this potential role of vanadium and mistakenly turned it into an anabolic steroid alternative that allegedly increases protein synthesis and reduces fat. Because vanadium is one of the more toxic minerals, its use as a supplement in high amounts should be avoided or minimized to a few weeks at a time. Vanadium amounts normally encountered in diets are about 10 to 20 mcg. If you choose to take supplements containing vanadium, vanadyl sulfate, or "vanadates." There are many athletes currently experimenting with vanadium and vanadyl sulfate supplementation taking amounts much higher than this range. Before playing around with vanadium supplements, you should implement the other supplementation and nutrition guidelines. First try the comprehensive approach presented in this book, and you will see that "magic bullet" approaches are not required.

The results of a study on vanadyl sulfate (J. Paul Fawcett et al., "The Effect of Oral Vanadyl Sulfate on Body Composition and Performance in Weight-Training Athletes," *International Journal of Sport Nutrition,* 1996, 6, 382–390) reported that vanadyl sulfate was ineffective in changing body composition in weight-training athletes. In this study 0.5 mg per kilogram of body weight were given to 11 males and four females for 12 weeks, and a placebo was given to 12 males and four females for the same amount of time. At the end of the study period there were no significant differences in body composition changes between the two groups.

No RDI value has been established for vanadium.

VITAMIN A—RETINOL AND PRO-VITAMIN A (Beta-carotene)

The principal vitamin A compound is retinol and it belongs to a class of chemicals called retinoids, which have varying degrees of vitamin A activity. Retinol is the standard against which the other compounds that display vitamin A activity are rated. The retinoids occur in animals. The carotenoids are another class of chemicals that display vitamin A activity. They are made by plants, but can also be stored in animal fat. They occur in the precursor form of vitamin A. The body converts carotenoids to vitamin A, mostly retinol. The carotenoids can build up in the body, but do not appear to develop signs of toxicity. Persons desiring to maintain high vitamin A intake will usually combine a moderate amount of vitamin A with a higher intake of beta-carotene. Beta-carotene is the most popular carotenoid and has about one-sixth the biological vitamin activity of retinol. The carotenoids are yellow-red plant pigments, and taking high amounts of them may affect a person's skin color with a yellow tint due to accumulation in subcutaneous fat. This condition is called carotenemia. Coloration disappears when the high dosages are discontinued. If carotenemia develops, just cut back on your dosage of beta-carotene.

Vitamin A has many functions and is essential for vision; cellular growth and development; testicular and ovarian function; integrity of the immune system; formation and maintenance of healthy skin, hair, and mucous membranes; and promotion of bone growth, tooth development, and anticancer functions. Low intake of the carotenoids, particularly beta-carotene, is associated with increased risk of lung cancer. This suggests that maintaining proper intake will help reduce the risk of lung cancer in persons susceptible to that disease. Some less conclusive studies indicate that vegetable and fruit intake may reduce the risk of cancer in the mouth, pharynx, larynx, esophagus, stomach, colon, rectum, bladder, and cervix. Scientists speculate that this anti-cancer function is due in part to vitamin A's role in promoting normal epithelial cells, like those found in the lungs and digestive system.

In addition to these important functions of vitamin A, beta-carotene functions as an antioxidant, having the ability to quench the free radicals, particularly singlet oxygen. This helps reduce cellular, molecular, and tissue damage caused by free radicals, which are greatly increased by exercise and increased oxygen uptake.

Deficiency signs of vitamin A include development of night blindness; glare blindness; rough, dry skin; dry mucous membranes; loss of appetite; increased susceptibility to infections; and slow growth. Toxic effects include headaches, vomiting, dryness of mucous membranes, bone abnormalities, and liver damage. Signs of toxicity in adults seem to appear after prolonged daily intakes of 15,000 mcg (50,000 IU) of retinol and 6,000 mcg (20,000 IU) of retinol in children and infants. The vitamin A that is most commonly used in supplements is vitamin A acetate and palmitate. These are effective and economical synthetic forms of retinol. Natural vitamin A retinol forms are available but are more expensive because they are concentrated and extracted from natural animal sources, such as fish liver oil. Beta-carotene, while of plant origin, comes in a synthetic form used mostly in supplements. Beta-carotene is several more times expensive than vitamin A. Both vitamin A and beta-carotene are found in gel caps, capsules, and tablets. The dry forms tend to be more stable than those suspended in oils. Taking a combination of vitamin A and beta-carotene is recommended, along with a diet rich in vegetables that are high in beta-carotene.

The performance-fitness intake guidelines for men and women who are healthy and actively training are vitamin A 5,000 IU to 25,000 IU per day and beta-carotene 15,000 IU to 60,000 IU, 20,000 IU to 80,000 IU for long distance athletes from food and supplements. The RDI for vitamin A is 5,000 IU for adults. The estimated safe range of vitamin A: 5,000 IU to 50,000 IU (25,000 IU to 50,000 IU in some cases). No toxicity has been observed for beta-carotene. Note that ingestion of over 25,000 IU of beta-carotene may lead to yellow or orange coloration of the subcutaneous fat. However, the coloration is reported to be harmless. Additionally, a note of caution to women who are pregnant or planning on becoming pregnant. High amounts of vitamin A have been associated with the incidence of certain birth defects. Consult your doctor about supplementation before and during pregnancy.

VITAMIN B_{12}

Vitamin B_{12} has been regarded in athletic circles as the primary energy vitamin. In fact, it is a common practice for athletes to get vitamin B_{12} shots during the season. Vitamin B_{12} is only part of the nutrition picture, but it does play a very essential role in maintaining performance. Vitamin B_{12} and cobalamin are terms used to describe a group of cobalt-containing compounds that display vitamin B_{12} activity. In the body, the predominant forms of B_{12} include hydroxocobalamin, enosylcobalamin, and methylcobalamin. Vitamin B_{12} forms essential coenzymes that are necessary for neural tissue development, folate metabolism, DNA synthesis (along with folacin), energy metabolism, new cell growth, and red blood cell synthesis. Studies conducted on nonathletes experiencing tiredness are credited with prompting widespread mega-dosing and B_{12} injections among athletes. These studies used injections of B_{12}. However, mega-dosing B_{12} by athletes is not supported by studies. Various studies examining strength and endurance effects of B_{12} have not demonstrated apparent immediate increases in performance. Thus far, B_{12}'s role is in promoting its essential metabolic functions. Recent attention has focused on a coenzyme form of B_{12} called cobamamide, or dibencozide. This has recently been touted as an anabolic nutrient form of B_{12} comparable to anabolic steroids. A study was conducted on children with growth deficiency disorders, and cobamamide improved growth. Direct comparison to anabolic steroids and an anabolic growth effect in healthy adults has not been proven. However, cobamamide has been reported by athletes to increase perceived energy levels and increase appetite. Use of coenzyme B_{12} by athletes is recommended, along with B_{12}.

Deficiency symptoms of B_{12} include a disease called pernicious anemia, fatigue, irritability, loss of appetite, constipation, headache, and sore tongue. B_{12} deficiency in the diet is rarely seen, and most deficiencies are attributed to poor B_{12} absorption. Pernicious anemia is actually a disease that develops from inhibited absorption of B_{12}.

Vitamin B_{12} must be activated before it can be absorbed. This is the job of a substance that is secreted by the stomach, called intrinsic factor. Vitamin B_{12} injections are needed in treatment of pernicious anemia because increasing the amount of B_{12} taken orally still needs intrinsic factor for activation and absorption. Excessive intakes of B_{12} do not appear to cause side effects. The performance-fitness intake guideline for men and women who are healthy and actively training is 12 mcg to 200 mcg per day from food and supplements. The RDI for vitamin B_{12} is 6 mcg. No toxic effects have been reported in adults taking amounts up to 500 mcg of vitamin B_{12} per day.

VITAMIN B_6

Vitamin B_6, also know as pyridoxine, is an essential vitamin and has become most noted by athletes for its role in amino acid metabolism. Vitamin B_6 actually occurs in nature as pyridoxine, pyridoxal, and pyridoxamine. In the body, B_6 is converted to its active forms, pyridoxal phosphate (PLP) and pyridoxamine phosphate (PMP), and serves primarily in many of the same types of transamination reactions that take place in amino acid metabolism. Due to its role in protein/amino acid metabolism, the need for vitamin B_6 increases as the intake of protein increases. Vitamin B_6 is also involved in conversion of the essential fatty acid linoleic acid to arachidonic acid; glycogen breakdown; energy production; and synthesis of red blood cells. Studies with athletes indicate results similar to those of niacin, due to B_6's tendency to increase utilization of glycogen stores and decrease fatty acid energy substrate use. So, for endurance athletes, high dosages of vitamin B_6 should be avoided. However, short-term anaerobic activity may benefit from extra B_6 due to the glycogen-liberating action. In sports such as weight lifting, sprinting, shot put, etc., the primary energy source is glycogen. It is possible that extra B_6 will promote greater glycogen utilization and result in greater power output. Coincidentally, strength-power athletes are on higher protein diets and their B_6 requirements therefore increase. Athletes undergoing glycogen depletion as part of a carbohydrate-loading program may expect more rapid depletion of glycogen stores, with as little as 8 mg of B_6 per day. This can be useful during the first glycogen depletion days of a carbohydrate loading cycle. Vitamin B_6 intake has also been reported to increase the exercise-induced rise in growth hormone, which is another potential benefit for strength athletes.

The performance-fitness intake guideline for men and women who are healthy and actively training is 25 mg to 100 mg per day from food and supplements. The RDI for vitamin B_6 is 2 mg. Levels up to 2000 mg do not seem to produce side effects when vitamin B_6 is taken for short periods of time. However, large amounts taken over several months may cause problems with the nervous system. Do not take high dosages unless directed by your doctor.

VITAMIN C

Vitamin C is an antioxidant and has multiple functions as a cofactor or coenzyme. It is involved in the formation and maintenance of collagen, which is an important constituent of connective tissues and intercellular substances. Collagen is a protein and an important component of skin, ligaments, and bones. Vitamin C promotes healthy capillaries, gums, and teeth; aids in intestinal iron absorption; blocks the production of nitrosamines—carcinogens; prevents the oxidation of folacin; helps heal wounds; may provide resistance against infections; aids in the metabolism of tyrosine and phenylalanine; and protects cells from free-radical damage. Vitamin C has been touted as a general cure-all by many. It gained great attention when the esteemed Nobel prize–winning biochemist Dr. Linus Pauling advocated its use to help prevent the onset of the common cold. As with the other antioxidants, vitamin C may play an important role in the prevention and correction of many dietary diseases. For athletes, these functions of vitamin C are very important, especially its antioxidant properties. Studies have also indicated vitamin C's role in increasing muscular strength, reducing lactate blood levels, and sparing glycogen. Endurance athletes need higher amounts of this and other antioxidants. Mega-dosing vitamin C above the PDI is not reported to cause any improvements in athletic performance. However, some individuals find that taking several grams of vitamin C a day when they feel a cold or flu developing may help reduce the duration. The primary form of vitamin C used in supplements is synthetic ascorbic acid. Other forms include buffered vitamin C and mineral ascorbates, such as calcium and magnesium ascorbate. Natural supplemental form of vitamin C is supplied by rose hips and is a very expensive ingredient when compared to the synthetic form. Supplements that contain a combination of ascorbic acid and vitamin C from rose hips are preferred. Also, bioflavonoids may increase the vitamin C absorption. There is also a patented form of vitamin C, called Ester C™. The company that manufactures it ran independent studies which indicate that it may have a higher bioavailability then other forms of vitamin C. The performance-fitness intake guideline for men and women who are healthy and actively training is 800 mg to 3,000 mg from food and supplements. The RDI for vitamin C is 60 mg. The estimated safe range of vitamin C is 60 mg to 5,000 mg per day.

VITAMIN D

Vitamin D was originally revealed as the active nutrient in cod liver oil that was used for the treatment of rickets and other disorders. Later, researchers also determined that ultraviolet light from sunlight or lamps could cure rickets. We know that vitamin D occurs in high amounts in cod liver oil and that the body can make vitamin D when exposed to ultraviolet light. There are several compounds that exert vitamin D activity. The most commonly encountered are calciferol, cholecalciferol, and ergocalciferol. Cholecalciferol is the major form of vitamin D that is made in the body. Ultraviolet light induces the conversion of a compound called 7-dehydrocholesterol into vitamin D_3 (cholecalciferol). Vitamin D_2, ergocalciferol, is produced commercially by ultraviolet irradiation of the plant sterol, ergosterol. The body can utilize these forms of vitamin D in the body by converting them to the biologically active form, 25-hydroxycholcalciferol. Vitamin D has several important functions and is essential for normal growth and development. Its main function is the metabolism of calcium and phosphorus to support normal mineralization (hardening) of bone. Vitamin D is involved in many aspects of calcium and phosphorus metabolism, including mediating intestinal absorption and utilization. Maintenance of the appropriate level of serum calcium is also necessary to promote proper functioning of the neuromuscular system and heart action. There is also some evidence that vitamin D functions to improve muscle strength. For athletes, there does not appear to be any added benefits of ingesting mega-doses of vitamin D. The performance-fitness intake guidelines for men and women who are healthy and actively training is 400 IU to 1,000 IU per day from food and supplements. The RDI is 400 IU per day.

VITAMIN E

Vitamin E is an antioxidant that protects cell membranes against oxidation, inhibits coagulation of blood by preventing blood clots, retards oxidation of the other fat-soluble vitamins, participates in cellular respiration, and treats and prevents vitamin deficiency in premature or low-birth-weight infants. A recent study has shown that adults taking 100 IUs of vitamin E per day had a reduced risk of cardiovascular disease. Of interest to athletes, vitamin E supplementation has been shown to lower blood lactate levels, decrease lipid peroxidation products formed during exercise, reduce oxidative cell damage, maintain muscle tissue, and play a possible role in testosterone production. High experimental intakes of vitamin E (200 IU to 1,200 IU) have been found to benefit athletes by improving energy functioning, reducing cellular damage, and stabilizing membranes. Supplementation has also had noticeably beneficial effects on physical performance and tissue protection at high altitudes (over 5,000 feet above sea level) during the athletic season. Higher than normal intakes of vitamin E are also indicated when recovering from an injury or surgery.

Both natural and synthetic forms of Vitamin E are found in supplements. The natural form, D-alpha tocopheryl succinate, is generally preferred due to its higher rate of absorption. The DL-alpha tocopheryl appears to be less bioactive. A combination of the two forms is also recommended (mixed tocopherols). Vitamin E is found in gel caps, in oil, or as a solid. All delivery systems are okay, but the dry form is likely to be more stable. The performance-fitness guidelines for vitamin E intake from food and supplements for men and women who are healthy and actively training are 200 IU to 1,000 IU, and for high altitude and injury recovery

600 IU to 1,200 IU for short periods of time (several weeks). The RDI for vitamin E is 30 IU. The estimated safe range of vitamin E is 20 IU to 1,200 IU per day.

VITAMIN K

Vitamin K's major function is the formation of prothrombin, which is vital for blood clotting. Without vitamin K, the entire blood-clotting process cannot be initiated. Vitamin K is therefore essential for maintenance of prothrombin levels and blood clotting. As athletes undergoing strenuous training are constantly damaging tissue, a supplemental amount of vitamin K is warranted to insure adequate vitamin K daily intake. Deficiency of vitamin K is rarely encountered in healthy individuals eating a balanced diet. However, deficiency can develop if green vegetables are restricted from the diet or drugs are taken that inhibit the formation of vitamin K by intestinal bacteria. Most instances of vitamin K deficiency are encountered with infants.

Vitamin K is sometimes given to patients before surgery to aid in blood clotting. Ingestion of too much aspirin can interfere with the metabolic pathways vitamin K is involved in and prevent normal blood clotting. The performance-fitness guideline for men and women who are healthy and actively training is 80 to 180 mcg per day from food and supplements. The RDI established for vitamin K is 80 mcg. The estimated safe range of vitamin K is 80 to 600 mcg.

WHEAT GERM OIL AND OCTACOSANOL

Octacosanol is a component of wheat germ oil, and both have been used by athletes for improved performance effects. Wheat germ also contains vitamin E, essential fatty acids, and plant sterols. Studies on humans have used amounts of octacosanol ranging from 1,000 to 2,000 or more mcg per day. Benefits include improved neuromuscular function, increased reaction time, improved endurance, improved muscle glycogen storage, and reduced effects of stress. Daily use of octacosanol along with wheat germ oil is recommended during the season and preseason.

ZINC

In athletic circles, zinc has developed a reputation as one of the primary "healing" nutrients and one of the prime contributors to male fertility. Zinc has many important metabolic roles in the body, and is part of various metalloenzymes that play roles in growth, testosterone production, DNA synthesis, cell replication, fertility, reproduction, and prostate gland function. Zinc functions as a free ion in cells, as a part of the synthesis of biomolecules, and as a part of enzymes. For the athlete, maintaining proper zinc intake is vital, especially for growth and repair of muscle tissue to meet the recovery demands of training. Dietary surveys on athletes report that low zinc intake is common. This occurs especially in endurance athletes, athletes on low-calorie diets, strength athletes, bodybuilding athletes, and female athletes. There are very few studies examining the actual effects of zinc supplementation on performance, but one study did show increased muscle endurance with zinc-supplemented athletes. But, be advised that too much zinc may impair performance. The role that zinc plays in healing and testosterone production should not lead you to think that more is better; it's not. The performance-fitness intake guidelines for men and women who are healthy and actively training is 15 mg to 60 mg from food and supplements. The RDI value is 15 mg. The estimated safe range of intake is up to 80 mg per day.

For more information about these and new supplement ingredients found to be useful for athletes, visit the following websites: *www.supplementfacts.com* and *www.dynatrition.com*.

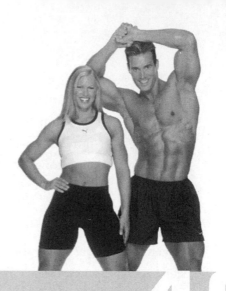

How to Be a
Natural Champion

Now that you know what nutritional supplements can do to maximize your health and performance, let's take a look at some of the drugs (doping substances) that have inevitably crept into sports to further enhance performance. We'll look at the drugs and supplements that are banned by sports organizations so you won't inadvertently take medications that are restricted. We list the main categories of banned drugs in sports, based on the International Olympic Committee and International Federation of Bodybuilders rules. If you compete in organized sports, your best bet is to report to your coach, trainer, or team doctor any prescription and nonprescription drugs you may be using, including nutritional supplements and special foods, to make sure that they do not contain substances that may be banned by your sporting organization. Even caffeine, a common ingredient in beverages, foods, and herbal dietary supplements, is sometimes considered a banned substance. Your first step to becoming a natural champion is to follow the Weider Triangle Method. This alone will improve your physical and mental performance by increasing strength and reducing excess body fat. Natural dietary supplements provide your body with the raw materials it needs for maximum growth, recovery, and maintenance of the structure and function of your body tissues and systems.

In this chapter we also review the primary doping substance categories to help you understand how these drugs work. Most importantly, we offer some nutritional solutions to stimulate your natural potential, where feasible. Banned categories include stimulants, narcotics, anabolic agents, diuretics, peptide hormones (such as growth hormones and insulin), and alcohol.

Are sports supplements drugs?

In general, no, but it's your responsibility to make sure they do not contain substances that have been made illegal by your sport's governing organization. Many sports, for example, ban the supplements that contain androstenedione, DHEA, and ephedrine from the plant ephedra.

What about creatine? Is it a drug? Creatine is a nutrient found in the food you eat, and your body makes its own supply to survive. Creatine is not a drug, although some journalists have mistakenly compared creatine to anabolic steroids in its function. The truth is that creatine is a nutrient that can improve your strength and aid in muscle growth. Refer to chapter 11 for more information about creatine.

In addition we'll show you how to increase your body's production of testosterone with proper training, rest, and nutrition. In fact, when you follow the Weider Triangle Method, your anabolic potential will be improved.

COMMON CLASSES OF BANNED DOPING SUBSTANCES

Let's look at some alternatives to the common classes of doping substances.

ANABOLIC STEROIDS

Technically speaking, anabolic steroids are synthetic derivatives of testosterone, a hormone your body produces naturally. Anabolic steroids mimic many of the functions of natural testosterone such as the development of male characteristics, like changes in the skin, distribution of body hair, enlargement of the larynx, development of testicles and sexual glands, and deepening of the voice (androgenic effects). Testosterone also stimulates the constructive phase of the metabolism, called *anabolism*. Metabolism is a general term that encompasses both the processes of repair and breakdown of tissues continually occurring in your body. Tissue and substance breakdown is called *catabolism,* and while this sounds hazardous, catabolism is just as important to the way your body functions as anabolism. The goal is for your body to be more anabolic then catabolic. If you don't eat properly, your body's metabolism will quickly become disrupted, and you can develop a catabolic metabolism, or at the very least a dysfunctional one. Your training program also affects metabolism. For example, if it is too strenuous, your metabolism becomes more catabolic because you are not giving your body enough time to recover. If it is too easy, then your body will not be stimulated to turn on its own anabolic growth and recovery systems, and your improvements in strength will be slow. Balance and complete nutrition are the key to building a strong training foundation.

In producing synthetic anabolic steroids, manufacturers attempt to modify the structure of testosterone so that the anabolic effects (to stimulate muscle growth) are increased, and the androgenic effects (male sexual characteristics) are reduced.

Effects of Doping with Anabolic Steroids

Athletes use anabolic steroids to increase protein synthesis, which in turn leads to an increase in muscle mass. Anabolic steroids also seem to reduce muscle breakdown from exercise and help speed the rate of recovery after exercise. Testing positive for anabolic steroid use can carry a stiff penalty that can range from disqualification to a lifetime sanction. Additionally, anabolic steroids have a number of dangerous side effects that can continue long after you stop taking them. Steroids shorten normal life span and can cause abnormal growth of the heart, which will lead to premature heart failure.

Most people turn to anabolic steroids with the illusion that the drugs will quickly and easily make them into champions. Nothing could be further from the truth. If all it took to make a champion was anabolic steroids, then more champions would be taking them. The fact is that today's athletes are turning away from steroids and other doping substances. In fact, sadly, the vast majority of illegal anabolic steroid users are junior level athletes or recreational bodybuilders looking to build up their biceps.

Major side effects of anabolic steroids

In women:

- Masculinizing effects, including deepening of the voice, growth of facial and body hair, and enlargement of the clitoris

- Menstrual cycle problems

- Breast reduction

- Male pattern baldness

In adolescents:

- Acne, rough and dry skin

- Cessation of growth process

In men:

- Reduced sperm count

- Decreased testicle size

- Acne

- Irreversible loss of hair

- Development of breast tissue

- Difficulty or pain while urinating

- Enlargement of prostate gland

General:

- Decrease of HDL (good) cholesterol

- Bloating

- Premature heart attacks and strokes

- Weakened tendons

- Kidney disease

- Abnormal liver function and liver damage

- Increase of aggressiveness and irritability—"Roid Rage"

- Abnormal growth of organs

- Increased injuries due to over aggressiveness and weakened tendons

- Decreased aerobic performance

Natural Alternatives to Anabolic Steroids

Power athletes and other top-level athletes who want to get an ergogenic edge without the use of illegal anabolic steroids have turned their attention to nutritional supplements and herbal products called natural anabolics. This is a catch-all term for nutritional supplements that promote tissue growth or increase the body's testosterone levels. Like their synthetic counterparts, these supplements maximize the body's anabolic-tissue-building capacity, while decreasing the body's catabolic-tissue-breakdown capacity. Recently, there has been an emphasis on the supplements that are anticatabolic—those that reduce substance and tissue breakdown. This has been and continues to be an important strategy in improving repair.

In the United States some dietary supplements called *metabolites* actually contain hormone substances. Metabolites are made in the body, and while the term often refers to common metabolite supplement ingredients such as carnitine, creatine, and coenzyme Q_{10}, it also encompasses androstenidione and DHEA. While these substances may be useful to help boost anabolism, they are banned by most sports organizations.

Note: If you are more than 40 years of age and are not competing in sports with these regulations, you may want to consult with your health-care provider about using these supplements as a form of hormone replacement therapy. There are possible side effects, especially for women, which include masculinization.

Here are some of the things you should focus on to boost your anabolism and decrease your catabolism.

- Follow the Dynatrition plan.

- Make sure to maintain adequate protein intake.

- Follow an effective weight-training program.

- Set realistic goals and develop a plan to achieve them, keeping in mind that it may take several years to do so.

What follows is a list of anabolic and anticatabolic supplement ingredients to consider including in your sports supplement program. See chapter 11 (Nutritional Supplement Review) for details on many of these ingredients.

- Protein Supplements

- Glutamine

- Branched-chain amino acids

- Zinc monomethionine aspartate

- Beta-hydroxy beta-methylbutyrate

- Alanine

- Ornithine alphaketoglutarate

- Beta-ecdysterone

- Tribulus

- Glucosamine

- Chondroitin sulfate

- SAMe

- Ferulic Acid

- Gamma oryzanol/beta-sitosterol

- Creatine monohydrate

- Panax ginseng (Chinese, Korean, Asian ginseng)

- Cordyceps

- Siberian ginseng

Below are supplements that may be beneficial for strength athletes, but either are banned by sports organizations or may result in unhealthy side effects if not used properly under medical supervision or if used for too long a time period.

- Androstenedione

- 4-androstenediol

- 19-norandrostenediol

- DHEA (Dehydroepiandrosterone)

- Pregnenelone

HUMAN GROWTH HORMONE

Human growth hormone (HGH) is a polypeptide hormone synthesized and stored inside the pituitary gland whose function is to control protein synthesis in the muscle, the growth in length of bones in legs and arms, the metabolism of fatty acids, and other effects as summarized below. Lower than normal levels during adolescence can result in a disease called dwarfism, and overproduction during adolescence and adulthood causes gigantism or acromegaly. As we progress through early adulthood, production of the growth hormone begins to decrease, which is a normal part of the aging process. But in an attempt to either boost HGH levels or delay the effects of aging, athletes and aging nonathletic adults sometimes take the drug HGH.

Major effects of human growth hormone

- Increase of the cellular reception of amino acids

- Increase of protein synthesis

- Increase in connective tissue growth

- Stimulation of glucose uptake in muscle and liver in the short term

- Decomposition of triglycerides and mobilization of free fatty acids

In recent years some athletes have begun to inject themselves with synthetic HGH with the hopes of increasing muscle strength and size and reducing body fat. This use of synthetic HGH is illegal, banned by all sports organizations, and is highly dangerous. The best known and most dreaded side effect of taking synthetic HGH is *acromegalia,* a condition in which adult bones begin to thicken. This leads to grotesque disfigurement of the face, joints, and entire body. Organs are also stimulated to continue to grow and, in rare instances, leukemia can develop.

Dangers of taking HGH

- Acromegalia

- Edema (inflammation of the soft tissues)

- Increased hair growth

- Fibroma moluscus (fibrous tumor of the superficial tissues)

- Increased sweating

- Increase of the oleaginous secretion of the skin

- Excessive growth of bones, hands, feet, and head

- Arthritis

- Joint pain

- Decreased libido

- Impotence

- Irregular menstruation

- Myopathia (degeneration of muscle tissue)

- Peripheral neuropathy (degeneration of the nerves)

- Abnormal growth of organs and glands, including salivary glands, liver, spleen, kidneys, and heart

- Cardiomyopathy (degeneration of the heart)

- Heart disease

- High blood pressure

- Hyperinsulinism

- Diabetes

- Polyps in the colon

- Leukemia

- Artherosclerosis (hardening of the arteries)

Natural Alternatives to HGH

There are ways to stimulate your body's natural secretion of growth hormone. Simply engaging in regular exercise will increase growth hormone production, and studies have shown that the higher the intensity of exercise, the greater the increase in production. Supplementation with certain amino acids also improves growth hormone production, as does adequate sleep. Consumption of too much fat in your diet and alcoholic beverages can reduce growth hormone, so use moderation.

Natural Alternatives to the Use of HGH

The following list shows some of the dietary supplements that have been shown to maintain and improve your natural production of HGH. Refer to chapter 11 for details on how to best use these supplements. Note that some of the supplements have multiple functions and may be included in other parts of this chapter.

- Arginine

- Glutamine

- Glycine

- Lysine

- Ornithine

- Orithine alphaketoglutarate

DIURETICS

Drugs that increase urine flow are called diuretics. While diuretics have some medical uses (to reduce hyperhydration and swelling, peripheral edema, and pulmonary congestion) they usually deplete water and some electrolytes—obviously an undesirable condition for anyone involved in sports.

So why would athletes use diuretics?

Diuretics are sometimes used for three main purposes:

- To dilute the urine in an attempt to pass drug tests. In the past this method was sometimes used because it was more difficult to detect some drugs such as steroids with a diluted sample. However, with modern methods of analytical detection, this doesn't work anymore.

- To eliminate excess water from the body, which may be causing bloatedness or problems with body function.

- To get into a lower weight category in sports like boxing, bodybuilding, judo, wrestling, etc., in a short period of time. Unfortunately, using diuretics as a drastic dehydration method to "make weight" is harmful to your health, and always results in decreased athletic performance.

The Dangers of Diuretics

Diuretics can deplete sodium, potassium, chlorine, and magnesium; increase uric acid, urea, and creatinine; and cause alterations in calcium balance, hypotension, allergic reactions, and hyperglycemia. Nutrient fluctuations like these are often accompanied by symptoms ranging from sleepiness, confusion, and vomiting, to life-threatening bradycardia, or coma due to acidosis or alkalosis.

Natural Alternatives to Diuretics

One of the best ways to maintain optimal fluid levels is to follow the nutrition and weight-training advice already discussed and drink plentiful amounts of pure water. As you get in better condition and your nutrition improves, problems with bloating should correct themselves. If you are experiencing repeated water retention, check with your doctor, as there may be a medical condition that needs specific treatment.

INSULIN

Insulin is another hormone made in your body that helps reduce blood-sugar levels. Made of a long chain of amino acids, insulin is crucial in helping the body turn the food we eat into energy. After a meal, insulin production increases, signalling your cells to let in nutrients such as glucose, amino acids, and fatty acids. Muscle cells are a primary target for these nutrients. Any excess glucose that is not used by the cells passes to the liver, where it is stored in the form of glycogen that will be used for energy later, perhaps during a long training session. Amino acids and glucose are then used to begin the anabolic process of muscle repair and growth. The greater the concentration of insulin, the greater the muscle anabolism will be.

If insulin is not functioning properly, then these nutrients circulate back to the liver and are turned to fat. Poor insulin functioning can actually reduce your energy and growth at the cellular level. Diabetes will develop in cases where the body does not make enough insulin, or does not properly use the insulin it makes.

As we age, the concentration and the quality of the insulin our bodies produce diminish, as does our capacity of protein synthesis and regeneration. This is one reason why we lose lean muscle mass as we get older.

Effects of Doping with Insulin

Some athletes experiment with insulin injections to boost muscle development. They mistakenly believe the extra insulin will have an anabolic effect, but insulin only produces an anabolic effect when it is in balance with the rest of the body's systems and hormones. The injection of excess of insulin in an otherwise healthy individual is perhaps one of the most dangerous performance-enhancing gimmicks you could attempt. It could eliminate almost all your blood sugar, causing severe hypoglycemia, which may lead to a complete shutdown of your brain and central nervous system, causing unconsciousness or sudden death. Injecting insulin will eventually stop your body's natural production of this important hormone.

Natural Alternatives to Insulin Doping

Many studies on diabetics demonstrate that improved blood sugar control and increased insulin function come from a proper diet and supplementation (see below). Even studies on healthy people show that supplements improve nutrient absorption resulting in improved energy levels, reduction of body fat, and increased lean body mass. Note that dietary fiber is another natural blood-level stabilizer. Here are some of the dietary supplements that research has shown can improve insulin production and function:

- Chromium

- Vanadium

- Taurine

- Glucosol (colosolic acid)

- Fenugreek seeds (4-hydroxyisoleucine)

- Dietary fiber

- Vitamin E

- Asian ginseng (Panax ginseng)

- Bioflavonoids

- Antioxidants

- Gymnema sylvestre

ERYTHROPOIETIN (EPO)

EPO is a hormone that occurs naturally in the body. It is produced by certain kidney cells and regulates blood-cell development in the bone marrow. Blood cells, in turn, are responsible for transporting oxygen in the bloodstream. EPO is used medically to treat people with anemia from kidney dysfunction and other causes.

Effects of Doping with EPO

In an attempt to increase blood cells and improve their oxygen-carrying capacity, some athletes inject themselves with EPO. The theory is that by increasing blood cells and the oxygen-carrying ability of the blood, EPO will reduce the onset of fatigue. EPO is very dangerous, and it has already caused the deaths of elite athletes.

Dangers of EPO

- Aggressiveness

- Skin rashes

- Fever

- Renal damage

- Formation of blood clots

- Headaches

- Arterial hypertension

- Convulsions

- Thickening of blood

- Abnormal blood clotting

- High blood pressure

Natural Alternatives to Erythropoietin

Currently there are no natural alternatives to EPO, but there are dietary supplements that can be used to improve circulatory system health. By maintaining healthy blood and improving the circulatory system you will also improve blood flow, delivery of oxygen to cells, and elimination of waste products. Here are some supplements that help improve circulatory system structure and function:

- Ginkgo

- Garlic

- Ginseng

- Grape seed extract

- Pycnogenol

- Gotu kola

- Green tea extract

- Horse chestnut seed extract

AMPHETAMINES AND DERIVATIVES

Amphetamines stimulate the central nervous system, causing sensations of well-being, euphoria, mental alertness, and increased energy. The effects of amphetamines are said to be similar to those of cocaine. They are highly addictive and dangerous for both physical and mental health, which is why their medical use is strictly controlled.

Effects of Doping with Amphetamines

Stimulants have been used as performance-enhancing aids for many years in sports, especially those that require prolonged effort. None of these substances are legal in competition at any level. These potent stimulants override your body's natural control systems and create an overload that can lead to collapse and, in the worst cases, death. People use the amphetamines for the following reasons:

- to increase athletic performance by means of physical or psychological stimulation

- to reduce appetite, for weight loss

- to increase muscle reserves of glycogen (muscle sugar)

- to reduce body fat

Amphetamines can be tempting because they allow you temporarily to train harder, eat less, burn body fat, and achieve more definition, but your tolerance develops so quickly that higher and higher doses are needed to achieve the same effects. The numerous side effects of amphetamines certainly outweigh any benefits. They are among the most dangerous and harmful substances that athletes sometimes abuse.

Dangers of amphetamines and other stimulants

- Skin rash or hives

- Chills or excessive sweating

- Increased heart beat/cardiac overload

- High blood pressure

- Arrhythmia

- Headache

- Shortness of breath

- Nausea, vomiting, abdominal cramps, diarrhea

- Kidney dysfunction

- Addiction

- Anxiety, aggressiveness, trembling

- Insomnia

- Weakness, dizziness, hyperactivity

- Confusion, delerium, suicidal tendencies

Natural Nutritional Alternatives to Amphetamines

It is possible to increase feelings of well-being and energy through nutritional means. While you may not feel the intense high that comes from amphetamines, your body will ultimately reach a natural high that will improve your athletic performance without the dangerous side effects. The list below offers some dietary supplements as alternatives to amphetamines.

- Tyrosine

- L-phenylalanine

- Ribose

- Branched-chain amino acids

- Vitamin B complex

- Energy sports drinks

- Ginseng

Note: There are many botanical supplements that are stimulants, but most of them contain caffeine or ephedrine. Of these, caffeine has the safest record, but it also has side effects if overused. Many sporting authorities ban the use of caffeine during competition. Read labels carefully to make sure products do not contain these ingredients.

CORTICOSTEROIDS

Corticosteroids are divided into two main types—glucocorticoids and mineralo-corticoids. Glucocorticoids, such as cortisol or cortisone, are best known for their anti-inflammatory and anti-stress actions. Athletes take them to alleviate pain and promote feelings of well-being. They are also prescribed to treat allergies, so if you take medication for allergies, you should confirm that it is not a banned substance.

Mineralocorticoids, such as dihydroepiandrosterone or aldosterone, regulate the balance of water and electrolytes and are not readily abused by athletes.

Effects of Doping with Corticosteroids

Corticosteroids have numerous side effects. In particular, the glucocorticoids will have catabolic effects if used for long periods of time. This means that they destroy your body, slowly breaking it down over time. Some of the undesirable side effects of these substances include:

- Retention of water

- High blood pressure

- Increased sensitivity to infections

- Slow wound healing

- Calcium imbalance and osteoporosis

- Impaired collagen production

- Muscular atrophy

- Increased appetite

- Peptic ulcer

- Sexual impotence

- False euphoria or psychoses

Natural Alternatives to Corticosteroids

The supplements listed below have been shown to improve connective tissue, growth, and healing, and even reduce pain and inflammation.

- Glucosamine, condroitin sulfate, MSM, and SAMe

- Ornithine alpha-ketoglutarate

- Anti-inflammatory botanicals, such as turmeric (curcumin) and boswellia

- Fatty acids, such as GLA, EPA, and DHA, from borage oil, evening primrose oil, hemp oil, and flaxseed oil

- Bromelian for short-term use, 2 to 3 weeks after an injury occurs

- Bioflavonoids

- Vitamin C

- Glutamine

SUMMARY

The following chart is not meant to be a comprehensive guide to every banned doping substance. Rather, it lists the main classes of substances most often abused by athletes and fitness exercisers, and offers natural alternatives when they are feasible. Each athletic organization has its own classes of banned doping substances, so check with yours to make sure.

LIST OF PROHIBITED DOPING SUBSTANCES AND METHODS

I. Prohibited Classes of Doping Substances

CLASS A: STIMULANTS: amineptine, amfepramone, amiphenazole, amphetamine, bambuterol, bromantan, caffeine, carphedon, cathine, cocaine, cropropamide, crotethamide, ephedrine, etamivan, etilamphetamine, etilefrine, fencamfamin, fenetylline, fenfluramine, formoterol, heptaminol, mefenorex, mephentermine, mesocarb, methamphetamine, methoxyphenamine, methylenedioxyamphetamine, methylephedrine, methylphenidate, nikethamide, norfenfluramine, parahydroxyamphetamine, pemoline, pentetrazol, phendimetrazine, phentermine, phenylephrine, phenylpropanolamine, pholedrine, pipradrol, prolintane, propylhexedrine, pseudoephedrine, reproterol, salbutamol, salmeterol, selegiline, strychnine, terbutaline, . . . and related substances.

CLASS B: NARCOTICS: buprenorphine, dextromoramide, diamorphine (heroin), methadone, morphine, pentazocine, pethidine, . . . and related substances.

CLASS C:

1. ANABOLIC AGENTS: androstenediol, androstenedione, bambuterol, boldenone, clenbuterol, clostebol, danazol, dehydrochlormethyltestosterone, dehydroepiandrosterone (DHEA), dihydrotestosterone, drostanolone, fenoterol, fluoxymesterone, formebolone, formoterol, gestrinone, mesterolone, metandienone, metenolone, methandriol, methyltestosterone, mibolerone, nandrolone, 19-norandrostenediol, 19-norandrostenedione, norethandrolone, oxandrolone, oxymesterone, oxymetholone, reproterol, salbutamol, salmeterol, stanozolol, terbutaline, testosterone, trenbolone, . . . and related substances.

2. BETA-2 AGONISTS: bambuterol, clenbuterol, fenoterol, formoterol, reproterol, salbutamol, salmeterol, terbutaline, . . . and related substances.

LIST OF PROHIBITED DOPING SUBSTANCES AND METHODS

CLASS D: DIURETICS: acetazolamide, bumetanide, chlortalidone, etacrynic acid, furosemide, hydrochlorothiazide, mannitol, mersalyl, spironolactone, triamterene, . . . and related substances.

CLASS E: PEPTIDE HORMONES, MIMETICS, AND ANALOGUES

1. Chorionic gonadotrophin (hCG); prohibited in males only
2. Pituitary and synthetic gonadotrophins (LH); prohibited in males only
3. Corticotrophins (ACTH, tetracosactide)
4. Growth hormone (hGH)
5. Insulin-like Growth Factor (IGF-1)
6. Erythropoietin (EPO)
7. Insulin; permitted only to treat athletes with certified insulin-dependent diabetes. Written certification of insulin-dependent diabetes must be obtained from an endocrinologist or team physician.

II. Prohibited Methods

The following procedures are prohibited:

1. Blood doping
2. Administering artificial oxygen carriers or plasma expanders
3. Pharmacological, chemical, and physical manipulation

III. Classes of Prohibited Substances in Certain Circumstances

1. ALCOHOL: Where the rules of a responsible authority so provide, tests will be conducted for ethanol.

2. CANNABINOIDS: Where the rules of a responsible authority so provide, tests will be conducted for cannabinoids (e.g. marijuana, hashish). At the Olympic Games, tests will be conducted for cannabinoids. A concentration in urine of 11-nor-delta 9-tetrahydrocannabinol-9-carboxylic acid (carboxy-THC) greater than 15 nanograms per millilitre constitutes doping.

3. LOCAL ANAESTHETICS: Injectable local anaesthetics are permitted under the following conditions:

List of Prohibited Doping Substances and Methods

3. Local anaesthetics *(continued)*

    a. Bupivacaine, lidocaine, mepivacaine, procaine, and related substances can be used, but not cocaine. Vasoconstrictor agents may be used in conjunction with local anaesthetics.

    b. Only local or intra-articular injections may be administered.

    c. Only when medically justified.

    Where the rules of a responsible authority so provide, notification of administration may be necessary.

4. Glucocorticosteroids: The systemic use of glucocorticosteroids is prohibited when administered orally, rectally, or by intravenous or intramuscular injection.

5. Beta-blockers: acebutolol, alprenolol, atenolol, betaxolol, bisoprolol, bunolol, carteolol, celiprolol, esmolol, labetalol, levobunolol, metipranolol, metoprolol, nadolol, oxprenolol, pindolol, propranolol, sotalol, timolol, and related substances. Where the rules of a responsible authority so provide, tests will be conducted for beta-blockers.

Exercise Log

Use photocopies of this sheet to plan your exercise sessions and keep track of your progress. List the muscle group, name of exercise performed, and the weight (Wt) of the workload and number of repetitions (Reps) performed for each set. Warm up with several minutes of aerobic exercise, followed by stretching, and 1 or 2 warm-up sets for each weight-lifting exercise. Also, on your last set of each muscle group, spend several seconds stretching the muscles you just worked.

Variable Weight Training / Exercise Log Sheet

Date:

Body Weight:

Percentage Body Fat:

Percentage Lean Body Mass:

Aerobic Exercise Performed:

Duration of Aerobic Exercise:

Muscle Group	Name of Exercise	Set 1 Wt/Reps	Set 2 Wt/Reps	Set 3 Wt/Reps	Set 4 Wt/Reps	Set 5 Wt/Reps	Set 6 Wt/Reps	Set 7 Wt/Reps	Set 8 Wt/Reps

Food Log

To keep track of your eating habits, use photocopies of this sheet to record the foods, beverages, and supplements you consume each day. Or use the log for advance meal planning.

DYNATRITION DAILY FOOD AND SUPPLEMENT LOG		
Morning	**Afternoon**	**Evening**
Breakfast:	Lunch:	Dinner:
Snack:	Snack:	Snack:
Supplements:	Supplements:	Supplements:

Related Websites

www.fitnessonline.com

The Fitness Online Network is the leading health and fitness content destination on the World Wide Web, and the online home of the Weider family of magazines: *Shape, Men's Fitness, Muscle & Fitness, Flex, Natural Health,* and *Fit Pregnancy*. Whether your goal is to lose weight, gain muscle, become a bodybuilder, or get in shape for bikini season, you'll find helpful information on this website. There's advice on diet and nutrition, exercise, "must-have" gear, and what's a waste of money. The goal of Fitness Online is to provide the user with tools and information to support personal health and fitness goals.

www.muscle-fitness.com

Muscle & Fitness is a lifestyle magazine for dynamic, active men and women who are passionate about improving their bodies and their health. Each issue includes detailed programs on exercise, strength training, and nutrition, as well as articles on fitness, physiology, performance psychology, sports medicine, weight management, relationships, and personal appearance.

www.flexonline.com

Published in nine languages and distributed in 14 countries, *Flex* is the leading bodybuilding magazine in the world. Training demonstrations by world-class champions, cutting-edge nutritional information, and behind-the-scenes stories from bodybuilding events all over the globe inform the publicaton. *Flex* is known for its inspirational and dramatic photography, as well as up-to-the-minute reports on the latest bodybuilding contests and events.

www.mensfitness.com

From carbs to khakis, supplements to sex, and great abs to great gear, *Men's Fitness* keeps its readers on top of their game, with the latest active lifestyle service information on fitness, health, relationships, and sports activities, from mainstream to extreme.

www.naturalhealthmag.com

For 30 years, *Natural Health* has been the leading healthy lifestyle magazine. *Natural Health* readers are a growing audience of new natural-health enthusiasts who have adopted the natural-health lifestyle.

Other Weider Publications include *Shape Magazine* (*www.shapemag.com*), *Muscle & Fitness Hers* (*www.muscleandfitnesshers.com*) and *Fit Pregnancy* (*www.fitpregnancy.com*).

References

Abumrad, N., and P. Flakoll. "The Efficacy and Safety of CaBHBM (Beta-Hydroxy Beta-Methylbutyrate) in Humans." Vanderbilt University Medical Center Annual Report (1991).

Adams, R. *The Big Family Guide to All the Vitamins.* New Canaan, CT: Keats Publishing, 1995.

Almada, A., et al. "Effects of B-BHBM Supplementation With and Without Creatine During Training on Strength and Sprint Capacity." *Federation of American Societies of Experimental Biology Journal,* Vol. 11 (1997), p. A374.

American College of Sports Medicine Position Stand. "The Recommended Quantity and Quality of Exercise for Developing and Maintaining Cardiorespiratory and Muscular Fitness, and Flexibility in Healthy Adults." *Med Sci Sports Exerc* Vol. 30 (June 1998), No. 6, pp. 975–91.

Anderson, Helen L., Mary Belle Heindel, and Hellen Linkswiler. "Effect on Nitrogen Balance of Adult Man of Varying Source of Nitrogen and Level of Calorie Intake." *Journal of Nutrition* (1969), pp. 82–90.

Anderson, M., et al. "Pre-Exercise Meal Affects Ride Time to Fatigue in Trained Cyclists." *Journal of the American Dietetic Association,* Vol. 94 (1994), pp. 1152–53.

Anderson, M. E., C. R. Bruce, S. F. Fraser, N. K. Stepto, R. Klein, W. G. Hopkins, and J. A. Hawley, "Improved 2000-meter rowing performance in competitive oarswomen after caffeine ingestion." *Int J Sport Nutr Exerc Metab,* Vol. 10 (Dec 2000), No. 4, pp. 464–75.

Apfelbaum, Marian, Jacques Fricker, and Lawrence Igoin-Apfelbaum. "Low and Very Low Calorie Diets." *American Journal of Clinical Nutrition,* Vol. 45 (1987), pp. 1126–34.

Armstrong, R. B. "Mechanisms of Exercise-Induced Delayed Onset Muscular Soreness: A Brief Review." *Medicine and Science in Sports and Exercise,* Vol. 16 (1984), No. 6, pp. 529–38.

Armstrong, R. B. "Muscle Damage and Endurance Events." *Sports Medicine,* Vol. 3 (1986), pp. 370–81.

Ashizawa N., R. Fujimura, K., Tokuyama, and M. Suzuki. "A Bout of Resistance Exercise Increases Urinary Calcium Independently of Osteoclastic Activation in Men." *Journal of Applied Physiology,* Vol. 83 (1998), pp. 1159–63.

Baker, O., et al. "Absorption and Excretion of L-Carnitine During Single or Multiple Dosings in Humans." *International Journal of Vitamin and Nutrition Research,* Vol. 63 (1993), pp. 22–26.

Ball, T., et al. "Periodic Carbohydrate Replacement During 50 Minutes of High-Intensity Cycling Improves Subsequent Sprint Performance." *International Journal of Sport Science* (1995), pp. 151–58.

Bamman, M. M., et al. "Changes in Body Composition, Diet, and Strength of Bodybuilders During the 12 Weeks Prior to Competition." *Journal of Sports Medicine and Physical Fitness,* Vol. 33 (1993), p. 383.

Beam, W. C. "The Effect of Chronic Ascorbic Acid Supplementation on Strength Following Isotonic Strength Training." *Medicine and Science in Sports and Exercise,* Vol. 30 (1998), p. S219.

Belanger, A. Y., and A. J. McComas. "A Comparison of Contractile Properties in Human Arm and Leg Muscles." *European Journal of Applied Physiology,* Vol. 54 (1985), pp. 26–33.

Bell, D. G., et al. "Effects of Caffeine, Ephedrine and the Combination on Time to Exhaustion During High-Intensity Exercise." *European Journal of Applied Physiology,* Vol. 77 (1998), pp. 427–33.

Bell, R. D., J. D. MacDougall, R. Billeter, and H. Howald. "Muscle Fiber Types and Morphometric Analysis of Skeletal Muscle in Six-Year-Old Children." *Medicine and Science in Sports and Exercise,* Vol. 12 (1980), No. 1, pp. 28–31.

Beniamini, Y., et al. "High-Intensity Strength Training of Patients Enrolled in an Outpatient Cardiac Rehabilitation Program. *J Cardiopulm Rehabil,* Vol. 19 (Jan-Feb 1999), No. 1, pp. 8–17.

Bergstrom, Jonas, and Eric Hultman. "Nutrition for Maximal Sports Performance." *Journal of the American Medical Association,* Vol. 221 (1972), No. 9, pp. 999–1004.

Berning, J. R. "The Role of Medium-Chain Triglycerides in Exercise." *International Journal of Sport Nutrition,* Vol. 6 (1996), No. 3, pp. 121–33.

Bier, Dennis M., and Vernon R. Young. "Exercise and Blood Pressure: Nutritional Considerations." *Annals of Internal Medicine,* Part 2 (1983), pp. 864–69.

Bonde-Petersen, Flemming, Knuttgen, Howard G., and Jan Henriksson. "Muscle Metabolism During Exercise with Concentric and Eccentric Contractions." *Journal of Applied Physiology,* Vol. 33 (1972), pp. 792–95.

Bonke, D., and B. Nickel. "Improvement of Fine Motoric Movement Control by Elevated Dosages of Vitamin B_1, B_6 and B_{12} in Target Shooting." *International Journal of Vitamin and Nutrition Research,* Vol. 30 (1989), p. 198.

Borum, Peggy R. "Carnitine." *Annual Reviews of Nutrition,* Vol. 3 (1983), pp. 233–59.

Boyne, P. S., and H. Medhurst. "Oral Anti-inflammatory Enzyme Therapy in Injuries in Professional Footballers." *The Practitioner,* Vol. 198 (April 1967), pp. 543–46.

Brilla, L. R., and T. E. Landerholm. "Effect of Fish Oil Supplementation and Exercise on Serum Lipids and Aerobic Fitness." *Journal of Sports Medicine and Physical Fitness,* Vol. 30 (1990), No. 2, pp. 173–80.

Brodan, V., E. Kuhn, J. Pechar, Z. Placer, and Z. Slabochova. "Effects of Sodium Glutamate Infusion on Ammonia Formation During Intense Physical Exercise in Man." *Nutrition Reports International,* Vol. 9 (1974), No. 3, pp. 223–32.

"Bromelain and Musculoskeletal Injuries." *Research Reviews,* Herbal Gram No. 39 (1997), p. 17.

Brown, C. Harmon, and Jack H. Wilmore. "The Effects of Maximal Resistance Training on the Strength and Body Composition of Women Athletes." *Medicine and Science in Sports,* Vol. 6 (1974), No. 3, pp. 174–77.

Bucci, L. *Nutrients as Ergogenic Aids for Sports and Exercise.* Boca Raton, FL: CRC Press, 1993.

Bucci, L. *Nutrition Applied to Injury Rehabilitation and Sports Medicine.* Boca Raton, FL: CRC Press, 1995.

Buono, Michael J., Thomas R. Clancy, and Jeff R. Cook. "Blood Lactate and Ammonium Ion Accumulation During Graded Exercise in Humans." *The American Physiological Society* (1984), pp. 135–39.

Burke, D. G., S. Silver, L. E. Holt, T. Smith, T. Palmer, C. J. Culligan, and P. D. Chilibeck. "The Effect of Continuous Low Dose Creatine Supplementation on Force, Power, and Total Work." *Int J Sport Nutr Exerc Metab,* Vol. 10 (Sep 2000), No. 3, pp. 235–44.

Burke, Edmond R., Frank Cerny, David Costill, and William Fink. "Characteristics of Skeletal Muscle in Competitive Cyclists." *Medicine and Science in Sports,* Vol. 9 (1977), No. 2, pp. 109–12.

Burke, L. M., and S. D. Read. "Dietary Supplements in Sport." *Sports Medicine,* Vol. 15 (1993), pp. 43–65.

Buskirk, Elsworth R., and José Mendez. "Sports Science and Body Composition Analysis: Emphasis on Cell and Muscle Mass." *Medicine and Science in Sports and Exercise,* Vol. 16 (1984), No. 6, pp. 584–93.

Butterfield, G. "Ergogenic Aids: Evaluating Sport Nutrition Products." *International Journal of Sport Nutrition,* Vol. 6 (1996), No. 3, pp. 191–97.

Butterfield, Gail E., and Doris H. Calloway. "Physical Activity Improves Protein Utilization in Young Men." *British Journal of Nutrition,* Vol. 51 (1984), pp. 171–84.

Calles-Escandon, Jorge, John J. Cunningham, Peter Snyder, Ralph Jacob, Gabor Huszar, Jacob Loke, and Philip Felig. "Influence of Exercise on Urea, Creatinine, and 3-Methylhistidine Excretion in Normal Human Subjects." *The American Journal of Physiology* (1984), pp. E334–E338.

Campbell, C. J., A. Bonen, R. L. Kirby, and A. N. Belcastro. "Muscle Fiber Composition and Performance Capacities of Women." *Medicine and Science in Sports,* Vol. 11 (1979), pp. 260–65.

Campbell, M. J., A. J. McComas, and F. Petitio. "Physiological Changes in Aging Muscles." *Journal of Neurology, Neurosurgery, and Psychiatry,* Vol. 36 (1973), pp. 174–82.

Carlson, Bruce M., and John A. Faulkner. "The Regeneration of Skeletal Muscle Fibers Following Injury: A Review." *Medicine and Science in Sports and Exercise,* Vol. 15 (1983), No. 3, pp. 187–98.

Carter, J. E. Lindsay, and William H. Phillips. "Structural Changes in Exercising Middle-Aged Males During a 2-Year Period." *Journal of Applied Physiology,* Vol. 27 (1969), pp. 787–94.

Casanueva, F. F., L. Villanueva, J. A. Cabranes, J. Cabezas-Cerrato, and A. Fernandez-Cruz. "Cholinergic Mediation of Growth Hormone Secretion Elicited by Arginine, Clonidine, and Physical Exercise in Man." *Journal of Clinical Endocrinology and Metabolism,* Vol. 59 (1984), No. 3, pp. 526–30.

Celejowa, I., and M. Homa. "Food Intake, Nitrogen and Energy Balance in Polish Weight Lifters, During Training Camp." *Nutrition and Metabolism,* Vol. 12 (1970), pp. 259–74.

Chang, Tse Wen, and Alfred L. Goldberg. "The Metabolic Fates of Amino Acids and the Formation of Glutamine in Skeletal Muscle." *Journal of Biological Chemistry,* Vol. 253 (1978), No. 10, pp. 3685–95.

Cheng, W., et al. "Beta-Hydroxy Beta-Methylbutyrate Increases Fatty Acid Oxidation by Muscle Cells." *Federation of American Societies of Experimental Biology Journal,* Vol. 11 (1997): p. A381.

Chin, S. "Dietary Sources of Conjugated Dienoic Isomers of Linoleic Acid, a Newly Recognized Class of Anticarcinogens." *Journal of Food Composition and Analysis,* Vol. 5 (1992), pp. 185–95.

Chin, S., J. Storkron, K. Albright, M. Cook, and M. Pariza. "Conjugated Linoleic Acid is a Growth Factor for Rats as Shown by Enhanced Weight Gain and Improved Feed Efficiency." *Journal of Nutrition,* Vol. 124 (1994), pp. 2344–49.

Christensen, H. "Muscle Activity and Fatigue in the Shoulder Muscles During Repetitive Work." *European Journal of Applied Physiology,* Vol. 54 (1986), pp. 596–601.

Clarkson, P., and E. Haymes. "Trace Mineral Requirements for Athletes." *International Journal of Sports Nutrition,* Vol. 4 (1994), p. 104.

Clarkson, Priscilla M., Walter Kroll, and Thomas C. McBride. "Plantar Flexion Fatigue and Muscle Fiber Type in Power and Endurance Athletes." *Medicine and Science in Sports and Exercise,* Vol. 12 (1980), pp. 262–67.

Colker, C. M. "Immune Status of Elite Athletes: Role of Whey Protein Concentrate: A Review." *Medicine and Science in Sports and Exercise,* Vol. 30 (1998), p. S17.

Conlay, L. A., R. J. Wurtman, J. K. Blusztajn, et al. "Decreased Plasma Choline Concentrations in Marathon Runners" (letter). *New England Journal of Medicine,* Vol. 175 (1986), p. 892.

Conzolazio, C. Frank, Herman L. Johnson, Richard A. Nelson, Joseph G. Dramise, and James H. Skala. "Protein Metabolism During Intensive Physical Training in the Young Adult." *American Journal of Clinical Nutrition,* Vol. 28 (1975), pp. 29–35.

Cook, James D., and Elaine R. Monsen. "Vitamin C, the Common Cold, and Iron Absorption." *American Journal of Clinical Nutrition* (1977), pp. 235–41.

Cook, M. "Immune Modulation by Altered Nutrient Metabolism: Nutritional Control of Immune-Induced Growth Depression." *Poultry Science,* Vol. 72 (1993), pp. 1301–5.

Copinschi, Georges, Laurence C. Wegienka, Satoshi Hane, and Peter H. Forsham. "Effect of Arginine on Serum Levels of Insulin and Growth Hormone in Obese Subjects." *Metabolism,* Vol. 16 (1967), pp. 485–91.

Cossack, Zafrallah T., and Ananda Prasad. "Effect of Protein Source on the Bioavailability of Zinc in Human Subjects." *Nutrition Research,* Vol. 3 (1983), pp. 23–31.

Costill, D. L., A. Barnett, R. Sharp, W. J. Fink, and A. Katz. "Leg Muscle pH Following Sprint Running." *Medicine and Science in Sports and Exercise,* Vol. 15 (1983), pp. 325–29.

Costill, D. L., and M. Hargreaves. "Carbohydrate Nutrition and Fatigue." *Sports Medicine,* Vol. 13 (1992), p. 86.

Costill, D. L., R. Bowers, et al. "Muscle Glycogen Utilization During Prolonged Exercise on Successive Days." *Journal of Applied Physiology,* Vol. 31 (1971), pp. 834–838.

Costill, D. L., W. M. Sherman, et al. "The Role of Dietary Carbohydrate in Muscle Glycogen Synthesis After Strenuous Running." *American Journal of Clinical Nutrition,* Vol. 34 (1981), pp. 1831–36.

Costill, David L., Michael G. Flynn, John P. Kirwan, Joseph A. Houmard, Joel B. Mitchell, Robert Thomas, and Sung Han Park. "Effects of Repeated Days of Intensified Training on Muscle Glycogen and Swimming Performance." *Medicine and Science in Sports and Exercise,* Vol. 20 (1987), No. 3, pp. 249–54.

Coyle, Edward F., and Andrew R. Coggan. "Effectiveness of Carbohydrate Feeding in Delaying Fatigue During Prolonged Exercise." *Sports Medicine* (1984), pp. 446–58.

Craig, B. "The Influence of Fructose on Physical Performance." *American Journal of Clinical Nutrition,* Vol. 58 (1993), p. S819.

Davidson, M. H., C. E. Weeks, H. Lardy, et al. "Safety and Endocrine Effects of 3-Acetyl-7-Oxo DHEA (7-Keto DHEA)." Paper presented at the Experimental Biology National Meetings, 1998.

Davies, Kelvin J. A., Alexandre T. Quintanilha, George A. Brooks, and Lester Packer. "Free Radicals and Tissue Damage Produced by Exercise." *Biochemical and Biophysical Research Communications,* Vol. 107 (1982), No. 4, pp. 1198–1205.

Davis, J. M., R. S. Welsh, and N. A. Alerson. "Effects of Carbohydrate and Chromium Ingestion During Intermittent High-Intensity Exercise to Fatigue." *Int J Sport Nutr Exerc Metab,* Vol. 10 (Dec 2000) No. 4, pp. 476–85.

Davis, Teresa A., Irene E. Karl, Elise D. Tegtmeyer, Dale F. Osborne, Saulo Klahr, and Herschel R. Harter. "Muscle and Protein Turnover: Effects of Exercise Training and Renal Insufficiency." *The American Physiological Society* (1985), pp. E337–345.

Despres, J. P., C. Bouchard, A. Tremblay, R. Savard, and M. Marcotte. "Effects of Aerobic Training on Fat Distribution in Male Subjects." *Medicine and Science in Sports and Exercise,* Vol. 17 (1985), No. 1, pp. 113–18.

Despres, J. P., C. Bouchard, R. Savard, A. Tremblay, M. Marcotte, and G. Theriault. "Level of Physical Fitness and Adipocyte Lipolysis in Humans." *The American Physiological Society* (1984), pp. 1157–61.

DiPrampero, P. Enrico. "Energetics of Muscular Exercise." *Biochemical Pharmacology,* Vol. 89 (1981), pp. 143–209.

Dohm, G. Lynis, George J. Kasperek, Edward B. Tapscott, and Gary R. Beecher. "Effect of Exercise on Synthesis and Degradation of Muscle Protein." *Biochemical Journal,* Vol. 188 (1980), pp. 255–62.

Dray, F. "Role of Prostaglandins in Growth Hormone Secretion." *Advanced Prostaglandin and Thromboxane Research,* Vol. 8 (1980), p. 1321.

Dyner, T., W. Lang, J. Geaga, et al. "An Open-Label Dose-Escalation Trial of Oral Dehydroepiandrosterone Tolerance and Pharmacokinetics in Patients With HIV Disease." *Journal of Immune Deficiency Syndromes,* Vol. 6 (1993), pp. 459–65.

Ebben, W. P., and D. O. Blackard. "Strength and Conditioning Practices of National Football League Strength and Conditioning Coaches." *Journal of Strength and Conditioning Research,* Vol. 15 (2001), No. 1, pp. 48–58.

Ehn, Lars, Bjorn Carlmark, and Sverker Hoglund. "Iron Status in Athletes Involved in Intense Physical Activity." *Medicine and Science in Sports and Exercise,* Vol. 12 (1980), No. 1, pp. 61–64.

Einzig, S., J. St. Cyr, R. Bianco, J. Schneider, E. Lorenz, and J. Foker. "Myocardial ATP Repletion With Ribose Infusion." *Pediatric Research,* Vol. 19 (1985), No. 4, p. 127A.

Engelhandt, M., G. Neumann, A. Berbalk, et al. "Creatine Supplementation in Endurance Sports." *Medicine and Science in Sports and Exercise,* Vol. 30 (1998), pp. 1123–29.

Erickson, Mark A., Robert J. Schwarzkopf, and Robert D. McKenzie. "Effects of Caffeine, Fructose, and Glucose Ingestion on Muscle Glycogen Utilization During Exercise." *Medicine and Science in Sports and Exercise,* Vol. 19 (1987), No. 6, pp. 579–83.

Erling, T. A. "Pilot Study With the Aim of Studying the Efficacy and Tolerability of CLA (Tonalin) on the Body Composition in Humans." *Medstat Research Ltd.,* Liilestrom, Norway, July 1997.

Essen, B. E., J. Jansson, J. Henriksson, A. W. Taylor, and B. Saltin. "Metabolic Characteristics of Fibre Types in Human Skeletal Muscle." *Acta Physiolgica Scandinavica,* Vol. 19 (1975), pp. 153–65.

Fahey, T.D., and M. Pearl. "Hormonal Effects of Phosphatidylserine During 2 Weeks of Intense Training." Abstract presented at the national meeting of the American College of Sports Medicine, June 1998.

Fahey, Thomas D., Lahsen Akka, and Richard Rolph. "Body Composition and VO2 Max of Exceptional Weight-Trained Athletes." *Journal of Applied Physiology,* Vol. 19 (1975), No. 4, pp. 559–61.

"Fatigue and Underperformance in Athletes." *British Journal of Sports Nutrition,* Vol. 32 (1998), pp. 107–10.

Ferreira, M., R. Kreider, M. Wilson, and A. Almada. "Effects of Conjugated Linoleic Acid (CLA) Supplementation During Resistance Training on Body Composition and Strength." *Journal of Strength and Conditioning Research,* Vol. 11 (1997), p. 280.

Fleck, S. J. "Cardiovascular adaptations to resistance training." *Med Sci Sports Exerc,* Vol. 20 (Oct 1988), No. 5 Suppl., pp. S146–51.

Food and Nutrition Board. Recommended Dietary Allowances, 9th Edition. Washington, D.C.: *National Academy of Sciences,* 1980.

Forbes, Gilbert B. "Body Composition as Affected by Physical Activity and Nutrition." *Metabolic and Nutritional Aspects of Physical Exercise: Federation Proceedings,* Vol. 44 (1985), No. 2, pp. 334–52.

Forbes, Gilbert B. "Growth of the Lean Body Mass in Man." *Growth,* Vol. 36 (1972), pp. 325–38.

Forbes, Richard M., and John W. Erdman Jr. "Bioavailability of Trace Mineral Elements." *Annual Reviews of Nutrition,* Vol. 3 (1983), pp. 213–31.

Fournier, Mario, Joe Ricci, Albert W. Taylor, Ronald J. Ferguson, Richard R. Montpetit, and Bernard R. Chaitman. "Skeletal Muscle Adaptation in Adolescent Boys: Sprint and Endurance Training and Detraining." *Medicine and Science in Sports and Exercise,* Vol. 14 (1982), No. 6, pp. 453–56.

Fox, Edward L., Robert L. Bartels, James Klinzing, and Kerry Ragg. "Metabolic Responses to Interval Training Programs of High and Low Power Output." *Medicine and Science in Sports,* Vol. 9 (1977), No. 3, pp. 191–96.

Franke, W. W, and B. Berendonk. "Hormonal Doping and Androgenization of Athletes: A Secret Program of the German Democratic Republic Government." *Clinical Chemistry,* Vol. 43 (1997), pp. 1262–79.

Friedman, J. E., et al. "Regulation of Glycogen Resynthesis Following Exercise." *Sports Medicine,* Vol. 11 (1991), p. 232.

Galton, David J., and George A. Bray. "Studies on Lipolysis in Human Adipose Cells." *Journal of Clinical Investigation,* Vol. 46 (1967), No. 4, pp. 621–29.

Gao, J. P., D. I. Costill, C. A. Horswill, and S. H. Park. "Sodium Bicarbonate Ingestion Improves Performance in Interval Swimming." *European Journal of Applied Physiology,* Vol. 58 (1988), pp. 171–74.

Garza, C., N. S. Scrimshaw, and V. R. Young. "Human Protein Requirements: The Effect of Variations in Energy Intake Within the Maintenance Range." *American Journal of Clinical Nutrition,* Vol. 29 (1976), pp. 280–87.

Gastelu, Daniel. *The Complete Nutritional Supplements Buyer's Guide.* New York: Random House, 2000.

Gastelu, Daniel, and Fred Hatfield. *Dynamic Nutrition for Maximum Performance.* Garden City Park, NY: Avery Publishing Group, 1997.

Gastelu, D. L. "Developing State-of-the-Art Amino Acids." *Muscle Magazine International,* May (1989), pp. 58–64.

Gleeson, M., et al. "Effect of Low- and High-Carbohydrate Diets on the Plasma Glutamine and Circulating Leukocyte Responses to Exercise." *International Journal of Sports Nutrition,* Vol. 8 (1998), pp. 49–59.

Goldberg, Alfred L., Joseph D. Etlinger, David F. Goldspink, and Charles Jablecki. "Mechanism of Work-Induced Hypertrophy of Skeletal Muscle." *Medicine and Science in Sports,* Vol. 7 (1975), No. 3, pp. 185–98.

Goldspink, David F. "The Influence of Activity on Muscle Size and Protein Turnover." *Journal of Physiology,* Vol. 264 (1976), pp. 283–96.

Gollnick, P. D., R. B. Armstrong, B. Saltin, C. W. Saubert IV, W. L. Sembrowich, and R. E. Shepherd. "Effect of Training on Enzyme Activity and Fiber Composition of Human Skeletal Muscle." *Journal of Applied Physiology,* Vol. 34 (1973), No. 1, pp. 107–11.

Gollnick, Philip D. "Metabolism of Substrates: Energy Substrate Metabolism During Exercise and as Modified by Training." *Metabolic and Nutritional Aspects of Physical Exercise: Federation Proceedings,* Vol. 44 (1985), No. 2, pp. 353–68.

Gontzea, I., P. Sutzescu, and S. Dumitrache. "The Influence of Muscular Activity on Nitrogen Balance and on the Need of Man for Proteins." *Nutrition Reports International*, Vol. 10 (1974), pp. 35–43.

Goss, F., et al. "Effect of Potassium Phosphate Supplementation on Perceptual and Physiological Responses to Maximal Graded Exercise." *International Journal of Sport Nutrition and Exercise Metabolism*, Vol. 11 (2001), pp. 53–62.

Graudal N. A., A. M. Galloc, and P. Garred. "Effects of Sodium Restriction on Blood Pressure, Rennin, Aldosterone, Catecholamines, Cholesterols, and Triglycerides: A Meta-Analysis." *Journal of the American Medical Association*, Vol. 279 (1998), pp. 1383–91.

Green, Jerry Franklin, and Alan P. Jackman. "Peripheral Limitations to Exercise." *Medicine and Science in Sports and Exercise*, Vol. 16 (1984), No. 3, pp. 299–305.

Greenhaff, P., et al. "Effect of Oral Creatine Supplementation on Skeletal Muscle Phosphocreatine Resynthesis." *American Journal of Physiology*, Vol. 266 (1994), pp. E725–730.

Gross, M., R. Kormann, and N. Zollner. "Ribose Administration During Exercise: Effects on Substrates and Products of Energy Metabolism in Healthy Subjects and a Patient with Myoadenylate Deaminase Deficiency." *Klinische Wochenschrift*, Vol. 69 (1991), pp. 151–55.

Haff, G. G. "Roundtable Discussion: Low Carbohydrate Diets and Anaerobic Athletes." *Strength and Conditioning Journal*, Vol. 23 (June 2001), No. 3, pp. 42–61.

Haff, G. G., et al. "A Brief Review: Explosive Exercises and Sports Performance." *Strength and Conditioning Journal*, Vol. 23 (June 2001), No. 3, pp. 13–20.

Hagerman, F. C., et al. "Effects of High-intensity resistance training on untrained older men. I. Strength, cardiovascular, and metabolic responses." *J Gerontol A Biol Sci Med Sci*, Vol. 55 (July 2000), No. 7, pp. B336–46.

Hamilton, K. L., M. C. Meyers, W. A. Skelly, and R. J. Marley. "Oral Creatine Supplementation and Upper Extremity Anaerobic Response in Females." *Int J Sport Nutr Exerc Metab*, Vol. 10 (Sep 2000), No. 3, pp. 277–89.

Haralambie, G., and A. Berg. "Serum Urea and Amino Nitrogen Changes With Exercise Duration." *European Journal of Applied Physiology* (1976), pp. 39–48.

Hargreaves, M., David L. Costill, A. Katz, and W. J. Fink. "Effect of Fructose Ingestion on Muscle Glycogen Usage During Exercise." *Medicine and Science in Sports and Exercise*, Vol. 17 (1985), pp. 360–63.

Harmsen, Eef, Peter P. DeTombe, Jan Willem DeJong, and Peter W. Achterberg. "Enhanced ATP and GTP Synthesis From Hypoxanthine or Inosine After Myocardial Ischemia." *The American Physiological Society* (1984), pp. H37–43.

Harper, M.J.K. "Effects of Androstenedione on Pre-implantation Stages of Pregnancy in Rats." *Endocrinology*, Vol. 81 (1967), pp. 1091–98.

Hartog, M., R. J. Havel, G. Copinschi, J. M. Earll, and B. C. Ritchie. "The Relationship Between Changes in Serum Levels of Growth Hormone and Mobilization of Fat During Exercise in Man." *Quarterly Journal of Experimental Physiology*, Vol. 52 (1967), pp. 86–96.

Heeker, A. L., and K. B. Wheeler. "Protein: A Misunderstood Nutrient for the Athlete." *National Strength and Conditioning Association Journal*, Vol. 7 (1985), pp. 28–29.

Helie, R., J. M. Lavoie, and D. Cousineau. "Effects of a 24-Hour Carbohydrate-Poor Diet on Metabolic and Hormonal Responses During Glucose-Infused Leg Exercise." *European Journal of Applied Physiology*, Vol. 54 (1985), pp. 420–26.

Hellsten-Westling, Y., B. Norman, P. Balsom, and B. Sjodin. "Decreased Resting Levels of Adenine Nucleotides in Human Skeletal Muscle After High-Intensity Training." *Journal of Applied Physiology*, Vol. 74 (1993), No. 5, pp. 2523–28.

Henneman, Dorothy, and Philip H. Henneman. "Effects of Human Growth Hormone on Levels of Blood and Urinary Carbohydrate and Fat Metabolites in Man." *Journal of Clinical Investigation*, Vol. 39 (1960), pp. 1239–45.

Hermansen, Lars, Eric Hultman, and Bengt Saltin. "Muscle Glycogen During Prolonged Severe Exercise." *Acta Physiolgica Scandinavica*, Vol. 71 (1967), pp. 129–39.

Heymsfield, Steven B., Carlos Arteaga, Clifford McManus, Janet Smith, and Steven Moffitt. "Measurement of Muscle Mass in Humans: Validity of the 24-Hour Urinary Creatinine Method." *American Journal of Clinical Nutrition*, Vol. 37 (1983), pp. 478–94.

Hickson, James F., Jr., and Klaus Hinkelmann. "Exercise and Protein Intake Effects on Urinary 3-Methylhistidine Excretion." *American Journal of Clinical Nutrition*, Vol. 41 (1985), pp. 32–45.

Hickson, Robert C., and Maureen A. Rosenkoetter. "Reduced Training Frequencies and Maintenance of Increased Aerobic Power." *Medicine and Science in Sports and Exercise*, Vol. 13, No. 1 (1981), pp. 13–16.

Hill, J. O., and R. Commerford. "Physical Activity, Fat Balance, and Energy Balance." *International Journal of Sport Nutrition*, Vol. 6 (1996), No. 3, pp. 80–92.

Hofman, Z., et al. "Glucose and Insulin Responses After Commonly Used Sport Feedings Before and After a 1-Hour Training Session." *International Journal of Sport Nutrition*, Vol. 5 (1995), pp. 194–205.

Holloszy, John O. "Adaptation of Skeletal Muscle to Endurance Exercise." *Medicine and Science in Sports*, Vol. 7 (1975), No. 3, pp. 155–64.

Holloszy, John O. "Exercise, Health, and Aging: A Need for More Information." *Medicine and Science in Sports and Exercise*, Vol. 15 (1983), No. 1, pp. 1–5.

Holt, Henry T. "Carica Paypaya as Ancillary Therapy for Athletic Injuries." *Current Therapeutic Research*, Vol. 11 (Oct 1969), pp. 621–24.

Horn, M. E. "Improved Sprint Cycle Performance Following Consumption of a Chromium-Carbohydrate Beverage During Prolonged Exercise." *Medicine and Science in Sports and Exercise*, Vol. 30 (1998), p. S288.

Horton, E., and R. Terjung. *Exercise, Nutrition, and Energy Metabolism*. New York: Macmillan Publishing Company, 1988.

Horton, Edward S. "Metabolic Aspects of Exercise and Weight Reduction." *Medicine and Science in Sports and Exercise*, Vol. 18 (1986), p. 10.

Hostler, D., et al. "The Effectiveness of 0.5-lb Increments in Progressive Resistance Exercise. *Journal of Strength and Conditioning Research*, Vol. 15 (2001), No. 1, pp. 86–91.

Ivy, J. L., R. T. Withers, P. J. Van Handel, D. L. L. Elger, and D. L. Costill. "Muscle Respiratory Capacity and Fiber Type as Determinants of the Lactate Threshold." *American Physiological Society* (1980), pp. 523–27.

Jacobs, Ira, Mona Esbjornsson, Christer Sylven, Ingemar Holm, and Eva Jansson. "Sprint Training Effects on Muscle Myoglobin, Enzymes, Fiber Types, and Blood Lactate." *Medicine and Science in Sports and Exercise,* Vol. 19 (1987), No. 4, pp. 369–74.

Jakeman, P., and S. Maxwell. "Effect of Antioxidant Vitamin Supplementation on Muscle Function After Eccentric Exercise." *European Journal of Applied Physiology,* Vol. 67 (1993), p. 426.

Jezova, D., M. Vigas, P. Tatar, R. Kvetnansky, K. Nazar, H. Kaciuba-Uscilko, and S. Kozlowski. "Plasma Testosterone and Catecholamine Responses to Physical Exercise of Different Intensities in Men." *European Journal of Applied Physiology,* Vol. 54 (1985), pp. 62–66.

Kaats, G. R., D. Blum, D. Pullin, et al. "A Randomized, Double Blind, Placebo Controlled Study of the Effects of Chromium Picolinate Supplementation on Body Composition: A Replication and Extension of a Previous Study." *Current Therapy Research,* Vol. 59 (1998), pp. 379–88.

Kamber, M., et al. "Nutritional Supplements As a Source for Positive Doping Cases?" *International Journal of Sport Nutrition and Exercise Metabolism,* Vol. 11 (2001), pp. 258–63.

Kanter, M. "Free Radicals, Exercise, and Antioxidant Supplementation." *International Journal of Sports Nutrition,* Vol. 4 (1994), p. 205.

Karagiorgos, Athanase, Joseph F. Garcia, and George A. Brooks. "Growth Hormone Response to Continuous and Intermittent Exercise." *Medicine and Science in Sports,* Vol. 11 (1979), No. 3, pp. 302–7.

Karlsson, Jan, and Bengt Saltin. "Diet, Muscle Glycogen, and Endurance Performance." *Journal of Applied Physiology,* Vol. 31 (1971), No. 2, pp. 203–6.

Karlsson, Jan, and Bengt Saltin. "Lactate, ATP, and CP in Working Muscles During Exhaustive Exercise in Man." *Journal of Applied Physiology,* Vol. 29 (1970), No. 5, pp. 598–602.

Karlsson, Jan, Lars-Olof Nordesjo, and Bengt Saltin. "Muscle Glycogen Utilization During Exercise After Physical Training." *Acta Physiolgica Scandinavica,* Vol. 90 (1974), pp. 210–17.

Kasai, Kikuo, Hitoshi Suzuki, Tsutomu Nakamura, Hiroaki Shiina, and Shin-Ichi Shimoda. "Glycine Stimulates Growth Hormone Release in Man." *Acta Endocronologica,* Vol. 90 (1980), pp. 283–86.

Kasai, Kikuo, Masami Kobayashi, and Shin-Ichi Shimoda. "Stimulatory Effect of Glycine on Human Growth Hormone Secretion." *Metabolism,* Vol. 27 (1978), pp. 201–8.

Kasperek, George J., and Rebecca D. Snider. "Increased Protein Degradation After Eccentric Exercise." *European Journal of Applied Physiology,* Vol. 54 (1985), pp. 30–34.

Katch, F. "U.S. Government Raises Serious Questions About Reliability of U.S. Department of Agriculture's Food Composition Database." *International Journal of Sport Nutrition,* Vol. 5 (1995), pp. 62–67.

Katch, Victor L., Frank I. Katch, Robert Moffatt, and Michael Gittleson. "Muscular Development and Lean Body Weight in Body Builders and Weight Lifters." *Medicine and Science in Sports and Exercise,* Vol. 12 (1980), No. 5, pp. 340–44.

Kellis, J.T., and L. E. Vickery. "Inhibition of Estrogen Synthetase (Aromatase) by Flavones." *Science,* Vol. 225 (1984), pp. 1032–33.

Kelly, V. G., and D. G. Jenkins. "Effect of Oral Creatine Supplementation on Near-Maximal Strength and Repeated Sets of High-Intensity Bench Press Exercise." *Journal of Strength and Conditioning Research,* Vol. 12 (1998), pp. 109–15.

Kidd, P. M. *Phosphatidylserine (PS): A Remarkable Brain Cell Nutrient.* Decatur, IL: Lucas Meyer, 1995.

Kies, C. V., and J. A. Driskell. *Sports Nutrition: Minerals and Electrolytes.* Boca Raton, FL: CRC Press, 1995.

Killingsworth, R., et al. "Hyperthermia and Dehydration-Related Deaths Associated with Intentional Rapid Weight Loss in Three Collegiate Wrestlers." *Morbidity and Mortality Weekly Report,* Vol. 47 (1998), pp. 105–8.

Kirkendall, D. "Effect of Nutrition on Performance in Soccer." *Medicine and Science in Sports and Exercise,* Vol. 25 (1993), pp. 1370.

Kirwan, John P., David L. Costill, Michael G. Flynn, Joel B. Mitchell, William J. Fink, P. Darrell Neufer, and Joseph A. Houmard. "Physiological Responses to Successive Days of Intense Training in Competitive Swimmers." *Medicine and Science in Sports and Exercise,* Vol. 20 (1988), No. 3, pp. 255–59.

Klissouras, Vassilis, Freddy Pirnay, and Jean-Marie Petit. "Adaptation to Maximal Effort: Genetics and Age." *Journal of Applied Physiology,* Vol. 35 (1973), No. 2, pp. 288–93.

Knopf, R. F., J. W. Conn, S. S. Fajans, J. C. Floyd, E. M. Guntsche, and J. A. Rull. "Plasma Growth Hormone Response to Intravenous Administration of Amino Acids." *Journal of Clinical Endocrinology,* Vol. 25 (1965), pp. 1140–44.

Koeslag, J. H. "Post-Exercise Ketosis and the Hormone Response to Exercise: A Review." *Medicine and Science in Sports and Exercise,* Vol. 14 (1982), No. 5, pp. 327–34.

Kraemer, W. J. et al. "Resistance Training Combined with Bench-Step Aerobics Enhances Women's Health Profile." *Med Sci Sports Exerc,* Vol. 33 (Feb 2001), No. 2, pp. 259–69.

Kreider, R., et al. "Effects of B-BHBM Supplementation With and Without Creatine During Training on Body Composition Alterations." *Federation of American Societies of Experimental Biology Journal,* Vol. 11 (1997), p. A374.

Kreider, R. B., et al. "Effects of Creatine Supplementation on Body Composition, Strength, and Sprint Performance." *Medicine and Science in Sports and Exercise,* Vol. 30 (1998), pp. 73–82.

Kurkin, V. A., and G. G. Zapesochnaya. "Chemical Composition and Pharmacological Properties of Rhodiola Rosea." *Chemical-Pharmaceutical Journal,* Vol. 20 (1986), No. 10, pp. 1231–44.

Kurzman, I. D., D. L. Panciera, J. B. Miller, et al. "The Effect of Dehydroepiandrosterone Combined With a Low-Fat Diet in Spontaneously Obese Dogs: A Clinical Trial." *Obesity Research,* Vol. 6 (1998), No. 1, pp. 20–28.

Lander, Jeffrey E., Barry T. Bates, James A. Sawhill, and Joseph Hamill. "A Comparison Between Free-Weight and Isokinetic Bench Pressing." *Medicine and Science in Sports and Exercise,* Vol. 17 (1985), No. 3, p. 344.

Lardy, H. A., N. Kneer, M. Bellei, et al. "Induction of Thermogenic Enzymes by DHEA and Its Metabolites." *Annals of the New York Academy of Sciences,* Vol. 774 (1995), pp. 171–79.

Lee, H., R. Graeff, and T. Walseth. "Cyclic ADP-Ribose and Its Metabolic Enzymes." *Biochimie,* Vol. 77 (1995), pp. 345–55.

Lemon, P. W. R., and D. Proctor. "Protein Intake and Athletic Performance." *Sports Medicine,* Vol. 12 (1991), No. 5, p. 313.

Lemon, P. W. R., and F. J. Nagle. "Effects of Exercise on Protein and Amino Acid Metabolism." *Medicine and Science in Sports and Exercise,* Vol. 13 (1981), No. 3, pp. 141–49.

Lemon, P. W. R., and J. P. Mullin. "Effect of Initial Muscle Glycogen Levels on Protein Catabolism During Exercise." *The American Physiological Society* (1980), pp. 624–29.

Lemon, P. W. R., et al. "Protein Requirements and Muscle Mass/Strength Changes During Intensive Training in Novice Bodybuilders." *Journal of Applied Physiology*, Vol. 73 (1992), pp. 767–75.

Lewis, Steven M. A., William L. Haskell, Peter D. Wood, Norman M. A. Manoogian, Judith E. Bailey, and MaryBeth B. A. Pereira. "Effects of Physical Activity on Weight Reduction in Obese Middle-Aged Women." *American Journal of Clinical Nutrition*, Vol. 29 (1976), pp. 151–56.

Linderman, J., and T. D. Fahey. "Sodium Bicarbonate Ingestion and Exercise Performance." *Sports Medicine*, Vol. 11, No. 9, p. 71.

Lucke, Christoph, and Seymour Glick. "Experimental Modification of the Sleep-Induced Peak of Growth Hormone Secretion." *Journal of Clinical Endocrinology and Metabolism*, Vol. 32 (1971), pp. 729–36.

McBride, J. M., et al. "Effect of Resistance Exercise on Free Radical Production." *Medicine and Science in Sports and Exercise*, Vol. 30 (1998), pp. 67–72.

MacDougall, J. D., D. G. Sale, G. C. B. Elder, and J. R. Sutton. "Muscle Ultrastructural Characteristics of Elite Power-lifters and Bodybuilders." *European Journal of Applied Physiology*, Vol. 48 (1982), pp. 117–26.

MacDougall, J. D., D. G. Sale, J. R. Moroz, G. C. B. Elder, J. R. Sutton, and H. Howald. "Mitochondrial Volume Density in Human Skeletal Muscle Following Heavy Resistance Training." *Medicine and Science in Sports and Exercise*, Vol. 11 (1979), No. 2, pp. 164–66.

MacDougall, J. D., D. G. Sale, S. E. Alway, and J. R. Sutton. "Muscle Fiber Number in Biceps Brachii in Bodybuilders and Control Subjects." *The Journal of Applied Physiology* (1984), p. 1399.

McGuigan, M. R. M., et al. "Resistance Training for Patients with Peripheral Arterial Disease: A Model of Exercise Rehabilitation." *Strength and Conditioning Journal*, Vol. 23 (June 2001), No. 3, pp. 26–32.

Mackova, Eva V., Jan Melichna, Karel Vondra, Toivo Jurimae, Thomas Paul, and Jaroslav Novak. "The Relationship Between Anaerobic Performance and Muscle Metabolic Capacity and Fibre Distribution." *European Journal of Applied Physiology*, Vol. 54 (1985), pp. 413–15.

MacLean, William C., Jr., and George G. Graham. "The Effect of Level of Protein Intake in Isoenergetic Diets on Energy Utilization." *American Journal of Clinical Nutrition* (1979), pp. 1381–87.

Mahesh, V. B., and R. B. Greenblatt. "The In Vivo Conversion of Dehydroepiandrosterone and Androstenedione to Testosterone in the Human." *Acta Endocrinology*, Vol. 41 (1962), pp. 400–6.

Malina, Robert M., William H. Mueller, Claude Bouchard, Richard F. Shoup, and Georges Lariviere. "Fatness and Fat Patterning Among Athletes at the Montreal Olympic Games, 1976." *Medicine and Science in Sports and Exercise*, Vol. 14 (1982), No. 6, pp. 445–52.

Manore, M. "Vitamin B_6 and Exercise." *International Journal of Sports Nutrition*, Vol. 4 (1994), p. 89.

Marable, N. L., J. F. Hickson Jr., M. K. Korslund, W. G. Herbert, R. F. Desjardins, and F. W. Thye. "Urinary Nitrogen Excretion as Influenced by a Muscle-Building Exercise Program and Protein Intake Variation." *Nutrition Reports International*, Vol. 19 (1979), No. 6, pp. 795–805.

Maresh, C., et al. "Dietary Supplementation and Improved Anaerobic Performance." *International Journal of Sport Nutrition*, Vol. 4 (1994), p. 387.

Marriott, B. *Food Components to Enhance Performance.* Washington, D.C.: National Academy Press, 1994.

Marsit, Joseph, et al. "Effects of Ascorbic Acid on Serum Cortisol and the Testosterone: Cortisol Ratio in Junior Elite Weightlifters." *Journal of Strength and Conditioning Research*, Vol. 12 (1998), pp. 179–84.

Maughan, Ronald. "Creatine Supplementation and Exercise Performance." *International Journal of Sport Nutrition* (1995), pp. 94–101.

Mayer, Jean, Roy Purnima, and Kamakhya Prasad Mitra. "Relation Between Caloric Intake, Body Weight, and Physical Work: Studies in an Industrial Male Population in West Bengal." *American Journal of Clinical Nutrition*, Vol. 4 (1956), No. 2, pp. 169–75.

Merimee, T. J., D. Rabinowitz, and S. E. Fineberg. "Arginine-Initiated Release of Human Growth Hormone." *New England Journal of Medicine* (1969), pp. 1434–38.

Merimee, Thomas J., David Rabinowitz, Lamar Riggs, John A. Burgess, David L. Rimoin, and Victor A. McKusick. "Plasma Growth Hormone After Arginine Infusion." *New England Journal of Medicine*, Vol. 23 (1967), pp. 434–38.

Mertz, Walter. "Assessment of the Trace Element Nutritional Status." *Nutrition Research* (1985), pp. 169–74.

Meydani, M., et al. "Protective Effect of Vitamin E on Exercise-Induced Oxidative Damage in Young and Older Adults." *American Journal of Physiology*, Vol. 264 (1993), pp. R992–98.

Mikesell, Kevin A., and Gary A. Dudley. "Influence of Intense Endurance Training on Aerobic Power of Competitive Distance Runners." *Medicine and Science in Sports and Exercise*, Vol. 16 (1984), No. 4, pp. 371–75.

Mitchell, J. B., D. L. Costill, J. A. Houmard, M. G. Flynn, W. J. Fink, and J. D. Beltz. "Effects of Carbohydrate Ingestion on Gastric Emptying and Exercise Performance." *Medicine and Science in Sports and Exercise*, Vol. 20 (1988), No. 2, pp. 110–15.

Mittleman, K. D., M. R. Ricci, and S. P. Bailey. "Branched-Chain Amino Acids Prolong Exercise During Heat Stress in Men and Women." *Medicine and Science in Sports and Exercise*, Vol. 30 (1998), pp. 83–91.

Monteleone, P., L. Beinat, C. Tanzillo, M. Maj, and D. Kemali. "Effects of Phosphatidylserine on the Neuroendocrine Response to Physical Response in Humans." *Neuroendocrinology*, Vol. 52 (1990), pp. 243–48.

Monteleone, P., M. Maj, L. Beinat, M. Natale, and D. Kemali. "Blunting by Chronic Phosphatidylserine Administration of the Stress-Induced Activation of the Hypothalamo-Pituitary-Adrenal Axis in Healthy Men." *European Journal of Clinical Pharmacology*, Vol. 43 (1992), pp. 385–88.

Morgan, William P. "Affective Beneficence of Vigorous Physical Activity." *Medicine and Science in Sports and Exercise*, Vol. 17 (1985), No. 1, pp. 94–100.

Morrissey, S. "Evaluation of the Effects of a Complex Herbal Formulation on Lactate Metabolism." *Medicine and Science in Sports and Exercise*, Vol. 30 (1998), p. S277.

Morrissey, S., R. Wang, and E. R. Burke. "Evaluation of the Effects of a Complex Herbal Formulation on Lactate Metabolism." Paper presented at the national meeting of the American College of Sports Medicine, Orlando, Florida, June 6, 1998.

Murphy, T., et al. "Performance Enhancing Ration Components Project: U.S. Army." Abstract presented at the 11th Annual Symposium of Sports and Cardiovascular Nutritionists, Atlanta, April 22–24, 1994.

Murray, Robert; Dennis E. Eddy, Tami W. Murray, John G. Seifert, Gregory L. Paul, and George A. Halaby. "The Effect of Fluid and Carbohydrate Feedings During Intermittent Cycling Exercise." *Medicine and Science in Sports and Exercise*, Vol. 19 (1987), No. 6, pp. 597–604.

Mutch, B. J. C., and E. W. Banister. "Ammonia Metabolism in Exercise and Fatigue: A Review." *Medicine and Science in Sports and Exercise*, Vol. 15 (1983), No. 1, pp 41–50.

Nishizawa, N., M. Shimbo, S. Hareyama, and R. Funabiki. "Fractional Catabolic Rates of Myosin and Actin Estimated by Urinary Excretion of N-Methylhistidine: The Effect of Dietary Protein Level on Catabolic Rates Under Conditions of Restricted Food Intake." *British Journal of Nutrition*, Vol. 37 (1976), pp. 345–421.

Nissen, S., et al. "Effect of Leucine Metabolite Beta-Hydroxy Beta-Methylbutyrate on Muscle Metabolism During Resistance Training." *Journal of Applied Physiology*, Vol. 81 (1996), pp. 2095–104.

Nissen, S., et al. "Effects of Feeding Beta-Hydroxy Beta-Methylbutyrate (BHBM) on Body Composition in Women." *Federation of American Societies of Experimental Biology Journal*, Vol. 11 (1997), p. A290.

"Nutrition, Exercise, and Bone Status in Youth." *International Journal of Sports Nutrition*, Vol. 8 (1998), pp. 124–42.

Okano, Goroh, Hidekatsu Takeda, Isao Morita, Mitsuru Katoh, Zuien Mu, and Shosuke Miyake. "Effect of Pre-Exercise Fructose Ingestion on Endurance Performance in Fed Men." *Medicine and Science in Sports and Exercise*, Vol. 20 (1987), No. 7, pp. 105–9.

Oscai, Lawrence B., and John O. Holloszy. "Effects of Weight Changes Produced by Exercise, Food Restriction, or Overeating on Body Composition." *Journal of Clinical Investigation*, Vol. 48 (1969), pp. 2124–28.

Ostaszewski, P., et al. "The Effect of Leucine Metabolite Beta-Hydroxy Beta-Methylbutyrate (BHBM) on Muscle Protein Synthesis and Protein Breakdown in Chick and Rat Muscle." Abstract in *Journal of Animal Science* (1996).

Paddon-Jones, D. J., and D. Pearson. "Cost-Effectiveness of Pre-Exercise Carbohydrate Meals and Their Impact on Performance." *Journal of Conditioning Research*, Vol. 12 (1998), pp. 90–94.

Palmer, Warren K. "Introduction to Symposium: Cyclic AMP Regulation of Fuel Metabolism During Exercise." *Medicine and Science in Sports and Exercise*, Vol. 20 (1988), No. 6, pp. 523–24.

Pariza, M. "Mechanism of Body Fat Reduction by Conjugated Linoleic Acid." *Federation of American Societies of Experimental Biology Journal*, Vol. 11 (1997), p. A139.

Pariza, M. U.S. Patent 5,385,616, "A Method of Enhancing Weight Gain and Feed Efficiency in an Animal Which Comprises Administering to the Animal a Safe and Effective Amount of a Conjugated Linoleic Acid."

Parkhouse, W. S., and D. C. McKenzie. "Possible Contribution of Skeletal Muscle Buffers to Enhanced Anaerobic Performance: A Brief Review." *Medicine and Science in Sports and Exercise,* Vol. 16 (1984), No. 4, pp. 328–38.

Pavlou, Konstantin N., William P. Steffee, Robert H. Lerman, and Belton A. Burrows. "Effects of Dieting and Exercise on Lean Body Mass, Oxygen Uptake, and Strength." *Medicine and Science in Sports and Exercise,* Vol. 17 (1974), No. 4, pp. 466–71.

Piehl, Karin. "Time Course for Refilling of Glycogen Stores in Human Muscle Fibres Following Exercise-Induced Glycogen Depletion." *Acta Physiologica Scandinavica,* Vol. 90 (1974), pp. 297–302.

Pizza, F., et al. "A Carbohydrate Loading Regimen Improves High Intensity, Short Duration Exercise Performance." *International Journal of Sport Science* (1995), pp. 110–16.

Prasad, Ananda S. "Role of Trace Elements in Growth and Development." *Nutrition Research* (1985), pp. 295–99.

Prud'homme, D. C. Bouchard, C. Leblanc, F. Landry, and E. Fontaine. "Sensitivity of Maximal Aerobic Power to Training Is Genotype-Dependent." *Medicine and Science in Sports and Exercise,* Vol. 16 (1984), No. 5, pp. 489–93.

Robertson, R. J., R. T. Stanko, F. L. Goss, et al. "Blood Glucose Extraction as a Mediator of Perceived Exertion During Prolonged Exercise." *European Journal of Applied Physiology,* Vol. 61 (1990), pp. 100–5.

Romieu, Isabelle, Walter C. Willett, Meir J. Stampfer, Graham A. Colditz, Laura Sampson, Bernard Rosner, Charles Hennekens, and Frank E. Speizer. "Energy Intake and Other Determinants of Relative Weight." *American Journal of Clinical Nutrition,* Vol. 47 (1988), pp. 406–12.

Rubin, M. A., et al. "Acute and Chronic Resistive Exercise Increase Urinary Chromium Excretion in Men as Measured with an Enriched Chromium Stable Isotope." *Journal of Nutrition,* Vol. 128 (1998), pp. 73–78.

Rudofsky, G. "The Effect of Intra-Arterial Infusion Treatment With Prostaglandin E1 in a Model of Ischemia in Healthy Volunteers." In H. Sinzinger H, Ed., *Prostaglandin E1 in Atherosclerosis.* New York: Springer Verlag, 1986, p. 49.

Saitoh, Shin-ichi, Yutaka Yoshitake, and Masahige Suzuki. "Enhanced Glycogen Repletion in Liver and Skeletal Muscle With Citrate Orally Fed After Exhaustive Treadmill Running and Swimming." *Journal of Nutritional Science and Vitaminology,* Vol. 29 (1983), pp. 45–52.

Salleo, Alberto, Guiseppe Anastasi, Guiseppa LaSpada, Guiseppina Falzea, and Maria G. Denaro. "New Muscle Fiber Production During Compensatory Hypertrophy." *Medicine and Science in Sports and Exercise,* Vol. 12 (1980), No. 4, pp. 268–73.

Sandage, B. W., L. A. Sabounjian, R. White, et al. "Choline Citrate May Enhance Athletic Performance." *Physiologist,* Vol. 35 (1992), p. 236a.

Satabin, Pascale, Pierre Portero, Gilles Defer, Jacques Bricout, and Charles-Yannick Guezennec. "Metabolic and Hormonal Responses to Lipid and Carbohydrate Diets During Exercise in Man." *Medicine and Science in Sports and Exercise,* Vol. 19 (1987), No. 3, pp. 218–23.

Saudek, Christopher D. "The Metabolic Events of Starvation." *American Journal of Medicine,* Vol. 60 (1976), pp. 117–26.

Schalch, Don S. "The Influence of Physical Stress and Exercise on Growth Hormone and Insulin Secretion in Man." *Journal of Laboratory and Clinical Medicine,* Vol. 69 (1967), No. 2, pp. 256–67.

Schauss, A. G. "Colloidal Minerals: Clinical Implications of Clay Suspension Products Sold as Dietary Supplements." *American Journal of Natural Medicine,* Vol. 4 (1997), pp. 5–10.

Schauss, A. G. *Trace Elements and Human Health,* 2nd Edition. Tacoma, WA: Life Sciences, 1996.

Scheett, T. P., et al. "Effectiveness of Glycerol As a Rehydrating Agent." *International Journal of Sport Nutrition and Exercise Metabolism,* Vol. 11 (2001), pp. 63–71.

Sen, C., et al. "Oxidative Stress After Human Exercise: Effect of N-Acetylcysteine Supplementation." *Journal of Applied Physiology,* Vol. 76 (1994), pp. 2570–77.

Serratosa Fernandez, L. and Fernandez Vaquero, A. "Arterial hypertension and exercise" *Rev Esp Cardiol,* Vol. 50 (1997), Suppl. 4, pp. 24–32.

Shanghai Compilation of New Drugs Confirmed in 1976. Shanghai: Sci-Tech Literature Publishing House, 1976.

Sharp, R. "Less Pain, More Gain for Distance Runners on HMB." Presented at the national meeting of Experimental Biology, San Francisco, 1998.

Shaw, P. C. "The Use of a Trypsin-Chymotrypsin Formulation in Fractures of the Hand." *British Journal of Clinical Practice,* Vol. 23 (January 1969), pp. 25–26.

Short, S. "Dietary Surveys and Nutrition Knowledge." In Hickson, J. F., and I. W. Wolinsky, Eds., *Nutrition in Exercise and Sport.* Boca Raton, FL: CRC Press, 1989.

Simon-Schnass, I., and H. Pabst. "Influence of Vitamin E on Physical Performance." *International Journal of Vitamin Nutrition Research* (1987), pp. 49–54.

Simoneau, J.-A., G. Lortie, M. R. Boulay, M. Marcotte, M. C. Thibault, and C. Bouchard. "Human Skeletal Muscle Fiber Type Alteration with High-Intensity Intermittent Training." *European Journal of Applied Physiology,* Vol. 54 (1985), pp. 250–53.

Skolnik, A. A. "Old Chinese Herbal Medicine Used for Fever Yields Possible New Alzheimer Disease Therapy." *Journal of the American Medical Association,* Vol. 277 (March 1997), No. 10, p. 776.

Soares, M. J., et al. "The Effect of Exercise on Riboflavin Status of Adult Men." *British Journal of Nutrition,* Vol. 69 (1993), pp. 541–551.

Spector, S. A., M. R. Jackman, L. A. Sabounjian, et al. "Effects of Choline Supplementation on Fatigue in Training Cyclists." *Medicine and Science in Sports and Exercise,* Vol. 27 (1995), pp. 669–73.

Spiller, G. A., C. D. Jensen, T. S. Pattison, C. S. Chuck, J. H. Whittam, and J. Scala. "Effect of Protein Dose on Serum Glucose and Insulin Response to Sugars." *American Journal of Clinical Nutrition,* Vol. 46 (1987), pp. 474–80.

Stanko, R. T., A. Mitrakou, et al. "Effect of Dihydroxyacetone and Pyruvate on Plasma Glucose Concentration and Turnover in Noninsulin-Dependent Diabetes Mellitus." *Clinical Physiology and Biochemistry* (1990), pp. 283–88.

Stanko, R. T., H. Reiss Reynolds, et al. "Pyruvate Supplementation of a Low-Cholesterol, Low-Fat Diet: Effects on Plasma Lipid Concentrations and Body Composition in Hyperlipidemic Patients." *American Journal of Clinical Nutrition,* Vol. 59 (1994), pp. 423–27.

Stanko, R. T., R. J. Robertson, R. J. Spina, et al. "Enhancement of Arm Exercise Endurance Capacity with Dihydroxyacetone and pyruvate." *Journal of Applied Physiology,* Vol. 68 (1990), pp. 119–24.

Stanko, R. T., R. J. Robertson, R. W. Galbreath, et al. "Enhanced Leg Exercise Endurance with a High Carbohydrate Diet and Dihydroxyacetone and Pyruvate." *Journal of Applied Physiology,* Vol. 69 (1990), pp. 1651–56.

Stone, M. H., et al. "Cardiovascular Responses to Short-Term Olympic Style Weight Training in Young Men." *Can J Appl Sport Sci,* Vol. 8 (Sep 1983), No. 3, pp. 134–39.

Stone, M. H., et al. "Health and Performance Related Potential of Resistance Training." *Sports Med,* Vol. 11 (Apr 1991), No. 4, pp. 210–31.

Street, C., et al. "Androgen Use by Athletes: Reevaluation of the Health Risks." *Canadian Journal of Applied Physiology,* Vol. 21 (1996), pp. 421–40.

Tarnopolsky, M. A., and MacLennan, D. P. "Creatine Monohydrate Supplementation Enhances High-Intensity Exercise Performance in Males and Females." *Int J Sport Nutr Exerc Metab,* Vol. 10 (Dec 2000), No. 4, pp. 452–63.

Tesch, Per, et al. "Skeletal Muscle Glycogen Loss Evoked by Resistance Exercise." *Journal of Strength and Conditioning Research,* Vol. 12 (1998), pp. 67–73.

Thomas, D., et al. "Plasma Glucose Levels After Prolonged Strenuous Exercise Correlate Inversely with Glycemic Response to Food Consumed Before Exercise." *International Journal of Sport Nutrition,* Vol. 4 (1994), p. 361.

Thompson, Deborah A., Larry A. Wolfe, and Roelof Eikelboom. "Acute Effects of Exercise Intensity on Appetite in Young Men." *Medicine and Science in Sports and Exercise,* Vol. 20 (1988), No. 3, pp. 222–27.

Thorland, William G., Glen O. Johnson, Thomas G. Fagot, Gerald D. Tharp, and Richard W. Hammer. "Body Composition and Somatotype Characteristics of Junior Olympic Athletes." *Medicine and Science in Sports and Exercise,* Vol. 13 (1981), No. 5, pp. 332–38.

Tipton, K. D., and Wolfe, R. R. "Exercise, Protein Metabolism, and Muscle Growth." *International Journal of Sport Nutrition and Exercise Metabolism,* Vol. 11 (2001), pp. 109–32.

Todd, Karen S., Gail E. Butterfield, and Doris Howes Calloway. "Nitrogen Balance in Men with Adequate and Deficient Energy Intake at Three Levels of Work." *Journal of Nutrition,* Vol. 114 (1984), pp. 2107–18.

Torun, B., N. S. Scrimshaw, and V. R. Young. "Effect of Isometric Exercises on Body Potassium and Dietary Protein Requirements of Young Men." *American Journal of Clinical Nutrition,* Vol. 30 (1977), pp. 1983–93.

Tric, I., and E. Haymes. "Effects of Caffeine Ingestion on Exercise-Induced Changes During High-Intensity, Intermittent Exercise." *International Journal of Sport Nutrition,* Vol. 5 (1995), pp. 37–44.

Trickett, P. "Proteolytic Enzymes in Treatment of Athletic Injuries." *Applied Therapeutics* (August 1964), pp. 647–52.

Tsintzas K. and C. Williams. "Human Muscle Glycogen Metabolism During Exercise. Effect Of Carbohydrate Supplementation." *Sports Medicine,* Vol. 25 (1998), pp. 7–23.

Tsomides, J., et al. "Controlled Evaluation of Oral Chymotrypsin-Trypsin Treatment of Injuires to the Head and Face." *Clinical Medicine* (November 1996), pp. 40–45.

Tullson, P., and R. Terjung. "Adenine Nucleotide Synthesis in Exercising and Endurance-Trained Skeletal Muscle." *American Journal of Physiology,* Vol. 261 (1991), pp. C342–47.

Tullson, P., D. Whitlock, and R. Terjung. "Adenine Nucleotide Degradation in Slow-Twitch Red Muscle." *American Journal of Physiology,* Vol. 258 (1990), pp. C258–65.

Tullson, P., J. Bangsbo, Y. Hellsten, and E. Richter. "IMP Metabolism in Human Skeletal Muscle After Exhaustive Exercise." *Journal of Applied Physiology,* Vol. 78 (1995), No. 1, pp. 146–52.

Tullson, P., P. Arabadjis, K. Rundell, and R. Terjung. "IMP Reamination to AMP in Rat Skeletal Muscle Fiber Types." *American Journal of Physiology,* Vol. 270 (1996), pp. C1067–74.

Udischev, S. N., and K. V. Yaremenko. "The Use of the Characteristic of the Rhodiola Rosea Extract to Stimulate Regenerative Processes for an Increase in the Selectivity of the Cyclophoshamide Anti-Tumor Action." In *New Medicinal Preparations from Plants of Siberia and the Far East.* Tomsk, Russia: Tomsk University Publishers, 1968, pp. 151–52.

Valeriani, A. "The Need for Carbohydrate Intake During Endurance Exercise." *Sports Medicine,* Vol. 12 (1991), No. 6, p. 349.

Van der Berg, J., N. Cook, and D. Tribble. "Reinvestigation of the Antioxidant Properties of Conjugated Linoleic Acid." *Lipids,* Vol. 73 (1995), pp. 595–98.

Van Erp-Baart, A. M., W. H. Saris, R. A. Binkhorst, J. A. Vos, and J. W. Elvers. "Nationwide Survey on the Nutritional Habits of Elite Athletes," part 1: "Energy, Carbohydrate, Protein, and Fat Intake." *International Journal of Sports Medicine,* Vol. 10 (1989), supplement, pp. S3–S10.

Verrill, D. E. and Ribisl, P. M. "Resistive Exercise Training in Cardiac Rehabilitation. An Update." *Sports Med,* Vol. 21 (May 1996), No. 5, pp. 347–83.

Viru, A. *Adaptation in Sports Training.* Boca Raton, FL: CRC Press, 1995.

Von Allworden, H. N., S. Horn, J. Kahl, et al. "The Influence of Lecithin on Plasma Choline Concentrations in Triathletes and Adolescent Runners During Exercise." *European Journal of Applied Physiology,* Vol. 67 (1983), pp. 87–91.

Walberg, Janet L., V. Karina Ruiz, Sandra L. Tarlton, Dennis E. Hinkle, and Forrest W. Thye. "Exercise Capacity and Nitrogen Loss During a High or Low Carbohydrate Diet." *Medicine and Science in Sports and Exercise,* Vol. 20 (1986), pp. 34–43.

Wang, R., and Q. Zheng. "Relationship Between Lactic Acid Metabolism and Exercise Performance Capacity Changes in Mice as a Result of Ingesting a Complex Herbal Formulation and Other Compounds." Report. Beijing, China: Academy of Medical Sciences, 1997.

Ward, P. S., and D.C.L. Savage. "Growth Hormone Responses to Sleep, Insulin Hypoglycemia and Arginine Infusion." *Hormone Research,* Vol. 22 (1985), pp. 7–11.

Weeks, C., H. Lardy, and S. Henwood. "Preclinical Toxicology Evaluation of 3-Acetyl-7-Oxo-Dehydroepiandrosterone (7-Keto DHEA)." Paper presented at the Experimental Biology National Meetings, 1998.

Weir, Jane, Timothy D. Noakes, Kathryn Myburgh, and Brett Adams. "A High Carbohydrate Diet Negates the Metabolic Effects of Caffeine During Exercise." *Medicine and Science in Sports and Exercise,* Vol. 19 (1986), pp. 100–5.

Weltman, Arthur, Sharleen Matter, and Bryant A. Stamford. "Caloric Restriction and/or Mild Exercise: Effects on Serum Lipids and Body Composition." *American Journal of Clinical Nutrition,* Vol. 33 (1980), pp. 1002–9.

West, D. "Reduced Body Fat With Conjugated Linoleic Acid Feeding in the Mouse." *Federation of American Societies of Experimental Biology Journal*, Vol. 11 (1997), p. A599.

Wilcox, Anthony R. "The Effects of Caffeine and Exercise on Body Weight, Fat-Pad Weight, and Fat-Cell Size." *Medicine and Science in Sports and Exercise*, Vol. 14 (1981), pp. 317–21.

Williams, M. H. "Vitamin Supplementation and Athletic Performance." *International Journal of Vitamin and Nutrition Research*, Vol. 30 (1989), p. 163.

Wolinsky, I. *Nutrition in Exercise and Sport*. Boca Raton, FL: CRC Press, 1998.

Wolinsky, I., and J. A. Driskell. *Sports Nutrition*. Boca Raton, FL: CRC Press, 1997.

Wolinsky, I., and J. Hickson. *Nutrition in Exercise and Sport*, 2nd Edition. Boca Raton, FL: CRC Press, 1994.

Wright, J. "Tribulus: A Natural Wonder." *Muscle and Fitness*, September 1996, pp. 140–42, 224.

Wu, F. C. "Endocrine Aspects of Anabolic Steroids." *Clinical Chemistry*, Vol. 43 (1997), pp. 1289–92.

Yan, W., et al. "Steroidal saponins from fruits of Tribulus terrestris." *Phytochemistry*, Vol. 42 (1996), No. 5, pp. 1417–22.

Yan, X. F., W. H. Lu, W. J. Lou, and X. C. Tang. "Effects of Huperzine A and B on Skeletal Muscle and Electroencephalogram." *Acta Pharmacologica Sinica*, Vol. 8, pp. 117–23.

Young, K., and C. T. M. Davies. "Effect of Diet on Human Muscle Weakness Following Prolonged Exercise." *European Journal of Applied Physiology*, Vol. 53 (1984), pp. 81–85.

Young, Vernon R., and Peter L. Pellett. "Protein Intake and Requirements with Reference to Diet and Health." *American Journal of Clinical Nutrition*, Vol. 45 (1987), pp. 1323–43.

Young, W., et al. "Risistance Training for Short Sprints and Maximum-Speed Sprints." *Strength and Conditioning Journal*, Vol. 23 (April 2001), No. 2, pp. 7–13.

Zawadzki, K. M., B. B. Yaspelkis, and J. L. Ivy. "Carbohydrate-Protein Complex Increases the Rate of Muscle Glycogen Storage After Exercise." *Journal of Applied Physiology*, Vol. 72 (1992), pp. 1854–59.

Index

About Gea Johnson and Michael O'Hearn

Gea Johnson is a distinguished weight-training athlete who is a world-class heptathlete and nationally ranked Olympic weight lifter. In addition to being a competitive athlete, Gea is a spokesperson for Weider Health & Fitness. She has appeared in many television commercials, infomercials, print advertisements, fitness videos, and magazine articles. Gea won America's first Miss Fitness contest in 1986. In the academic arena, Gea achieved the honorable titles of Nation's Most Outstanding Collegiate Scholar Athlete and Academic All-American of the Year. She has received more than 20 scholar athlete awards and scholarships from top athletic and business organizations nationwide. Gea makes frequent appearances to lecture about opportunities for women in sports.

Mike O'Hearn is a championship athlete and an important role model because he takes an active stand against the use of drugs in sports.

Mike began to develop his athletic potential at a young age and became a well-rounded athlete by participating in running, shot-put, discus, gymnastics, swimming, basketball, baseball, soccer, football, powerlifting, bodybuilding, and martial arts.

By his early 20s Mike's physique began to pay off with appearances in *Muscle & Fitness* magazine. He holds impressive titles in bodybuilding and weight-lifting competitions, including Mr. Universe, Mr. International, the NPC California Superheavyweight class, and the California Powerlifting Championships three times (he can deadlift more than 700 pounds). He was also the undisputed, undefeated champion of *Battledome,* a popular TV show. Mike is now building a career in movies and television.

To find out more about Mike O'Hearn you can visit his website at *www.mikeohearn.com,* or for appearances Mike can be contacted by writing to Mike O'Hearn, P.O. Box 2764, Venice, CA 90294–2764.

About the Authors

Since 1945, Ben Weider and his brother Joe have operated Weider Health & Fitness in Canada and the United States. The Weider organization has fostered the development of a strong and still-growing fitness and strength-conditioning industry. In addition, Ben and Joe Weider were instrumental in developing the vitamin, mineral, protein, and sports-nutrition industry.

Ben Weider, Ph.D., C.M., C.Q.

Ben Weider is the president of the International Federation of BodyBuilders (IFBB) which he founded in Montreal in 1946. There are presently 170 countries affiliated with the IFBB, and it now ranks as one of the top seven international sport federations in the world. On January 30, 1998, the International Olympic Committee (IOC) granted official recognition to the IFBB under rule 29. After 52 years of determination and persistence, this recognition is probably the most important of Ben Weider's accomplishments. The IFBB is a member of the General Association of International Sports Federations (GAISF). It is recognized by the Olympic Council of Asia and the Supreme Council for Sport in Africa. The IFBB is recognized and participates in the following games: the Pan American Games, the

Southeast Asia Games, the Asian Games, the South American Games, the Central American Games, the Caribbean Games, the Arab Games, the South Pacific Games, the African Games, and the World Games. To acknowledge Ben Weider's lifelong accomplishments in sports and fitness, he has been awarded honorary Ph.D.'s in Physical Education and Sports Sciences.

Joe Weider

A true pioneer in his efforts to bring strength and fitness consciousness to the public's attention, Joe Weider continues to use his expertise to help people the world over lead healthier, happier lives.

Joe oversees the Weider magazine publishing enterprise and is the dominant force in the fitness-publishing field because of an unyielding passion for what he does best—educating athletes and the public on the importance of physical development and nutrition.

Joe Weider has been recognized for his leadership, dedication, and outstanding contributions to the field of physical fitness. He was named Publisher of the Year in 1983 by the Periodical and Book Association; in 1992 the United States Sports Academy presented him with the Dwight D. Eisenhower Fitness Award; and in May 1995 he received the Lifetime Achievement Award from the Governor's Council on Physical Fitness and Sports from California Governor Pete Wilson. But the honor that Joe is perhaps most proud of is the Distinguished Citizen Award that was presented to him by the Boy Scouts of America in June 1991 that refers to him as "the father of fitness."

In recognition of women's dedication to the sport, Joe and Ben went on to create the Ms. Olympia contest in 1978. In 1995, a Fitness Olympia category was also added.

Daniel Gastelu

Daniel Gastelu, M.S., M.F.S., is founder of Supplementfacts International, a company devoted to providing reliable information about nutrition and dietary supplements. He serves as director of nutritional sciences for the International Sports Sciences Association, is a director of an international healthcare company, and is actively involved in many facets of the dietary supplement industry, including product development, manufacturing, and regulatory affairs. Gastelu developed and coauthored the ISSA's Specialist in Performance Nutrition certification program and course book, which is used to certify doctors, physical therapists, fitness trainers, strength coaches, and nutritionists. A graduate of Rutgers University, where he taught science courses, he is a Master Fitness Trainer, and Specialist in Performance Nutrition. He also creates and teaches continuing education courses about nutrition and dietary supplements for pharmacists.

During the past two decades Gastelu has developed hundreds of health-care products, including dietary supplements, sports nutritionals, nutraceutical foods, and over-the-counter drugs. He directed innovative research programs examining the effects of different nutrition programs on body composition, health, and physical performance. In recent years Mr. Gastelu has worked on numerous projects with prominent health experts such as: Shari Lieberman, Ph.D.; Cherie Calbom, M.S., C.N.; Stephen Gullo, Ph.D.; Ann Louise Gittleman, M.S.; Varro Tyler, Ph.D.; Frederick J. Vagnini, M.D.; Frederick C. Hatfield, Ph.D.; Richard Simmons; Jack La Lanne; Denise Austin; and Tony Little. His recent books include: *The Complete Dietary Supplements Buyer's Guide, Dynamic Nutrition for Maximum Performance, All About Sports Nutrition, All About Bioflavonoids, All About Carnitine, Avery's Sports Nutrition Almanac,* and *Performance Nutrition: The Complete Guide.*